SUPERCOMPUTATIONAL SCIENCE

SUPERCOMPUTATIONAL SCIENCE

Edited by

R. G. Evans

and

S. Wilson

Rutherford Appleton Laboratory
Oxfordshire, United Kingdom

PLENUM PRESS • NEW YORK AND LONDON

Library of Congress Cataloging-in-Publication Data

Supercomputational science / edited by R.G. Evans and S. Wilson.
       p.   cm.
    "Proceedings of a summer school on Supercomputational Science,
held September 18-29, 1989, at Abingdon, Oxfordshire, United
Kingdom"--T.p. verso.
    Includes bibliographical references and index.
    ISBN 0-306-43663-9
    1. Supercomputers--Congresses.   I. Evans, R. G. II. Wilson, S.
(Stephen), 1950-
QA76.5.S89437 1990
004.1'1--dc20   90-45241
                                                          CIP

Proceedings of a summer school on Supercomputational Science,
held September 18–29, 1989, at Abingdon, Oxfordshire, United Kingdom

ISBN 0-306-43663-9

© 1990 Plenum Press, New York
A Division of Plenum Publishing Corporation
233 Spring Street, New York, N.Y. 10013

Printed in the United States of America

Preface

In contemporary research, the supercomputer now ranks, along with radio telescopes, particle accelerators and the other apparatus of "big science", as an expensive resource, which is nevertheless essential for state of the art research. Supercomputers are usually provided as shared central facilities. However, unlike , telescopes and accelerators, they are find a wide range of applications which extends across a broad spectrum of research activity.

The difference in performance between a "good" and a "bad" computer program on a traditional serial computer may be a factor of two or three, but on a contemporary supercomputer it can easily be a factor of one hundred or even more! Furthermore, this factor is likely to increase with future generations of machines. In keeping with the large capital and recurrent costs of these machines, it is appropriate to devote effort to training and familiarization so that supercomputers are employed to best effect.

This volume records the lectures delivered at a Summer School held at The Coseners House in Abingdon, which was an attempt to disseminate research methods in the different areas in which supercomputers are used. It is hoped that the publication of the lectures in this form will enable the experiences and achievements of supercomputer users to be shared with a larger audience.

We thank all the lecturers and participants for making the Summer School an enjoyable and profitable experience. Finally, we thank the Science and Engineering Research Council and The Computer Board for supporting the Summer School.

R.G. Evans and S. Wilson

January 1990

Rutherford Appleton Laboratory
Oxfordshire.

Contents

Supercomputers in the Computational Sciences 1
    R.G. Evans and S. Wilson

Supercomputing on Conventional Architectures 3
    R.G. Evans

Supercomputing with Novel Architectures 13
    R.G. Evans and S. Wilson

Good Programming Techniques I:
    Testing and the Life Cycle of a Software
    Product 25
    J.B. Slater

Good Programming Techniques II:
    Test Case Design Methodologies 35
    J.B. Slater

Good Programming Techniques III:
    Non–Computer Based Testing 45
    J.B. Slater

Parallel Processing on Shared Memory Multi–User Systems 55
    V.R. Saunders

Running FORTRAN Programmes in an OCCAM Environment 65
    L. Heck

Numerical Recipes for Supercomputers 81
    S. Wilson

The NAG Library in a Supercomputing Environment 109
    J.J. Du Croz and P.J.D. Mayes

Computer Simulation of Plasmas 131
    A.R. Bell

Computational Implementation of the R–Matrix Method in
    Atomic and Molecular Collision Problems 147
    K.A. Berrington

Multitasking the Householder Diagonalization Algorithm
    on the CRAY X–MP/48 155
    K.A. Berrington

Relativistic Atomic Structure Calculations I:
Basic Theory and the Finite Basis Set
Approximation 159
H.M. Quiney

Relativistic Atomic Structure Calculations II:
Computational Aspects of the Finite Basis Set
Method 185
H.M. Quiney

Vector Processing and Parallel Processing in Many—Body Perturbation
Theory Calculations for Electron Correlation Effects in Atoms
and Molecules 201
D.J. Baker, D. Moncrieff and S. Wilson

Electron Correlation in Small Molecules and the
Configuration Interaction Method 211
P.J. Knowles

Energy Minimization and Structure Factor Refinement
Methods 235
I. Haneef

Molecular Dynamics Methods 243
I. Haneef

Molecular Dynamics of Protein Molecules 251
D.S. Moss and T.P. Flores

Supercomputers in Drug Design 269
W.G. Richards

Path Integral Simulations of Excess Electrons
in Condensed Matter 275
J.O. Baum and L. Cruzeiro—Hansson

Computational Methods in Electronic Structure
Calculations of Complex Solids 287
W.M. Temmerman, Z. Szotek, H. Winter and G.Y. Guo

Implementation of a Numerical Sea Model
on a CRAY X—MP Series Computer 319
A.M. Davies and R.B. Grzonka

River Flood Prediction:
A Study in FORTRAN Optimization 327
B.J. Ralston, F. Thomas and H.K.F. Yeung

Supercomputing — A Forward Look 333
B.W. Davies

Contributors 345

Index 347

SUPERCOMPUTERS IN THE COMPUTATIONAL SCIENCES

R.G. Evans and S.Wilson

Rutherford Appleton Laboratory, Chilton, Oxfordshire OX11 0QX

The digital computer is a major tool of research in almost every branch of contemporary science. It is widely recognized that computation is now an indispensible alternative to the traditional methods of scientific investigation — theoretical analysis and laboratory experiment. Over the last four hundred years, science has progressed by a symbiotic interaction between theory and experiment. Theory has suggested new experiments and then interpreted their results. Equally, experiment has tested existing theories and suggested new theories. Now theory provides the basic equations for the computational approach. The situation is summarized in Figure 1.

The computational approach can frequently afford solutions to scientific problems which are theoretically intractable because of their complexity. The computer can not only provide a route to information which is not available from laboratory experiments but can also afford additional insight into the problems being studied. Moreover, because it is often more efficient than the alternatives, the computational approach can increasingly be justified in economic terms.

The use of computing machines as a primary method of research now goes beyond the well established areas of application, the natural sciences, and includes medical and environmental sciences, engineering, the social sciences and humanities. The importance of advanced computing in contemporary research cannot be overstated and its future potential appears enormous.

Increasingly, modern high performance, general purpose computers depart from the serial architecture which has been in use since the dawn of the electronic computer age in the late 1940's. On these serial machines each of the operations which constitute the program are carried out sequentially and thus the speed of the computer is ultimately limited by performance of the electronic devices from which they are constructed. On the new generation of machines which have become widely available over the past decade, the hardware is designed for the efficient processing of vectors and for executing parts of the computation concurrently. With the advent of these supercomputers, we appear to be entering an era of massive computing power; an era in which computing power will no longer be the scarce resource it has been over the past forty years. However, to effectively tap this power in attacking new areas of scientific endeavour the algorithms and numerical methods we employ must exploit the hardware features of the target machine. Only by doing this can we

Supercomputational Science
Edited by R.G. Evans and S. Wilson
Plenum Press, New York, 1990

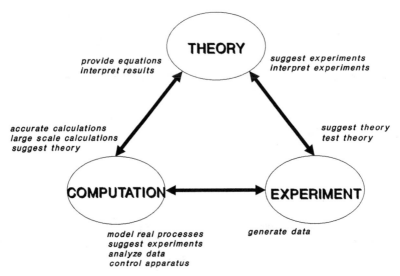

Figure 1. The relation between theory, experiment and computation.

exploit the full potential of *state−of−the−art* supercomputers in our research activities; only by doing this can we engage in **supercomputational science**.

As computers are employed in an increasingly wide range of research activities, there appears to be a growing body of techniques which are common to a number of fields. The following chapters are the work of experts in computing and the computational sciences, who use supercomputers in their research. It is hoped that the reader will find this volume, which records the lectures given at a summer school held at the Coseners House, Abingdon, during September, 1989, not only a useful insight into the effective exploitation of supercomputers in contemporary research but also find it of value in their own work.

SUPERCOMPUTING ON CONVENTIONAL ARCHITECTURES

R G Evans

Rutherford Appleton Laboratory, Chilton, Oxfordshire OX11 0QX

INTRODUCTORY DEFINITIONS

There is no accepted definition of the term "supercomputing" apart from the rather glib statement that it is 'the most powerful machine available'. For the purpose of this lecture we shall loosely extend the definition to include machines within a factor of about ten of the fastest available at any time so that the currently popular 'mini–supers' may also be discussed. It is also appropriate to reduce the discussion to computers of general applicability rather than include such special purpose machines as FFT engines for image and signal processing and computers that have been built for a single problem such as Lattice Gauge models.

As far as "conventional architecture" is concerned we shall assume that broadly speaking the machine has a large single memory that is shared between a handful of processors, and more importantly that the user sees a single memory space for programming. Conventional architectures will undoubtedly stray away from these definitions as time progresses.

EVOLUTION OF "CONVENTIONAL ARCHITECTURE".

The early days of electronic computing, say in the 1950's, were dominated by problems of complexity and reliability. Everyone has surely heard the stories of the computers with 10,000 vacuum tubes, each with a mean lifetime of a few thousand hours, and the men who were employed continuously in replacing failed devices. In the early machines there was a premium on reducing the device count in order to improve reliability and this meant that each sub–system was likely to be called into play for more than one function. Typically an adder would be used for address calculation as well as data processing, and register space was likely to be restricted.

At this early time there was a distinction into processors with "Harvard" and "von–Neumann" architecture (see Figure 1). The Harvard architecture machines had separate memories for program instructions and data, and separate pathways or busses for program and data to reach the central processor. The von–Neumann machine was simpler and conceptually more elegant in that it did not distinguish between program and data except in the way that individual elements were acted upon in the central processing unit (c.p.u.). Program and data could be and often were interleaved, existed in the same memory unit, and shared the same pathway to

Supercomputational Science
Edited by R.G. Evans and S. Wilson
Plenum Press, New York, 1990

and from the cpu. The elegance and simplicity of the von–Neumann architecture made it almost universally accepted until the present day.

The attraction of the simplicity of the von–Neumann architecture is also its limitation since the pathway between cpu and memory is a bottleneck in terms of trying to speed up the machine. The Harvard architecture with its dual pathways has in principle a greater throughput and has had a renaissance, particularly in high speed signal processing chips in recent years. The removal of the "von–Neumann bottleneck" is a continuing problem for supercomputer designers.

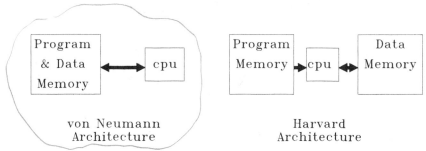

Fig.1. The von Neumann and Harvard architectures

In the 1960's and 1970's the reliability of semiconductor and particularly integrated circuit based computers became sufficiently good that separate functional units could be employed for each type of instruction, dedicated floating point adders and multipliers were feasible and register sets became large enough for compilers to optimise operation sequences for the minimum number of memory references. Machines such as the Ferranti ATLAS 1, the CDC 6600 and 7600 and the IBM 360/195 were generally considered to be the first supercomputers. Machines of this generation made use of "pipelining" particularly for instruction processing, while one instruction was being decoded and acted upon the next would be fetched from memory. The CDC 7600 and IBM 360/195 also made limited use of pipelining for floating point calculations, while waiting for a floating point result they would try to find something else to do.

In scientific terms the first supercomputers could make a reasonable effort at solving sets of non–linear coupled differential equations or matrix eigenvalue problems, and could tackle problems which were large enough to defy analytic theory and realistic enough to be of practical importance.

MEMORY SPEED LIMITATIONS

It is fairly obvious that as the ability to compute more numbers increases then for most applications it is also necessary to store an increasing amount of data. By the time of the CDC 7600 the speed of the central processors, even for floating point operations, had outrun the speed of memory units, at least on the scale of storage that was needed for real jobs. To get around the problem of needing rapid access to memory, but also to have a large amount of memory the CDC 7600 (and many other machines up to the present time) organised their memory into a hierarchy of small (fast, also called cache) memory and large (slow or main) memory. Those who remember programming the CDC 7600 will recall having to advise the compiler as to which data should reside in small memory, and making different choices for different subroutines.

The hierarchical organisation of memory has continued and present day machines such as the IBM 3090 have four (or five) levels of hierarchy:

Registers	typically 8 x 128 words
Cache	64 kByte
Main Memory	256 MByte
Expanded Memory	2 GByte
Disk (Virtual) Memory	100 GByte

The improvements in compiler technology over the years means that in most cases the user need not bother about memory allocation, but where the ultimate speed is required, for instance in accessing large matrices it can be useful to know how particular hardware will behave and tune the code accordingly.

VECTOR PROCESSING

Although the CDC 7600 and IBM 360/195 had used limited pipelining of the floating point arithmetic units the first machine to support vector instructions to obtain greater floating point speed was the rather unsuccessful CDC STAR–100 in 1974. The appearance of what most of us now consider to be the modern supercomputer was the Cray–1 in 1976. The machine was the brainchild of Seymour Cray who was one of the chief designers of the CDC 6600 and 7600 but left Control Data to form his own company dedicated to making the world's fastest computers. The evolution of the "vector processor" was one of the earliest attempts to get around the von–Neumann bottleneck − if both an instruction and data had to be fetched from memory for every arithmetic operation, and memory access was the limiting factor, then why not try to find circumstances when the same operation was perfomed on many data elements and eliminate the multiple fetches of the same instruction?

Performing exactly the same operation on many data elements also maximises the benefits of "pipelining", that is splitting the task up into pieces that are short enough to be performed in one clock cycle and then passing the intermediate answer on to the following section while simultaneously taking in the next data element. For instance a floating point add has several logical sub–sections (see Figure 2):

Choose the larger exponent

Normalise the smaller number to the same exponent

Add the mantissas

Renormalise the mantissa and exponent of the result

If these four tasks are done in one execution unit then the result is not available for four clock cycles and at any time three out of the four stages are idle. The vector or pipelined approach is to feed a new data element in on every clock cycle and after the initial four clock cycle delay a new result appears on each clock cycle.

This simple description of a vector pipeline brings out some of the more important concepts:

The pipeline does exactly the same thing to each data element.

There is a delay before any results appear equal to the number of stages in the pipeline.

Eventually there is one result per pipeline per clock period.

Hockney (1984) uses a formalism based on the above model to characterise the performance of vector processors in terms of two simple parameters:

$$t = r_\infty^{-1} \left(n + n_{1\,2} \right)$$

where t is the time to calculate n results. By re—arranging the formula it is easy to see that $n_{1\,2}$ is the number of stages in the pipe and r_∞ , the asymptotic speed for

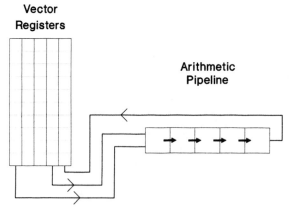

Vector Registers

Arithmetic Pipeline

Fig. 2. The logical sub—sections of a floating point addition.

long vectors is the reciprocal of the clock period. Hockney's formula has the advantage that it generically describes more complicated cases such as the chaining together of two functions (eg add and multiply in the Cray 1 and nearly all other vector processors) or the provision of multiple pipelines operating in parallel (Cyber 205, ETA 10 and most of the Japanese supercomputers).

Clearly chaining functions together increases the startup time and the value of $n_{1\,2}$ but Hockney's formula also shows that having two pipes is equivalent to having one pipe with twice the speed and twice the startup delay (in terms of clock cycles). One of the design trade—offs in a vector super—computer is balancing a long vector pipe with high peak speed against a shorter pipe with lower peak speed but better performance on typical programs.

The restriction that the pipe must carry out the same operations on each data element is one of the major restrictions of the vector architecture. Not only is there the requirement of similar operations, but in view of the delay before loading operands and obtaining the result there is also the problem of data dependency and recurrence. Fr instance the classical vector operation is:

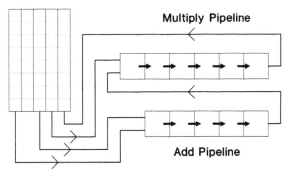

Fig. 3.

```
      DO 10 I = 1, 100
           X(I) = A(I)+ B(I)*C(I)
 10    CONTINUE
```

where there is clearly no dependency. However the loop :

```
      DO 10 I = 1, 100
           X(I) = A(I) + B(I)*X(I+K)
 10    CONTINUE
```

is very complicated for a compiler to analyse.

If $K > 0$ then there is no problem and the loop may vectorise. If $K < 0$ but $|K| >$ (number of stages in pipe), the loop may also vectorise since the result of the first operation will be available in time to be loaded into the Kth operation. Compilers do not usually work out the possible range of K themselves and need 'directives' if the programmer can guarantee that K is always in a given range. Some newer compilers will generate code for both a scalar and a vector loop and decide at run time which to execute based on the current value of K.

Simple conditional operations may be allowed within a loop, for instance the loop:

```
      DO 10 I = 1, 100
           IF (A(I) . GT. 0. 0)  X(I) = X(I) + A(I)
 10    CONTINUE
```

may be handled by special hardware which always calculates $X(I)+A(I)$ but only stores the result back to X(I) on the specified condition. Cray introduced a series of "vector merge" functions for the Cray 1 which returned one of two possible results depending on the value of the third argument. This was necessary only because the early compiler could not always spot the equivalent code sequence, and modern compilers from other vendors may not support the Cray functions since their compiler produces equivalent code automatically.

The flexibility of vector hardware continues to improve and most current machines also support the dynamic calculation of array indices within a loop, particularly important for table look up and most particle in cell methods:

```
      DO 10  I = ...
           IX = X(I) / DX              ! which cell is the particle in
           V(I) = V(I) + E(IX)*DT      ! accelerate the particle
           X(I) = X(I) + V(I)*DT       ! move the particle
 10    CONTINUE
```

AMDAHL'S LAW

Following the introduction of the early vector processors it was observed by many (particularly those who did not make vector processors!) that their performance was frequently disappointing. Gene Amdahl had in fact already formulated a very simple description of the performance of vector machines while they were still being designed:

Suppose the vector unit is V times the speed of the scalar unit and the code being run has a fraction of the code which is vector and $(1 - \alpha)$ which is scalar.

The time to run the program is:

$$T = (1-\alpha) + \alpha/V$$

If the vector unit is appreciably faster than the scalar unit then the second term is usually negligible and the perceived speed of the machine is its scalar speed divided by $(1-\alpha)$ *i.e.* it is the scalar speed and the quality of the code/compiler that govern the results!

LIMITATIONS OF VECTOR PROCESSING

Not surprisingly there are two separate threads to the problem of obtaining more speed from vector supercomputers, for code which is well vectorised there is the problem of how to make the vector units faster, and for code which is poorly vectorised the problem is to make the vector architecture more flexible so that more code is vectorised, and to speed up the scalar units.

1. Increased Vector Speed

Since the concept of the vector processor is simply that of the production line of simple individual tasks the limitations on its speed are equally simple but lead into different development strategies.

(a) Break the operation down into even smaller steps

There is little scope for improvement in this area since there are already only a couple of logic levels per pipeline stage. When the vector clock becomes faster than the scalar clock (*e.g.* Fujitsu VP, Cray–2) the manufacturer has already pushed this as far as is reasonable.

(b) Have more pipelines

There is theoretically no limit to which this can be increased and the practical limit is the cost, balanced against the useful performance improvement. Remember from Hockney's equation that more pipes imply a larger value of n 1/2 and the vector performance is only obtained for longer and longer vectors.

Most manufacturers have chosen to increase the number of cpu's rather than have multiple vector pipes per cpu. As will be discussed later there are other cost considerations that go along with peak performance, and the increased flexibility of having multiple independent cpu's is usually regarded as justifying the additional cost. If all cpu's share the same memory then the programmer's task is simplified but the control logic needed to route memory requests and resolve conflicts is rather complicated. It is generally regarded as a practical limit for about 16 cpu's to share a common memory although there have been novel suggestions such as the BBN butterfly switch to increase this limit.

(c) Reduce the clock cycle time

This is the obvious route to future improvements from all manufacturers. For the next decade the limitations will be cost and the technological limitations of integrated circuits. In most cases the route to greater speed is to make the devices smaller since capacitance scales as L2 but for constant thicknesses resistance is independent of L. Devices limited by carrier diffusion times also clearly benefit from smaller sizes. By the year 2000 most integrated circuit technologies will be approaching physical limits (usually quantum effects).

There are three different choices in terms of the technology of integrated circuit manufacture:

Silicon Emitter Coupled Logic (ECL) is the most popular choice since it is today the fastest technology that offers useful degrees of integration ($10000 - 50000$ gates per chip) so that the number of chips per processor is kept to a resonable level. The Cray Y–MP and C–90 ranges will be built in ECL as will some of the Japanese machines. ECL will probably allow clock speeds down to 1nsec (cf 8.5nsec Cray X–MP, 4.5nsec Cray 2) but dissipates a lot of heat and needs very complicated cooling which adds to the cost.

Silicon Complementary Metal Oxide Semiconductor (CMOS) technology is catching up with ECL in speed but currently has a penalty of about x5. It has the advantages of much higher levels of integration (up to a million gates per chip) and lower heat dissipation, which both help to reduce cost. CMOS is the usual choice for mini–supercomputers and the cost/ performance tradeoff of mini–super's versus state–of–the–art machines is one of the more "exciting" developments.

It is possible to make CMOS gates several times faster by cooling them to liquid nitrogen temperatures, in view of its lower heat dissipation per gate it is quite feasible to chill a complete supercomputer to these temperatures and the thermodynamic efficiency of the cooling remains about 20% (cf <1% at liquid helium temperatures). ETA used this technology for the ETA–10 series with the option of a cheaper, slower room temperature machine or the more expensive liquid nitrogen version. Several cooled machines were built and perform reasonably well at the hardware level. The range was let down largely by late delivery of operating system software.

The switching speed of silicon transistors is ultimately limited by the electron mobility and *Gallium Arsenide* promises a fundamentally faster device. However the development of GaAs is some years behind silicon but it is catching up due to military demand for its better radiation resistance as well as better speed. Currently the major problem for GaAs is the number of gates per chip, which is limited mostly by the inferior crystallographic structure of GaAs substrates. The Cray–3, due in 1990/91 will be GaAs but the level of integration per chip will be the same as the 1981 Cray–2.

2. Memory Bandwidth

As the vector speed is increased the main problem becomes the memory bandwidth needed in order to provide the operands to the processor. The access time of main memory will always be much slower than the vector cycle time and usually vector registers are provided to reduce the start up delay. For complicated loops the contents of the vector registers can be re–used rather than initiating another series of memory fetches.

If the vector register bandwidth is not matched by the register to main memory bandwidth then the processor will quickly exhaust the contents of the registers and will slow down, this was a criticism of the Cray–1 where the memory bandwidth was only 1/3 of that needed, and the Cray X–MP corrected the problem. Since the response time of the main memory will be fairly slow it is necessary to divide the memory into many "banks" with consecutive addresses in adjacent banks. Provided the memory references are to consecutive addresses then different banks will be accessed but if the addresses are with a large 'stride' then the same bank may be accessed before it has responded to (or recovered from if it is dynamic memory) the previous access.

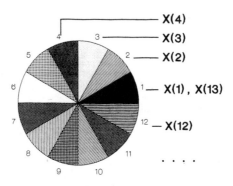

Fig. 4.

If the memory cycle time is M clock periods and there are P vector pipelines each requiring 4 (three loads and a store) references per clock cycle then there must be at least 4*M*P banks of memory. For the Cray X–MP/48 with four pipes and a memory response time of 4 clock cycles there must be 64 banks of memory. For machines such as the Fujitsu VP with a faster vector, more pipes and slower main memory there can be as many as 512 banks of main memory. The banking of main memory is very expensive since the data pathways have to be duplicated N times and the control logic needed to route the data and handle bank conflicts also gets very complicated.

MORE FLEXIBLE "VECTOR" UNITS

For those programs which achieve low levels of vectorisation or operate on short vectors there is little incentive to increase the peak speed of the machine (which is very expensive to achieve). It may instead be profitable to simplify the vector unit for modest speed (and cost) and to spend the money on multiple independent functional units or multiple cpu's. To some extent this is the approach of the IBM 3090 Vector Facility which does not have the flat out speed of some other supercomputers, but coupled to a fast scalar unit it performs very well on a wide range of code.

Taken to its extreme this line of argument replaces vector units by multiple scalar units each obeying different instructions. Pipelining still gives a large number of results per instruction, but in order to get the flexibility of multiple independent functional units the possible number of different instructions is much greater. This is most efficiently handled by increasing the length of the instruction word with specific bit positions corresponding to each functional unit for maximum decoding efficiency. Not surprisingly these machines are called Very Long Instruction Word (VLIW) designs. To get the best performance from them requires a very sophisticated compiler, able to schedule the different operations in the most efficient way.

Some of the most exciting developments in this area come from the realm of single chip processors. The latest generation of processors such as the Motorola 88000, the Intel i860 and the Intel 80486 have more than one million CMOS devices per chip. With on–chip cache memory, multiple functional units including pipelined floating point add/multipliers and 4GByte address space the i860 in particular has been described as a 'Cray on a chip'. The current device offers about 40Mflops peak performance but substantial development is likely as integrated circuit technology improves still further.

FUTURE TRENDS

For the foreseeable future there is a market for the "most powerful" computer almost independent of cost. The defence industries, oil companies and possibly aerospace have such a large cost/benefit from supercomputing that the capital cost of supercomputers is quickly recovered. In the academic market the price/performance is more critical and it would be a brave person who predicted the outcome between "mini–super" and "super" computers.

Given the need for the fastest machine, most manufacturers are pushing the multiple cpu, shared memory route to greater performance. Multiple vector pipes per processor are only marginally cheaper, since most of the cost is in providing the memory bandwidth for peak speed, but multiple cpu's are more flexible.

There is a practical limit, at about 8 or 16, of the number of processors which can sensibly share the same main memory, but expansion beyond this number is likely (Cray C–90 (?), Chen SS–1) by a looser level of coupling between clusters of 8 or 16 processors. Extension of this route closes the gap between "conventional" and "novel" architectures but the important distinction will probably be that from the programmers point of view the "conventional" machines will appear to have a single large memory.

In speed terms silicon and GaAs will be direct competitors for the next few years but ultimately GaAs must surely win. The cost penalty may however restrict it to the very upper echelons of the market.

For academic supercomputing there will be dramatic improvements in the power of desktop machines (eg based on the Intel i860) and the biggest threat to mini–super computers probably comes from the performance of the new generation of 'single user' or group machines. It is likely that more and more users will be satisfied by the performance of local machines but there will remain a few users who always need the ultimate the performance.

The "usability" of central supercomputers should improve dramatically with higher speed networks of better functionality and a more pervasive use of UNIX as the operating system for most scientific computing from desktop workstations to supercomputers. As systems such as X–windows become more popular the aim should be an environment where a scientist has a workstation on his (or her) desk and moving a job from the workstation to a supercomputer on campus or at a national centre should be as simple as pointing a mouse at another window!

How this desirable and technologically feasible state of affairs will be funded is another matter.

REFERENCE

Hockney R W, in "PDE Software: Modules, Interfaces and Systems", ed Engquist and Smedsaas, North Holland, Amsterdam 1984

SUPERCOMPUTING WITH NOVEL ARCHITECTURES

R.G. Evans and S. Wilson

Rutherford Appleton Laboratory, Chilton, Oxfordshire OX11 0QX.

INTRODUCTION

The increase in speed of electronic computing machines in the period 1950–90 was attributable to improvements in electronic engineering and to the use of parallel computation. Until the early seventies the parallel computation was to a large extent transparent to the computer user. Since that time, however, this has ceased to be the case and the user has found it necessary to familiarize himself with some of the details of the machine architecture in order to exploit the capabilities of the particular target machine effectively. "Conventional" architectures are typified by the CRAY range of machines, which have a small number of very powerful vector processors sharing a common memory. On the other hand, "novel" architectures usually have a large number of less powerful processors together with a distributed memory.

In this chapter, we briefly survey the use of novel architectures in supercomputing. We begin by outlining the technological and economic case for large scale parallelism. In using a large number of processors, it is essential to have a clear idea of the way in which the various processing units and the memory units are interconnected and we therefore describe some of the frequently used architectures. We then turn to the problem of programming for large scale parallelism.

TECHNOLOGICAL AND ECONOMIC ARGUMENTS FOR LARGE SCALE PARALLEL COMPUTING

It is obvious that the theoretical maximum power of any computational architecture can be raised by increasing the number of processing elements but less obvious that a given performance can often be achieved more economically by having a large number of processors. In the early days of computing the reliability problems of the increased number of components would have precluded the possibility of making a large number of cooperating processors, but the benefits of VLSI (Very Large Scale Integration) circuit technology in reducing the size, cost and component count of a processing element have reversed the situation.

The explosion of the personal computer and workstation market means that high performance processors, multi–megabyte memories and fast disk storage are now almost commodity items. The technology of building these machines is well suited

Supercomputational Science
Edited by R.G. Evans and S. Wilson
Plenum Press, New York, 1990

to robotic manufacture and the cost of MIPS (Millions of Instructions Per Second) or MFLOPS (Millions of FLoating–point OPerations per Second) on a desktop machine continues to fall at a dramatic rate. On the other hand, the fastest single processor machines demand exotic technology in their integrated circuits, board design, cooling, packaging and largely manual assembly. In many ways they are the "Ferraris" of the computing world.

Harnessing the power of many processors on the same calculation is a critical problem and is the area where it has not so far been possible to draw on mass market technology. The need to communicate rapidly and flexibly between processors is most elegantly solved by integrating the communications devices onto the processor chip, as in the Inmos transputer, but the present transputer hardware implementation supports only point to point communications. An attempt by Intel to use LAN (Local Area Network) technology, in the form of ethernet controllers, to perform inter processor communications was a failure due to excessive overheads on each data transfer.

Amdahl's Law for Parallel Processing

It is interesting to explore parametric models for the performance of parallel processing machines in which each of the processing elements is a vector processor (see, for example, Hack, 1989). According to "Amdahl's Law", the normalized performance of a vector processor may be written

$$S_v = [1 - \alpha[1 - R(l)]]^{-1}$$

where S_v is the improvement in performance due to vectorization, α is the fraction of vector operations and $R(l)$ is the ratio of the scalar unit performance to the vector unit performance for a vector of length l. For a parallel processor the normalized performance can be written

$$S_p = [1 - \beta[1 - g(p)]]^{-1}$$

where S_p is the improvement in performance due to parallelisation, β is the fraction of parallel work available, and p is the number of processors. g(p) is the sum of two terms

$$g(p) = P(p) + (\epsilon p)^{-1}$$

where $P(p)$ is the computational overhead associated with parallel computation and ϵ is the fractional utilization of the parallel configuration.

The most efficient use of a vector multiprocessor requires that the product of S_v and S_p be maximized. In Figure 1, we show the normalized performance surface $S_t = S_v.S_p$ as a function of the fraction of vector work (α) and the fraction of parallel work (β) for a 16 processor machine with $R(l)$=0.5, ϵ=1 and neglecting the computational overhead associated with parallel computation, $P(p)$=0. For this hypothetical case, quite large values of β are required in order to exploit a reasonable fraction of the theoretical capabilities of the system. In Figure 2, we show the normalized performance surface for a 256 processor machine with $R(l)$=0.1, ϵ=1 and again neglecting the computational overhead associated with parallel computation. This case requires an even larger value of β to achieve a reasonable fraction of the system's theoretical capabilities. In both Figure 1 and 2, the predicted performance lies well below the maximum for the majority of the surfaces. What is more the area for which performance is better than given fraction of the maximum is reduced when the number of processors is increased.

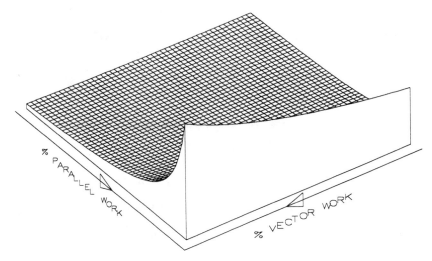

Figure 1. Parametric model for a computer with 16 vector processing units, with $R(\bar{l})=0.5$, $\epsilon=1$ and neglecting the computational overhead associated with parallel computation

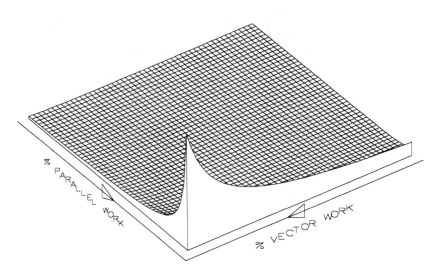

Figure 2. Parametric model for a computer with 256 vector processing units, with $R(\bar{l})=0.1$, $\epsilon=1$ and neglecting the computational overhead associated with parallel computation

NOVEL ARCHITECTURES

In practice, computational scientists have at least two concerns: the time taken to run a single job and the complexity of the implementation on the target machine. With each generation of computers, these two factors have become more tightly coupled. With the advent of highly parallel computing architectures, the time required for a single job has become a very strong function of the implementation, whilst at the same time the complexity of implementation has increased significantly.

In order to make effective use of highly parallel machines, it is essential to have a clear idea of the way in which the various processing units and the memory units are interconnected.

One of the first classification schemes for computers architectures is due to Flynn (1972). He divided machines into

(a) SISD – Single Instruction stream – Single Data stream

(b) SIMD – Single Instruction stream – Multiple Data stream

(c) MISD – Multiple Instruction stream – Single Data stream

(d) MIMD – Multiple Instruction stream – Multiple Data stream

As explained, for example, by Hockney and Jesshope (1981) this is only one of a number of schemes, none of which gives a unique classification of architecture and none of which is, therefore, totally satisfactory. However, Flynn's taxonomy is widely used.

The *serial computer* is the conventional von Neumann machine which would be designated SISD in Flynn's classification scheme. There is one stream of instructions and each instruction leads to one operation thus leading to a stream of logically related arguments and results. This is the type of machine architecture that has dominated computational science for the past forty years. It has had a significant influence on the design of the "traditional" algorithms employed in computational science.

The *vector processing computer* can be designated SIMD machine in Flynn's taxonomy. The CRAY 1 was the first commercially successful machine of this type.

Consider, in detail, the task of adding two floating point numbers. For simplicity we assume that each number is represented by a mantissa and a decimal exponent. The addition can be divided into the following subtasks :

(a) determine the shift of one mantissa relative to the other in order to line up the decimal point,

(b) actually shifting the mantissa to line up the decimal points,

(c) adding the mantissa to obtain the mantissa of the result,

(d) normalize the result by shifting the mantissa so that the leading digit is next to the decimal point

(e) calculation of the exponent.

Obviously, these five subtasks must be executed sequentially since each subtask is dependent on the result of one or more previous subtasks. However, if we wish to add two vectors then the subtasks can be executed in parallel. As we illustrate in Figure 3, whilst subtask (a) is being carried out for the n th. elements of the vectors, subtask (b) can be executed for the n−1 th. element, subtask (c) for the n−2 th. elements subtask (d) for the n−3 th element, and subtask (e) for the n−4 th. element. n is then increased by one and the whole process repeated. This process is known as pipelining and, after being initiated, continues until all elements of the vectors have been processed or the number of operand registers associated with the functional unit have been exhausted. A pipeline works at its maximum efficiency if the number of operations to be processed is equal to an integer multiple of the number of operand

registers. The "start up" of pipeline processing demands some extra time and the efficiency is, therefore, degraded for short vectors. Often it is necessary to rearrange randomly addressed data so that it is contiguous in memory.

Vector processors currently afford the most powerful single processor machines.

In Flynn's taxonomy *array processors* may, like the vector processors described above, be described as SIMD machines.

An example of this type of architecture is provided by the ICL Distributed Array Processor (DAP). The DAP 510, which is now marketed by AMT, consists of 1024 single–bit processor elements arranged as a 32 by 32 array. The DAP 610 has 4096 processing elements arranged in a 64 by 64 array. Each processing element simultaneously executes the same instruction. Nearest neighbours are connected and a bus connects processors by rows and columns. Such machines have been used quite extensively in, for example, statistical mechanics, molecular simulation and molecular graphics.

Parallel Processors are designated MIMD machines in Flynn's taxonomy. Implementations on such machines raise questions of interprocessor communications and connectivity. It is essential, therefore, to have a clear idea of the way in which the various processing units and the memory units are interconnected. Hockney (1988) has provided a useful structural taxonomy for parallel computers. He points out that parallel computers can, at the highest level, be basically divided into "networks" and "switched" systems.

Scalar processing

Vector processing

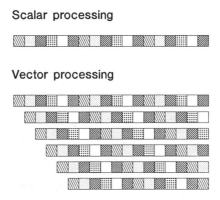

Figure 3. Floating point operations on scalar proccessing and vector processing machines. Each square represents a suboperation and time proceed accross the page.

A network system consists of a number of processors each with its own local memory which are connected together with an identifiable topology. Each processor and its local memory is referred to as a processing element. The processing elements can be connected together as a mesh, a cube, a hierarchical configuration or in a reconfigurable array. The mesh network, which is shown in Figure 4 contains some one–dimensional configurations, for example rings, and some multidimensional configurations, for example a square, hexagon and other geometries. Cube networks, which are illustrated in Figure 5, range from pure hypercubes to "cube–connected–cycle" networks. The hypercube has particularly interesting and interconnection features. The n processor hypercube, the n–cube, consists of 2^n nodes,

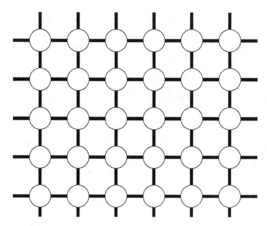

Figure 4. Mesh architecture. Each circle represents a processing element which consists of a processor and associated memory.

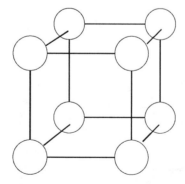

Figure 5. Cube architecture. Each circle represent a processing element which consists of a processor and associated memory.

each associated with a single processing element and numbered by an n–bit binary number between 0 and 2^{n-1}. The processing elements are interconnected so that there is a linked between two processors if and only if their binary representation differs by one and only one bit. For example, in the case n=3, the eight processing elements are labelled

000	001	010	011
100	101	110	111

and can be represented as the vertices of a three–dimensional cube. The hypercube architecture contains many classical topologies, such as two–dimensional and three–dimensional meshes, in fact, it contains meshes of arbitrary dimension. It has homogeneity and symmetrical properties since no single processing element plays a particular role. In "cube–connected–cycle" networks each node of a cube is replaced by a ring or cycle of processing elements. Heirarchical networks are defined in a recursive manner as we illustrate in Figure 6. This class of network architectures can be subdivided into tree networks, clusters of clusters, pyramids, etc. Finally, we can have reconfigurable networks for which the interconnection pattern between the processing elements can be changed during program execution.

In a switched system there is a distinct unit that connects the processors and the memory units. The switch unit is responsible for all interconnections between the attached units. Switched systems can be subdivided into "shared memory" systems and "distributed memory" systems. In a shared memory system a number of processing units are connected via the switch unit to a number of independent memory units forming a common shared memory. This is illustrated in Figure 7. Each processing unit has its own local memory in a distributed memory system and the switch unit interconnects these processing units. This is illustrated in Figure 8.

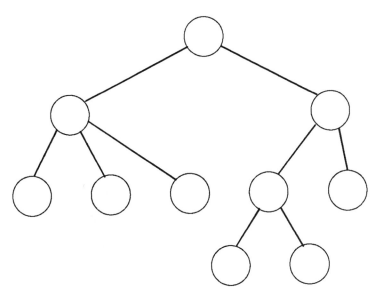

Figure 6. Hierarchical architecture. Each circle represent a processing element which consists of a processor and associated memory.

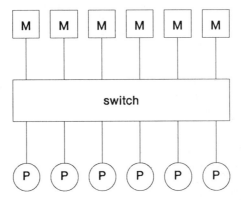

Figure 7. Shared memory achitecture.

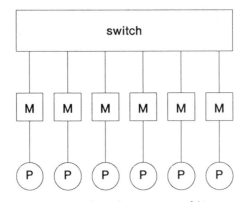

Figure 8. Distributed memory architecture.

PROGRAMMING MODELS FOR PARALLEL COMPUTING

Most of today's programmers have been so indoctrinated with the reduction of an abstract problem to a set of sequential tasks for the classical serial processor that there is a substantial "un–learning" process in making the most of parallel processors. Fortunately most of the processes in the real world are inherently parallel and provide useful analogies for parallel programming.

Data Driven Parallelism

The simple loop in many cases represents the same operation performed on the separate elements of a data structure. If a loop will vectorise on a conventional vector machine it is a good candidate to run individual iterations of the loop on separate processors. For all but the simplest loops where the iterations are independent the partitioning of the work on to different processors will depend on the architecture of the machine concerned. Consider the following code to compute gradients of a scalar variable:

```
      do 100 i = 1, 10000
      grad(i) = ( x(i) − x(i−1) ) / dx
100   continue
```

On a machine such as the AMT DAP with very efficient connection to nearest neighbours such a loop is implemented with each iteration on successive processors and some operating system software to handle the problem of matching the ends, assuming there are less than 10000 real processors. On the other hand a network of Inmos transputers takes much longer to exchange data on the serial links than to perform floating point operations and an optimal solution would be be to divide the computation such that processor 1 computes $i = 1..N$, processor 2 computes $i = N+1..2N$, and so on. Communications overheads then occur only at the boundaries of the data domains.

Data driven parallelism frequently requires a degree of correspondence between the geometry of the real world problem being tackled and the interconnection pattern of the processing elements. Taking the geometrical analogy further, the problem of dividing the data space into smaller elements for more processors is that there is an effective "surface to volume ratio" that determines the ratio of computing to communications. If this gets to be too large then the communications overheads dominate and the problem may actually run slower on more processors. Reconfigurable links or general message passing networks are desirable because they enable a wide variety of problems to be tackled efficiently on given hardware.

The extreme case of data driven parallelism is where the problem at hand requires successive largely identical computations to be performed for a series of input data sets. In this case each processing element can be assigned to perform one complete calculation cycle and when it is complete it looks for the next set of data on the input queue. This is very straightforward to program, has minimal communications overheads but requires that each processing element has the memory and other resources needed to perform a complete calculation. This method is frequently known as the "processor farm".

Process Parallelism

In contrast to the processor farm, which may be likened to a car factory where each worker has the skills to make a whole car himself, process driven parallelism is more akin to the production line where data flows through a succession of processes, each on separate processors on its way through the calculation. Mapping process driven parallelism on to a network of identical processors usually requires different numbers of processors to be assigned to each process to maintain load balancing. Consider the following highly idealised example:

```
        do 100 i = 1, 10000
        y(i) = exp( x(i) − x(i−1) )
100     continue
```

The processes are simply the calculation of the first difference

$$temp = x(i) − x(i−1)$$

and the natural exponential

$$y(i) = exp(temp)$$

The implementation of the exponential function will probably take several times longer than the subtraction so correspondingly more processors need to be allocated to the process. The distribution of tasks amongst them could either be handled by a form of data driven parallelism with each processor calculating the exponential of one input data element (as illustrated in Figure 9), or by further subdividing the exponential process into the calculation of a power series with each processor simply doing a multiply and add (as shown in Figure 10). As with data driven parallelism it is fruitless to assign too small a computational workload to each process as the communications overheads then dominate.

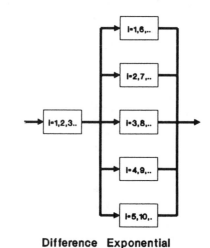

Difference   Exponential

Figure 9.

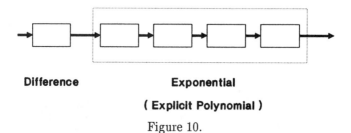

Difference   **Exponential**

(Explicit Polynomial)

Figure 10.

Languages for Parallel Programming

There are two quite distinct approaches to this problem, the vector supercomputer manufacturers, having to cope with only a few processors and shared main memory (ie data is global to all processes) have added Fortran subroutine calls to initiate new processes, wait on the completion of processes and guard access to data or system resources that can only be meaningfully used by one process at a time. These concepts are common to the major manufacturers but the implementation details, including the choice of compiler directives or language extensions are all different.

A similar approach has been adopted by most of the US manufacturers of distributed memory machines with Fortran routines for process initiation, synchronisation and message passing. In the UK a quite different approach has arisen out of Hoare's work on Communicating Sequential Processes and the inherently parallel language OCCAM is the preferred method of high level programming for the Inmos transputer. OCCAM provides an elegant if minimalist approach to parallel programming and has the great advantage of a sound theoretical basis so that the complicated locking structures of other language extensions are unnecessary. It is probably fair to say that OCCAM has proved very popular with new students in parallel programming but has been resisted by the established programmers particularly outside the UK.

Fortran 8X offers a great deal of standardisation of data driven parallelism on arrays and matrices and is very similar to the delightfully straightforward DAP Fortran originated many years ago by ICL. The necessity of matching the detailed algorithmic interpretation to specific machine architecture has fuelled a great increase in the popularity of portable libraries such as the various levels of BLAS (Basic Linear Algebra Subroutines) and general mathematical libraries such as NAG or IMSL. At least in the case of the major computer manufacturers it is possible to obtain highly optimised code for these libraries and guarantee good performance while maintaining portability.

CONCLUDING REMARK

Although the theoretical maximum power of a given computer architecture can be increased indefinitely by using more and more processing elements, the challenge of the novel architectures, described in this chapter, is to realise this power in practice. Whilst it is clear that this can be achieved in specific areas of application, e.g. image processing, it has yet to be convincingly demonstrated that novel architectures can provide an easily used, general purpose computer environment.

REFERENCES

Flynn, M.J., 1972, I.E.E.E. Trans. Comput. C 21 948.

Hack, J.J., 1989, Parallel Computing 10 261

Hockney, R.W., 1988, Parallel Computing 2 119

Hockney, R.W., & Jesshope, C.J., 1981, Parallel Computers, Adam Hilger, Bristol.

GOOD PROGRAMMING TECHNIQUES I:

TESTING AND THE LIFE CYCLE OF A SOFTWARE PRODUCT

John B Slater

Bath University Computing Service
University of Bath, Claverton Down, BATH, Avon BA2 7AY

These lectures are not about routine techniques such as Top—down—design and structured programming. They assume some knowledge of these techniques and attempt to build up testing and procedures which supplement these techniques.

These notes are based on those for the SERC Summer School held in Abingdon in July 1989. I am very grateful to Mr R.W.Paulson of Salford University and Mr P.Carr of Bath University for their work in helping devise those notes.

INTRODUCTION

Users want computing results as quickly as possible. Unfortunately they often confuse this with wanting each result as quickly as possible. This leads to the idea of writing programs for *now*. Code is temporary; it is understood only for long enough to get the required results; and even then only by its author. This phenomenon can be observed in almost all Ph.D. programs (the lecturer is unfortunately no exception to this rule).

During the 1970's, the problems associated with this way of doing things became increasingly apparent. These notes aim to help the reader move towards more effective ways of doing things which are more appropriate to a longer term view of software.

SERC supports many software packages on its hardware. Some of them are very large. Many have been modified for different machines or added to several times. Each modification seems harder than the last. Documentation and reality often part company. Versions get lost, go wrong, develop unaccountable bugs and take longer to run. Modifications do not always do quite what was intended. These phenomena are not unique to SERC. Manufacturers with operating systems that work have experienced them for some time. The problems arise in any evolving code environment when insufficient care is taken.

Very few packages last for ever! However, the need for major modification can often be foreseen at the time of initial creation, even if the nature of the modifications are unknown, and the initial work and all subsequent work should be designed to maximise overall efficiency.

Supercomputational Science
Edited by R.G. Evans and S. Wilson
Plenum Press, New York, 1990

25

Care must be taken in many regards. It is necessary to follow procedures, recognise the real problems, specify the work effectively, design and code the solutions effectively, test them rigorously, integrate them into the package, document them properly and follow a suitable acceptance procedure. To do this, it is necessary to respect the problem as being worthy of serious attention. It is also necessary to take account of the fact that the next modification will probably be done by someone else who is likely to have no previous knowledge of the problem.

There is a place for short throw—away programs. These appear in experiments, prototyping and above all testing. However, use should be carefully controlled and documented and above all they should be viewed as precisely what they are: pieces of planned obsolescence. Active discarding of machine— readable source can help with this approach.

"Comments" and "flow diagrams" are classical examples of techniques which many people think beneath them. University students, because they are taught easy programming first, often rapidly abandon both techniques. As a result, they are surprised when their programs cease to work after a few weeks of "real" FORTRAN or C programming.

Teamwork is a vital ingredient. Various team techniques for testing and developing code have been developed and these will be discussed in some detail.

Writing specifications should be an important part of working in the SERC software environment. These can be for either internal or external use. Deciding whether to accept revised code provided from elsewhere is a further area where expertise can assist. Viewing specification and acceptance interfaces from the other side can also assist in understanding some of the problems that can arise for coders. A sequence of specification, coding, testing, debugging, documenting and acceptance should be followed even in a supervisor/student situation. A very common area on which specifier and implementor have differing views is on error actions. This is usually the fault of an incomplete specification followed by a woolly implementation. Unacceptable products are seldom entirely the fault of the implementors.

Testing is not only used when the software is being finally accepted. It is of relevance to all phases of the software development cycle: to specifying, to designing, to coding and to maintaining as well as to acceptance testing.

Although seemingly trivial, it is vital to have an understanding of what testing means, as this fixes the tester's attitudes. Many people use definitions such as:—

> testing is the process of demonstrating that errors are not present

> the purpose of testing a program is to show that it performs its intended functions correctly

> testing is the process of establishing confidence that a program does what it is intended to do

These definitions describe the opposite of the way that testing should be regarded. The purpose of testing is to find errors so that they can be subsequently removed. Hence programs should not be tested to show that they work: rather the assumption should be made that the program contains errors and the purpose of the testing process is to find them. It is therefore more appropriate to define testing as:—

> testing is the process of doing things with a program (or system) with the intention of finding errors.

This has the implication that testing will be done better if a programmer does not test his own programs. It is very difficult for any of us to be destructive about something that we have created ourselves.

Errors can occur at any stage in the development of the software. In general, the later they occur the more expensive they are to correct, as the following table shows

Detection of Error	Relative cost
Preliminary Design	1.0
Detailed Design	1.1 − 1.5
Coding	1.5 − 3.0
Integration	2 − 6
Validation	4 − 18
Operation	10 − 80

The reasons for this are that, as a project progresses,

a) Testing becomes more complex and costly.

b) Documentation of changes becomes more widespread and costly.

c) Communication of problems and changes involves more people.

d) Repeating of previous tests becomes costly.

e) Once operation has started, the development team is reassigned.

Investment in extra checking and testing at the beginning of a program pays off later by reducing the number of costly after–deployment computer errors. The main effort at present, however, is to increase coding quality. Acceptance that high–level languages are superior to assembly languages for applications programming is widespread. Fourth generation languages in the commercial field are becoming much more widespread as are authoring languages in CAL. Package use is on the increase. The object is to write a smaller number of lines of code in order to have less to test. In the scientific area progress has been relatively slow although structured languages, notably C are making considerable inroads in some areas. In some cases a small amount of assembler may be warranted (input/output operations, timing loops in real time systems, micro–coding, small sections of high use code) but this is dwindling. The more intelligent approach is to use assembler routines callable from a high level program.

Language standardisation, leading to increased portability, has become accepted over the past decade. Most manufacturers will convert to ANSI or ISO standards. It appears likely that ADA and C will join FORTRAN and COBOL as widely used standard languages.

Evolution of structured programming techniques in recent years has also led to significant increases in programmer productivity. Software configuration control on large products and the requirement that design be documented adequately is the significant advance on the managerial side. Design representations are not standardised and nor are they likely to be − but the requirement that design be produced on paper or in a machine, rather than held in the minds of a few designers, is important.

Languages develop over the years, (witness FORTRAN and COBOL), to take account of new features. Concomitant with this, program developers have found it increasingly necessary to develop tools to aid them in the development process: tools for editing and storage, processing and preprocessing, configuration control, testing and debugging. IPSEs (Integrated Programming Support Environments) are now more widely available.

As more practitioners adapt the existing design techniques, a greater uniformity on the design process will evolve, resulting in the ability to collect information about their reliability and productivity. It will then be possible to compare and contrast the methods. One of the greatest needs is for measures of goodness of software. Software reliability models exist, but there is a requirement to know, by some means other than intuition, when there has been sufficient testing and redesigning to raise the software reliability to an acceptable level.

FEATURES OF PROGRAM TESTING

There are seven features of testing which should be considered. These are

a) independence of testing

b) definition of expected results

c) inspection and recording of all results

d) invalid and unexpected cases as test data

e) error clumping

f) effects of module complexity

g) testing time as a function of production time

a) Independence of Testing

It is very difficult to be completely detached when testing something that you have created yourself or that has been created under your direction. Other people test your code better than you do yourself. We all feel very defensive about our own creations. Standard practice should be to use test data obtained from the customer, to use test data provided by yourself while developing the code, but also to provide for testing by someone independent.

The form of testing should be that each module is tested separately (horizontal testing), that the entire package should be tested (either starting from the top or working from the bottom − or both), and that each module be tested both in logical order and in development order.

b). Definition of Expected Results

This is a part of testing which is often ignored, to the detriment of the finished code. Perhaps the reason for ignoring it is, in part, a continuation of the syndrome which is apparent in most people learning programming for the first time, that "if the computer gives these results, they must be right". It is of considerable importance to agree not only on suitable test cases, but also on the results expected from them. In the case of the testing of a modification of an existing assumed correct piece of code, a lot can easily be done by throwing the test data at the existing code and then considering what changes are to be expected as a result of the modification. For completely new code, agreement of expected results from test data is more difficult, since it is not always possible to reconcile it with the need to cover every logical path through the package.

If the code is to solve a numerical problem, the posing of test cases to which the analytic solution is known is a possibility. The problem is then to know whether the analytic solution should be produced by the numerical method chosen. Another possibility is to test using degenerate cases, except that many errors arise as a result of the interaction between various parameters of the problem and that this may not arise in the degenerate cases. It is also possible to compare with results obtained using a different numerical method. It should be noted that precision is often vital in numerical work, so that a knowledge of whether double or single precision is used may well be of importance when comparing with known results.

c) Inspection and Recording of All Results

The results of testing should be recorded and checked against any known results. This is true not only of tests of the entire code, but also of tests of individual modules. This procedure will result in towers of results, both in the physical sense and in the hierarchical sense, since the modules are interdependent. These should be recorded, either on backing store or on paper or (preferably) both.

Note that it is much easier to let the computer do your checking for you when the checking is against known results, so that, especially for numerical work, a reasonably sophisticated file comparison program is desirable. Checking visually is best done by two pairs of eyes, one of which should belong to someone with a 'feel' for the problem. Visual checking is not as hard work as may appear at first, since a 'feel' for patterns of errors soon comes to the checker.

Alternatives are not always optional; it is often necessary to use force in order to test them all. Inspection of results reassures that all logical paths have been covered. To do this, it is necessary to test with full knowledge of how the module being tested works (white box testing).

Part of the documentation of any data processing project should be the data used to test the code and the results obtained from the testing. If any modification of the code is done after acceptance, the original test data should be used with the package as well as any new test data designed to test the modification. The object is to bring to light any unwanted side effects which may arise as a result of the modification.

d) Invalid and Unexpected Cases as Test Data

It is important to take account of special cases, even if the only thing done is to print a warning message or to abort when one arises. This is particularly true when coding user interfaces. When users choose the parameters for the package in such a way that a problem is likely to arise, they should be told about it at the time that they choose the parameters. If they then choose to ignore the warning, that is their business. When supplying data to a user interface, the code should give users the opportunity to recover from their mistakes.

e) Error Clumping

An empirical law states that the probability of more errors increases with the number of errors found. If this approximates reality, the modular approach to programming is seen to be advantageous, since there is a chance that errors can then be isolated within a limited number of modules. These can then be tested independently.

Following from the empirical law, there is a point at which the decision to rewrite the code has to be taken, since there are so many errors that rewriting is cheaper than correction. If this course is taken, however, the rewritten code must be tested and debugged as thoroughly as the original. This may take considerable time and effort.

Quality assurance requires that the entire testing process is done thoroughly. The psychological effect of knowing that a program or a package has been tested thoroughly and independently is that confidence in it is increased considerably. Users tend to believe in the results from a package that they know has been tested thoroughly.

f) Effects of Module Complexity

Larger or more complex modules take longer to code and also have a greater testing/production ratio. Various papers have measured complexity and have shown that it depends on

(i) the number of variables in a module

(ii) the number of labels in a module

(iii) the depth of nesting

(iv) the sum of lengths of the (backward) jumps in the module

Since production time rises with complexity at a rate greater than one, simple economics dictate that it is desirable to keep complexity as low as possible. However, this should not be interpreted as advocacy of two–line subroutines. Over–simplicity is paid for by the corresponding increase in the complexity of the structure of the entire package. Modularity in the code should reflect modularity in the problem.

g) Testing Time as a Function of Production Time

The time allowed for testing should be at least as long as the time allowed for the production of the code. Failure to do this will result in higher costs at a later stage, since debugging after acceptance is usually done under considerable pressure and often results in introducing new "bugs" as a result of fixing the original one.

The tests should follow the design of the code. At each design stage the module should be tested immediately and independently.

DEVELOPMENT CYCLE

The stages to be gone through in the development cycle of a software product may be categorised in a number of ways. One way is to divide them into specification, analysis and design, construction and acceptance testing. For our purposes, it is preferable to subdivide these stages further as follows

a) Definition of Requirements

With any project, the first stage is to determine what the customer really wants, as opposed to what the customer says is required. The aim is to arrive at a functional specification for the proposed system.

b) Definition of Objectives

Having arrived at a definition of the requirements for the proposed system, the next step is for the person to do the work to assess the feasibility and the costs of the proposed system. The aim is for the contractor to arrive at specific objectives.

c) External Specification

At this stage, the specific objectives are translated into a precise specification. This is where testing starts. Included in the specification are timescale, conditions of acceptability, documentation standards, etc. This will be discussed more fully below. The specification forms the first part of the documentation of the system. A major interest is in specifying what crosses the interface rather than in what form it goes in and comes out. This phase should be fully documented and tested to make sure that all the required information is input and output.

d) System Design

The package being developed will consist either of a single program or of a set of programs which interact to form a system. In the latter case, the structure of the system should be considered at this stage. A "black box" approach should be followed. The processes being carried out by the individual programs in the system should be viewed in their entirety rather than their individual structure being considered.

The approach can be regarded as similar to that of an engineer. Different designs may be explored. Experience tells the designer which are the most likely to be fruitful. When a particular design is decided on, it is common for a prototype to be produced, which is then refined on the basis of discussion both internal and with the customer.

The main aim of this phase is to define interfaces between the programs in the package and also between the programs and humans where appropriate. In doing this, it is advisable to follow the structure of the overall problem.

e) Program Structure Design

The next phase is to design the structure of each program in the system. This is done by specifying the function of each program, together with the hierarchical structure of the modules of which it is composed and the interfaces between the modules.

Each program should be thoroughly documented and tested against the design and the specifications to make sure that the correct information is passed through the interfaces.

f) Module Interface Specification

The next phase is to be completely precise about the information passing between the modules. In FORTRAN terms, this is the place where decisions are taken as to what information is passed through COMMON and what information is passed by means of parameters. Strict attention should be paid to detail. Any restrictions on information should be clear, also when and where validation checks are to be made to avoid using peculiar values.

In addition to attention being paid to the interfaces between modules, care should also be taken to determine which modules are required by a particular module and by which modules a particular module is required. In fact, part of the documentation is to specify precisely this.

g) Coding

At this stage, the module interface specification is translated into source code, using whatever language is appropriate. Coding should be done to the ANSI or other standard appropriate for the language being used, for reasons of portability. The layout of the code should conform to the normal house practice (if there is one), and the code should be well commented. The main thing to remember is that understandability of the code matters.

h) Acceptance Testing

When the software has been developed to a suitable stage (or when the deadline for completion can no longer be postponed), a formal acceptance test should be held. The originator of the requirement plays the major part in this.

i) Use

It is commonly believed by those who have never written one that once a package is accepted, the composer can forget about it, apart from fixing bugs. In fact, the wise composer keeps a careful eye on how the package is used. It is sensible to generate a system which results in all peculiarities being recorded and reported. Bugs that "everyone" (except the composer) knows about do one's reputation no good at all.

A good monitoring method for the system helps when determining what modifications are required when the time comes for the package to be updated. Included in this should be its usage, any queries made about it, and also any areas where expected usage is less than was anticipated.

A list of known bugs in the package should be available to users. When bugs are fixed, the list of known bugs should be likewise amended. Due notification should be given of alterations before they are made, giving a date when the alteration is to be made.

A software package is there to be used. If users or prospective users do not have confidence in the package, or their complaints and comments are not dealt with in a reasonable time, they will not use the package. This will lead to the premature retirement of both the package and the composer.

j) Subsequent Perturbation

Once the package has been completed to the agreed specifications, and people have started to use it, the dreaded words "Wouldn't it be nice if ..." are always heard. The obvious thing to do is to ignore them in the hope that they will go away. This never happens, but it is inevitably tried. In fact, perturbations of the package are inevitable. They can be divided into two classes, bug fixes and enhancements.

Bug fixes are always needed. The temptation is always to adopt the fire–fighting approach to bug–fixing, that is for all hands to leap in, find the bug, fix it and go home. Unfortunately, this approach usually causes more trouble because of the inadequate testing of the modification that it causes.

When bugs are fixed, there are two separate problems; diagnosis and cure. Diagnosis is more suitable for the fire–fighting approach. If cure is attempted by similar means, the fix is likely to have unfortunate side effects. It is far better to carry through a proper change procedure. This involves carrying out tests on the amended system before putting it into service.

In the case of enhancement, changes should be regarded as a separate mini–project. Changes should be planned, controlled and tested. Finally, users of the system should be notified that the change is to be made and also when it is to happen. The old version of the system should be kept as a backup.

As far as possible, interfaces should not be altered as a result of changes made to the system. The aim is to keep the recoding necessary as localised as possible. Changes to user documentation should be made available to users at the time that the changes are released, and changes to system documentation likewise. The changes to the system documentation should be done, not by replacement, but by addition. Thus the amended documentation should consist of the original documentation, a list of alterations to it and, if the list be long, the amended documentation.

Any side effects that changes give rise to should be noted carefully. There should hopefully be none, but this is unlikely for a large package. The cause of the side effects should be found and, if they are detrimental, they should be fixed using the change procedure described above.

Above all, any changes made should be tested using not only test data designed to test the changes, but also previous test data. The altered package should not be released until this has been done. Note that a file comparison program is a useful tool in checking old results against the new results.

DOCUMENTATION

Documentation can be divided into system documentation and user documentation. System documentation consists of flow charts, a glossary, specifications for internal and external interfaces, resource requirements, limitations, references to the sources of algorithims used and a description (where appropriate) of how they have been applied.

The user documentation should be designed to make sure that anyone who knows nothing about the package finds starting to use it reasonably painless. It should also aim to provide a ready reference guide for the regular user with a bad memory. It should contain instructions concerning the input of parameters and data, giving typical values where appropriate for the parameters as well as any limits placed on them. If the format of the data is important, as it will probably be for a FORTRAN 77 package, this should be made clear. The user documentation should also contain a reasonable number of examples of using the package, illustrating its main features. Finally interpretation of output from the package is required. Any messages that the package may give should be listed, together with suggestions as to their use and advice as to what to do when they arise.

The user documentation should also contain an (honest) assessment of the limitations of the packages from the point of view of the user. Where the package has used a particular algorithm, an assessment of that algorithm together with discussion of the types of problem for which it is or is not suitable should be given. The information under the "HELP" facility should be regarded as part of the user documentation.

Aids to Documentation

Most modern machines have a text processing package available. This may vary from a fully functional word processor to something such as a DTP package. The fundamental object of such a package is to take a file of text which is arranged in arbitrary line lengths and to format it to have uniform line length and predetermined spacing between lines. Most packages have additional facilities, such as the ability to print text half a space up or down, but it is advisable to know the minimum about any particular text processing package, as otherwise the tendency is to become "locked in" to that package. This induces resistance to change.

GOOD PROGRAMMING TECHNIQUES II

TEST CASE DESIGN METHODOLOGIES

John B Slater

Bath University Computing Service, University of Bath
Claverton Down, BATH, Avon BA2 7AY

This lecture discusses the general problem of designing test cases. Not all test cases will feature in a non—computer—based test. Indeed, probably no more than half a dozen will be used. The tester will nevertheless want a lot more than that available, tests being chosen according to the direction the non—computer—based test takes. All tests will be used for computer based testing. It is with the total set of tests this lecture deals.

THE AIM OF TESTING

The aim of testing is to find a subset of all tests with the highest probability of detecting the most errors. Usually the subset has a finite size attached to it (e.g. 50 test cases) or more probably a finite time condition within which it has to be completed (e.g. until May 1st). The finite number condition makes the problem not dissimilar to that of selecting the England Cricket Team or a University Challenge Team. In the latter case, the objective is to find four people with the highest probability of answering the most questions between them (ignoring complications of starter and bonus). In the former case, the objective is to choose eleven people who perform together best as a team with the highest probability of winning. It is an unfortunate fact that program testers rarely do better than the England Cricket selectors and often even worse.

Time deadlines are nastier. Unless you can estimate better than most, the objective changes to that of providing up to "n" ordered tests such that, if you assume that the probability of getting "t" tests done is p(t), then

$$\sum_{t=1}^{n} p(t)\, q(t)$$

is maximal, where q(t) is an objective measure of the probability of detecting errors with "t" tests. As q(t) is rarely measurable and p(t) is a guess, this formula is not helpful. All that is really being said is that, if you know there is to be a cut off in the testing process, you should test as broadly as possible before you get there, then thicken out the testing gradually.

Supercomputational Science
Edited by R.G. Evans and S. Wilson
Plenum Press, New York, 1990

Four sorts of testing are used

(a) logic covering (white–box)

(b) case covering (black–box)

(c) monte carlo (as you go along)

(d) analogy (look where probability dictates for this problem/coder)

WHITE BOX TESTING

This assumes that you have knowledge of the design/code of the program. You can, for instance, attempt to ensure that your test cases cover

(i) all statements

(ii) all decisions

(iii) all conditions

(iv) all decisions/conditions

Making sure each statement is executed once in at least one test is unlikely to be sufficient. One would really want every possible path through a program to be tested, but the number of tests this is likely to engender becomes astronomic as soon as optional loops (or choice within a loop) are included.

All decisions being taken in all possible directions is a distinct improvement on every statement being executed once. For example, consider the following code

```
        .
        .
        .
        IF (A.GT.0.0) GOTO 61
        IF (B.GT.0.0) GOTO 62
        C=−B
61      D=E
62      CONTINUE
        .
        .
        .
```

To make sure each statement is executed, it suffices to have A non–positive and B non–positive in the test case, but this leaves a lot untested. In decision coverage, three cases are required. These are

(i)   A positive

(ii)   A non–positive with B positive

(iii)   A and B both non–positive

However it is clear that, once multiple entry points have been covered separately, decision coverage will imply statement coverage.

Decision coverage will, however, meet problems with complex decision criteria. As an example, consider

IF (A.GE.0.0 .OR. F(X).LT.1.0) GOTO 61

Only two cases need to be considered. These are

(i)   A non–negative

(ii)   A negative with F(X) greater than or equal to 1.0, so F(X) need never be less than 1.0

This problem is solved by moving to condition coverage which specifies that all conditions should take on all possible outcomes at least once. This gains over decision coverage in that, for instance, it forces F(X) to be less than 1.0 in at least one case. Unfortunately, only two test cases are still needed. These could be

(i)   A and F(X)–1 both non–negative

(ii)   A and F(X)–1 both negative

Control will now always move to label 61, so we have lost not only decision coverage but possibly statement coverage as well.

What is thus normally used is that combination in which every condition has all outcomes, every decision has all outcomes and each entry point is used. This is clearly strictly stronger than anything considered above. In our case, three examples would suffice to test the branch but may still not cover any side effects involved in evaluating F(X).

As a partial attempt to move towards complete path testing, some attempt at multiple coverage can be made using design techniques so as to test combinations of decisions being made in a fixed order. This is called multiple coverage. The problem is remarkably similar to that of the design of experiments, with appropriate Steiner systems and other well known techniques having a part to play. All of this is written up in many books on statistics. For full combinations of all decisions/conditions (analogous to all four cases in the above tests), other techniques for test case generation of a mechanised nature exist. These correspond to all subsets of a subset (Gray code), or all n–subsets of a subset (revolving door) with the least possible changes. These techniques are, however, relatively unlikely to play a significant part in the basic test case design process.

BLACK BOX TESTING

In this case, one stands back from the problem and asks where the errors are likely to occur by looking at the problem and at the potential solution.

Boundary Value Techniques

One answer to the question of where errors are most likely to occur is "at the limit". If a linear equation solver for up to 50 variables works for 49 variables, for 50 variables, for one variable, for two variables and for no variables, it is likely to work with all numbers of variables from none to fifty inclusive. On this basis, the idea of looking at extremes of the various parameters seems reasonable.

Boundary value testing is usually used in conjunction with equivalence partitioning (see below). It is not sufficient to test extremes of input. Extremes of output must also be tested assuming always that the appropriate input be known. As well as testing the extreme itself, it is worth while to test close to the extreme. This is because the extreme will frequently be a special case (possibly coded as such!). It is also advisable to test near and at extremes of an intermediate type within the problem. You can do this without knowing anything about the code.

As an example, suppose that

$$f(x) = x \sin(1/x) \text{ on } [-1,1]$$

is to be evaluated by a machine routine. Tests should be made at $x=-1.0$ and $x=1.0$, and at $x=-0.999$ and $x=0.999$. Tests should also be made at $x=0.0$, $x=.001$ and $x=-.001$ as parts of $f(x)$ are extreme at these points.

EQUIVALENCE PARTITIONING

Equivalence partitioning is thought by many to be the essence of black–box testing. The basic idea is to identify a number of test cases which include all the cases required. This is followed by identifying a much smaller set of cases which will test everything that the larger set tested.

To give a better feel for this idea, suppose that there are 64 test cases which "cover" all test cases. Suppose that it is possible to identify six criteria which are orthogonal (independent) so that performances under these six criteria determine the test case. Note that 64 is the sixth power of two. One then asks if it is possible to find twelve test cases which test the six criteria on each possible side in an independent fashion. This is a quasi–formal way of saying that we should choose test cases so that each case covers a large set of other possible test cases (when considered as part of a set), and which also presents a large set of actual cases.

Equivalence classes tend to be small and hence the number of equivalence classes large in the area of invalid cases, where this technique has most to show in halting the growth of the number of cases.

Working with equivalence classes can be hard without the use of some form of documentation aid. Various examples are given by Myers [1]. Again, the theory of the design of experiments has a part to play choosing test cases wisely from amongst a larger subset.

CAUSE EFFECT GRAPHING

The author has had little experience of the use of this technique. The idea is to establish a digraph of the causes and effects of the program. A cause is an input condition or an equivalence class of input conditions. An effect is either an output condition (eg the printing of specific message) or a change to the system (an update of a file etc). All causes and effects are assigned an identifier, and the total graph is configured. Intermediate states may be used to simplify logic.

Not all causes will be independent. A rule about potential input restrictions is called a constraint, and the graph is now annotated with constraints.

What follows is that, by tracing the cause effect operations, the graph can be converted into a finite decision table in which each column can be converted into a test case. Programs exist to help analyse the network. For further information see Myers [1].

MONTE–CARLO TESTING

To test a program, a further program of a random walk nature is written. It first makes a test using only very crude data, that is, random bits are first sent as data. This checks the program for faults connected with computer noise. The data is then slowly refined towards meaningful data in a Monte–Carlo fashion. As each refinement is made, new test data is generated to feed into the system. Eventually the program makes (mostly) legitimate demands on the system and tests the logic in a conventional fashion. The process is then repeated using a different walk. This method is used for important real time signal processing and related work where the effort of writing such a suite is considered worthwhile.

ERROR GUESSING

Some people are basically good at "smelling out" errors. Intuition and experience are used to detect likely errors and hence likely test cases. This experience can be of the type of problem, type of coder, actual problem or actual coder variety. The technique is not dissimilar to the compilation of checklists for the code inspection.

A STRATEGY FOR TESTING

No one technique or combination is preferred. A lot depends upon the type of problem and the way in which it is specified. Monte–Carlo techniques are specialised and apply mainly to real time vital programs. A good analogy to the testing process is that of someone given a new British Rail timetable and a detailed map of the tracks. The problem is to find the errors in the proposed procedures.

Some problems lend themselves to cause–effect graphing. If the specification is of the "if–then–else" variety, cause– effect graphing is likely to be very effective. The more complicated the logic, the more effective this technique will be, or rather the less effective all other techniques will be. Scientific problems rarely lend themselves to this approach except at the highest levels. Control of the flow through the routines of a crystallographic package is an example where the techniques might have value.

Boundary value tests should always be used. Input boundary values are usually easy to identify, but remember that this is true for the coder also. It is worth spending time on finding output boundary conditions. It is often worth a small white box "peep" at the code to see if the coder has identified the output boundaries and/or coded them as separate cases.

Many boundary value tests will coincide with cause–effect tests, especially when parameters have two values only. Boundary value tests can be thought of as the continuous equivalent of the discrete cause–effect tests. Scientific problems tend to have ranges of inputs or outputs rather than discrete sets, so boundary value analysis is vital in this area.

Error guessing is always a valuable supplement to other testing methods, but it should be thought of in that light. It can sometimes be used in advance of other testing with devastating effect. In this case, sort out the problems that arise before proceeding with the testing proper. Alternatively, late "hunch" error guessing is also useful in the testing process. A strange combination not thought to be possible (and hence excluded from cause–effect graphing) or the realisation of a new output boundary are good examples of the sort of thing that can occur.

The identification of equivalence classes for the input/output now follows. Often this will replicate test cases already chosen, but sometimes new classes of invalid data are added. It is in this area that the techniques have most to offer. Valid coverage will generally have already been achieved.

So far, all testing has been of a black (or at least a murky) box variety. Only now should the lid be taken off the box to examine the program logic. Decision/condition coverage, with all entry points tested with some multiple coverage where you suspect problems, is good. This must be achieved by building round the existing test cases. In all cases this building round process must be used to avoid unnecessary work.

When planning white box testing, it is vital that realism be practised. There is little point in devising several million test cases. However, having done this, and in any case, it is vital to record the test cases devised and then to use this as a basis for the documentation of the actual testing. Much subsequent work can be saved if test cases are known to have been carried out.

AN EXAMPLE

A good old chestnut is testing whether a set of three integers form an isosceles, equilateral or scalene triangle

Monte—Carlo techniques are not appropriate for this problem. Cause effect graphing is a reasonable technique here. The causes are such things as the first number being a positive integer etc. By no means does it tell the whole tale but the decision process is sufficiently simple to generate the whole cause—effect graph without too much trouble. Boundary value analysis adds some other cases — perhaps cases that are just not straight lines. It also adds large numbers, but here it is important to have large scalene as well as large isosceles and equilateral triangles. Equivalence classes add various examples of invalid data, characters in various places, including decimal points, commas and carriage returns.

Finally the use of white box testing will, along with a lot of repeated cases, complete the set. This will lead to a further set of examples, including the data in column 80 or 81 type. FORMAT statements and READ and WRITE statements are also the subject of white box testing to ensure the limits of the applicability are reached.

PRAGMATIC TESTING

The above description fits well a small program, or so one would think. What about the 3000 line (uncommented, undocumented) epics that other people write and you have to modify and to test. Or perhaps the 3000 line epic that you write. A first piece of advice is "don't". Hopefully, the use of structured techniques will lead you to design in sensible modules. The best thing that can be done with a single 3000 line program which is uncommented and undocumented is to leave well alone. If you can't leave well alone, rewriting is often the best long term solution, although sometimes "management" takes some convincing. Often, however, the use of various tools (see below) pinpoints the fact that the program really does have the form of a set of modules — it has just been coded in an obscure fashion.

We therefore concentrate on the case when the code is divided up into subunits in some fashion and ask what the best testing method is in these circumstances. The technique is called module testing. The idea is to test each module individually as a separate entity before configuring them. With a well written program modules will corresponds to pieces in a large to medium scale design, but this is not always the case. Thus module testing is not the same as structured testing, although it ought to be.

Having tested the modules individually it is necessary to recombine them. This is usually done in a steady build up fashion — one by one the pieces are assembled. If the module structure is a tall tree, this is usually done in a bottom up fashion. Modules at the bottom of the tree are put together with the next level up and tested as a whole. Then these groups are assembled to provide a group at the next level and so on. A top–down approach is sometimes used where the actual lower level routines are replaced by dummy calls or routines which give answers for the specific test cases used. This is not without danger, but it does avoid some pitfalls of the alternative approaches.

Testing modules individually is not always easy. A test may need to be constructed, consisting of a calling routine and a substitute for any routines that the module calls. One way round this is to follow the bottom–up strategy and to use the actual lower modules with only the calling routine a rig. Thus testing of higher level modules and the way in which they fit with their subservient modules occur simultaneously. This is not unreasonable, especially if the design has reduced the higher module to a set of calls with simple logic. The code of a major graphics package or any other professionally coded work often has this form.

Bottom–up testing of this form tends to use more resources but it has been found to be very effective. The alternatives have a number of basic flaws in them for general programming. However, in some pragmatic cases where "modules" cannot be decoupled, it may be necessary to follow other procedures.

Tests are actually best conducted neither by the coder nor the designer of the test. Forced to choose, the test designer is preferable, although he is also an "interested party".

DEBUGGING

A test has highlighted an error. This error must be removed. How do we set about removing it?

Experience shows that very few programmers employ a systematic technique for finding errors. Some try to explain the error away, if necessary by changing the specification. Others rush to a pot of tea and the code and cast around until they find it. Yet others cover their code liberally in PRINT statements wherever they are easy to put, then gradually home in on the error. Others start modifying the code where "they never liked it anyway". Eventually the error goes away and the problem is declared to be solved.

Thus, a naive form of divide and conquer is used to find bugs to some effect. A bug is discernable by a wolf howling in Alaska and it is necessary to find it. So, divide Alaska into two and choose the half from which the howling comes. Divide it into two etc and eventually you have your wolf. This technique can be very useful, but not all bugs correspond to wolves howling. Even if they do, the wolf is often the symptom not the cause. A wolf can travel a long way howling with poison in its stomach. It is the poison dump you need to detect and remove.

It is vital, on detecting a bug, to ensure that any "fixes" you devise do not have undesirable side effects. Strictly, a completely new set of tests must be run, the bug fix being treated as a new module. It is also important to have a good change control system. Always retain a "working" version and add to it incrementally so that you can revert to it if required. A worst case is to put lots of different "fixes" from a variety of sources, in at the same time on the only copy of the code. You then discover that the new version doesn't work at all!

The crucial thing when debugging is to keep calm, and to keep track of what you do, recording it in detail. Some people are much better at debugging than others. A healthy scepticism is a good start, also the ability to question everything as being a potential cause of the detailed problem. Lecturers seem to develop an aptitude for debugging, especially when dealing with student programs. Some trivial bugs, such as zero for letter O or vice versa shout at some people from the page. Others require sophisticated tools to find them.

Debugging is hard work. Another skill that you must acquire is knowing when to stop. Like mathematical proof, a sledgehammer approach, especially when you are tired, is unlikely to get you anywhere. You are probably a long distance from the correct nut–tree. Sleep can be helpful in finding bugs, especially when a direct method is being used.

Like mathematical proof, a number of different approaches are possible. Reasoning backed up by evidence at each stage is the preferred procedure. The computer should be thought of either as a last resort in debugging or as an evidence–providing tool. It should never be thought of as something which provides the answers. IKBS may change this. Although some powerful tools are now available, in particular when associated with compilers, these should be again thought of as supplying evidence rather than solutions. Bugs when found should normally be documented as such before being removed. Sometimes bugs can be left in code as comments to remind the future unwary.

The divide and conquer approach outlined above is an example of brute force. The idea is to make up in activity for what is lacking in thought. Manufacturers can be keen to present you with tools that assist with this approach. If you have compiled with a debugger present you may usually insert "check points" in your programs. On reaching a checkpoint, the program will pause if so directed. You can then look at the values of variables, change them, change the flow (if stuck in a loop, say), find the sequence of subprogram calls that got you there, check array bounds are not violated, etc, etc.

The cost of debugging is considerable however, so sometimes dumps are essential. Some compiling systems include direct options for checking on some things. These should not be thought of specifically as debugging tools, but as preventative rather than curative medicine. The following can be of use if present

CHECK ARRAY BOUNDS
CHECK OVERFLOW
CHECK UNDERFLOW
CHECK CARRY
CHECK ANSI (checks for standard conformation)

IMPLICIT LOGICAL (A–Z) (helps find misspelling errors)

CHECK ARGUMENTS (checks the number and type of all arguments passed
    in a FORTRAN call or function reference if this is possible)

PROFILE (this feature which is available on some systems, gives a count of the number of times
    each statement was executed during a run)

Splattering PRINT statements is another form of divide and conquer. This leads to enormous quantities of data and often to very long output files.

Recompilation is necessary each time and, with a large program, the time taken can be immense. In some cases of real time programming, the very act of putting in the PRINT statement makes the problem go away, so the technique fails completely.

THINKING TESTING

Thinking testing usually takes one or the other of the following four forms

Induction

After a test case gives rise to an error, the behaviour of a significant number of test cases with respect to that error is drawn up. An attempt is made to organise this data so as to deduce the likely error — good white—box testing should make this possible. Given a hypothesis, it is tested against all available evidence. Assuming it is consistent, an appropriate fix is made and testing recommences.

Deduction

In this case a list of possible hypotheses is drawn up. Other test cases are then used to eliminate some and to refine others. After a few steps of successive elimination and refinement, the remaining hypotheses can be tested and (hopefully) proved.

Backtracking

A point at which an error has occurred is identified. The program is then mentally executed backwards to a point at which there is demonstrably no error. The bug lies on this path, and the backwards execution process often finds it.

Testing Refinement

As with induction, test cases will hopefully give a clear indication of where the errors lie. A further set of test cases, increasing the coverage of this area of code, is devised. These are used to refine knowledge of the location of the error. The process is repeated until the error is located precisely.

DOCUMENTATION

The main piece of documentation is the program itself. It must be readable, follow house style, and have suitable naming conventions that are internally and externally consistent. To help achieve this, a number of things can be done, including comments, PRINT statements, supplementary notes, etc. Documenting tools exist and form part of Integrated Programing Software Environments (IPSEs).

Standards for coding and documentation have existed for some time. The NCC standard is well known, but it concentrates on the commercial aspects. Hence it is largely data—driven. Standard forms exist for file descriptions, flow charts (or their equivalents), "card" layouts, procedure documents, outline descriptions, output formats, parameter lists, control lists, instructions, user guides etc. SERC has a number of standards. As with other scientific organisations, they tend to be process driven with the emphasis on explanation, parameter lists and descriptions, guides for preparation of data and interpretation of results, and the ubiquitous "system documentation".

System documentation should contain many things. Parameters and their use at a technical level are vital. A discussion of the testing design, what was carried out with what results, bugs fixed, subsequent testing, human testing problems etc is very useful. Lists of calling routines as well as called routines are extremely useful, provided they are updated as a matter of routine. If this is not done, they are worse than useless.

If you are modifying a routine, it is important to fall into the original style and conventions. This will not only help you but subsequent workers. It is also essential not to destroy earlier documentation, but to supplement it. Old copies should be retained so that the ability to revert is retained in all senses.

It is vital in the documentation process that documentation be collected assiduously as the project proceeds. Details of tests carried out and the results should be filed carefully so that someone can take over at short notice. If possible, documentation should be structured in design levels, as is the project. In this way a modifier can pick up the work fairly quickly.

A short pause after completion of coding but before the documentation is finally structured can however be of value, as it permits minor modifications to be made in the light of experience. Documentation will continue to change as the program develops. Thus it should be machine readable as far as possible.

From a project management point of view, documentation should be addressed early and sufficient time allowed for it throughout the project. Both management pressure and programmer's instincts lead documentation to be left late and under–resourced. This is a bad strategy in the longer term.

System documentation must be done whilst the program is relatively fresh. NCC and other forms help jog the memory of the documentor, as do the utilities mentioned above. An update policy for documentation is likely to be required almost as soon as the documentation is complete, if not before. It should include how bugs and their fixes are to be included, testing strategy for alterations, and references to documentation in the machine that must also be modified.

User instructions and aids are vital. Clear instructions for the preparation and meaning of all data and the interpretation of all results, including unexpected ones, must be given. A "HELP" type facility for users in distress is a valuable asset for any major program which has a wide audience. Above all, the actual user interface is a vital part of the program (which is itself a piece of documentation). Questions must be clear, unambiguous and free from jargon. Output to screen should be timed correctly. Preferably, it should not be insulting. The study of user interfaces could be the subject of a whole lecture course, but that is not our current purpose. User documentation is often written before the project starts. This can be good practice, although it should be thought of as a first draft. Certainly a policy of agreeing user documentation with the customer and also agreeing any modifications as a matter of routine has many attractions, including the early identification of misunderstandings between customer and contractor. However, too rigid an adherence to the original user documentation is likely to be of little advantage to either party.

GOOD PROGRAMMING TECHNIQUES. III.

NON–COMPUTER BASED TESTING

John B Slater

Bath University Computing Service, University of Bath
Claverton Down, BATH, Avon BA2 7AY

DEVELOPMENT

In the early days of computing the programmer designer, numerical expert, etc spent a good deal of time checking through every single facet of a program before it was let near the computer. Computer time was so precious that any amount of human effort was considered to be worthwhile to avoid a wasted run on the machine. Dry running or desk checking — the technique of "playing computer" to real data — was an expected weapon in the armoury of all programmers, not merely as a means of avoiding bugs, but as the main means of finding them after an unsuccessful run. This phenomenon can be reproduced if you look at current GCSE syllabi, especially as taught at those few schools still relying on batch services for their computing.

Such a system led to an inevitable reaction when computing time became cheaper and more available. Quickly the idea of "throw it at the machine as soon as possible, so as to get typing and all other errors sorted out" caught on as programmers discovered that they were truly left alone if they went and hid at a VDU all day long.

Non–computer based testing was considered unusual, restricted to those few programs capable of being "proven" — intellectual curiosities mainly. Students still possess the ability to lash up something quickly, type it in and sort it out from there. It is often hard to convince them that this is not the best way. Undergraduates have often been severely restricted in usage when they were at school, so the temptation to over–react is irresistible.

Since the early 1970s, there has been a growing awareness that some types of test are currently done better by the human brain than by the machine. This has only been formalised in the current decade. Human testing can be applied throughout the design stage, but it has a further important role to play. This occurs after the completion of coding, but before computer based testing has commenced. Perhaps the encapsulation of the human processes into an expert system will subsequently permit a return of much of this domain to the machine.

The techniques we discuss below have become associated with structured programming, but are essentially independent. Indeed, structured programming is a necessary prerequisite for the techniques to be applicable without a very high complexity which makes them very long to complete rigourously.

Supercomputational Science
Edited by R.G. Evans and S. Wilson
Plenum Press, New York, 1990

45

The aim of structured programming is to make a formal "proof of correctness" of a program an easier task. This remains the ultimate goal for any program. The fact that full proof is rarely attainable is no reason not to strive for it. A large "proven" component in a program is a very useful asset in diminishing the complexity of the testing operation.

The methods below, are significantly less formal. These methods have been found to work well, particularly when allied to structured design. Errors are found earlier than in a computer based testing environment, so the costs of correction are substantially lower.

The knowledge that design or code is going to be subjected to human based testing seems to make the initial work better. Programmers dislike having their mistakes found by human beings, but, surprisingly, seem indifferent to a machine in this role. In addition, if code is on a machine when a mistake is found, there is a tendency to code round the true problem rather than to redesign or to recode the appropriate section. This is an unhealthy practice, both for the present and for the future life of a program product.

A kinder explanation of the psychological phenomenon noted in the last paragraph is that knowledge of human testing leads inherently kind programmers to design and code in a more readable fashion, so as to make the testing easier. In so doing, they write better code. Whatever the reason, there is considerable evidence for the fact that human based testing has an important role to play in the development of successful software even before the testing actually commences.

We now consider a number of techniques including inspections, walkthroughs, desk checking, double checking and peer reviews. These are all based about a number of common ideas, so we discuss these ideas first.

Reading is Easier than Writing

This obvious fact is known to any five year old schoolchild, to any scientist at University without any formal training in German, to any research worker in a scientific field and to any program author.

It is Easier to Knock Down Someone Else's Sandcastles

Writing or designing code is a creative process and, if flaws are present, the author is unlikely to be best at finding them. Again this phenomenon is noticeable in the scientific paper field. Thus, human based testing is best done by someone from a different group.

Knowledge is a Pre−requisite for Good Human−based Testing

The more a tester knows about both the problem that the work addresses and the detail of the attack at all levels of design and coding, the more likely he is to find mistakes. Yet again, the analogy of a reviewer of a scientific paper is a good one.

Testing must follow Structure

First test the top level design and then refine in a similar fashion until the tester is working at the detailed code level. Testing can only be restrained in complexity if this "rule" is followed.

Discussion is Valuable

Talking things through is a valuable approach to many problems. The very requirement to explain things to someone else often orders an individual's thinking and enables the detection of errors. This is even the case if the author is the explainer. "Mistakes found in seminars" is a possible analogy.

Role—Playing is important

The fact that someone is cast in the role of finding mistakes often makes them live up to that role. A person charged with 'rigourous testing as in the book' is more likely to find serious mistakes than someone asked to "check a program out". Often serious mistakes are first noticed as minor blemishes. It is the former instruction that leads to the blemishes being noted.

Management—free

When a management role is present, all other roles change, rarely for the better. As at a 'final trial' in physical sports, objectives change from 'doing the best for the team' to 'impressing the selectors'. Play moves unmistakably to the side of the field where the selectors are seated. Thus, whilst management is looking, lots of mistakes (or potential mistakes) are found by everybody. Once the managerial back is turned, however, interest diminishes.

Parallelism

Human based testing can exploit the parallelism of a situation, in particular in a modification exercise. It is possible to have several human based testing operations simultaneously active on the same code, testing out different aspects of a design.

WALKTHROUGHS

In a walkthrough, the emphasis is on testing with real data examples. All participants must familiarise themselves with the design and code in advance. The designer/coder should be present together with a moderator who is responsible for timing (internal and external), predistribution of materials, the organisation of the (up to two hour) session, and the achievement of the objectives.

The testing expert is expected to come equipped with a large number of test cases on which he wishes to try the design or code. The moderator will have had a brief meeting with the expert in advance of the walkthrough to review the cases to be covered (and not to conduct a prewalkthrough).

The designer/coder plays a fairly passive role. It is worth noting the walkthroughs can take place at any point in a structured design situation. Indeed, there is advantage in identifying high—level design problems before too much lower level work is wasted.

The process is a form of group task—checking, using the board or its equivalent as an interactive device and the program/designer as an available resource, to be used when all else fails. However, listening to discussion can cause the programmer to see errors more quickly than others. If this happens, he should not sit and watch everyone else struggle.

The objective is to locate errors rather than to solve them, but the true location must be found at the appropriate level of design. It is never correct to identify a symptom as the error and to proceed. Hopefully very rarely, this may lead to the re—examination of an already accepted piece of design.

Recording of errors is important, and the role of a secretary is one of those essential in a walkthrough team. This is a distinct role from that of the moderator, unlike in the inspection, where there is usually a set of preprinted forms which can be used to simplify the role. Sometimes two or three people take on the secretary's role because of the difficulties in recording errors. This is particularly true when a number of errors occur in concentrated form, as frequently happens.

Walkthroughs, pioneered by Weinberg [2], have been found to be one of the most profitable forms of human testing, provided that the psychological conditions are favourable.

DESK CHECKING

Traditional desk checking still has a minor role to play for the solitary programmer wanting to do some human based testing. Otherwise it has been found to be less effective.

DUPLICATION

Duplication of task followed by rigourous comparison is used in many of the fail—safe type of processes, especially in the aerospace industry. Techniques where many computers are coded and tested separately and majority decisions taken in the event of disagreement are not unknown.

PEER REVIEW

A final technique used to produce better code is the idea of peer review. Each program is a 'test' being 'marked' anonymously by someone else. Not only the efficiency, but also the clarity, documentation, style and modifiability are open for comment. It is thought by many that it is the threat of this that has effect, rather than the technique. Some commentators believe that the effect is likely to be resignation. Others remark that this is little different from management doing the reviewing, except that peers know a lot more. It is hardly used in the UK.

INSPECTIONS

Inspections differ from walkthroughs in that they are process— driven rather than data—driven. An inspection is a form of group code reading. The team is usually four or five in size with specific roles to be played. An inspection usually revolves about a check list approach with back—up forms and other documentation often providing the check lists. The inspection proceeds in a structured fashion through the design, but usually does not start until most code has been produced.

One member of the team takes the role of moderator with responsibility for distribution of preparatory materials, the timing of session (internal and external), and ensuring that decisions are reached and correctly recorded. The designer and coder are further team members with an inspection expert being a fourth member. In a large project with several levels of design, the team may expand or it may contract if one person is both the designer and the coder.

Appropriate preparatory work of design and code reading is essential to give all members of the team a working knowledge of the system. A substantial part of the session is spent with designers and/or coders explaining, statement by statement in the latter case, how their system works. The remainder of the team ask questions, and analyse the procedure with respect to check lists of common programming errors.

The moderator must ensure that the procedure does not become too destructive — or too constructive. As with a walkthrough, the objective is to find errors not to correct them. Proper recording of errors found can not only help this process, but also subsequent ones. In extreme cases, it can cause future additions to be made to the check lists themselves.

Checklists are a mixture of the general and the particular. In the latter case, there may be common errors in this type of work, or even with this specific program or coder. The following section, an example of some of the things that appear on detailed check lists, is taken from Myers. It should be thought of as a basis for the actual check list.

DATA–REFERENCE ERRORS

1. Is a variable referenced whose value is unset or uninitialised? This is probably the most frequent programming error; it occurs in a wide variety of circumstances. For each reference to a data item (eg variable, array element, field in a structure), attempt to "prove" informally that the item has a value at the point.

2. For all array references, is each subscript value within the defined bounds of the corresponding dimension?

3. For all array references, does each subscript have an integer value? This is not necessarily an error in all languages, but it is a dangerous practice.

4. For all references through pointer or reference variables, is the referenced storage currently allocated? This is known as the "dangling reference" problem.

5. When a storage area has alias names with differing attributes, does the data value in this area have the correct attributes when referenced via one of these names? Situations to look for are the use of the DEFINED attribute or based storage in PL/I, the EQUIVALENCE statement in FORTRAN, and the REDEFINES clause in COBOL. As an example, a FORTRAN program contains a real variable A and an integer variable B; both are made aliases for the same storage area by using an EQUIVALENCE statement. If the program stores a value into A and then references variable B, an error is likely to be present since the machine would use the floating–point bit representation in the storage area as an integer.

6. Does a variable's value have a type or attribute other than that expected by the compiler? This situation might occur where a PL/I or COBOL program reads a record into storage and references if by using a structure, but the physical representation of the record differs from the structure definition.

7. Are there any explicit or implicit addressing problems if, on the machine being used, the units of storage allocation are smaller than the units of storage addressability?

8. If pointer or reference variables are used, does the referenced storage have the attributes expected by the compiler?

9. If a data structure is referenced in multiple procedures or subroutines, is the structure defined identically in each procedure?

10. When indexing into a string, are the limits of the string exceeded?

11. Are there any "off by one" errors in indexing operations or in subsequent references to arrays? Many people start counting at 1 rather than 0 (or vice versa).

DATA—DECLARATION ERRORS

1. Have all variables been explicitly declared? A failure to do so is not necessarily an error, but it is a common source of trouble. For instance, if a FORTRAN subroutine receives an array (eg in a DIMENSION statement), a reference to the array ((eg X=A (I)) is interpreted as a function call, leading to the machine's attempting to execute the array as a program. If a variable is not explicitly declared in an inner procedure or block, is it understood that the variable is shared with the enclosing block?

2. If all attributes of a variable are not explicitly stated in the declaration, are the defaults well understood?

3. Where a variable is initialised in a declarative statement, is it properly initialised? In many languages, initialisation of arrays and strings is somewhat complicated and hence error prone.

4. In each variable assigned the correct length, type, and storage class (eg STATIC, AUTOMATIC, BASED, or CONTROLLED in PL/I)?

5. Is the initialisation of a variable consistent with its storage type? For instance, if a variable in a FORTRAN subroutine needs to be reinitialised each time the subroutine is called, it must be initialised with an assignment statement rather than a DATA statement.

6. Are there any variables with similar names (eg VOLT and VOLTS)? This is not necessarily an error, but it is a sign that the names may have been confused somewhere within the program.

COMPUTATION ERRORS

1. Are there any computations using variables having inconsistent (eg non—arithmetic) data types?

2. Are there any mixed—mode computations? An example is the addition of a floating—point variable to an integer variable. Such occurrences are not necessarily errors, but they should be explored.

3. Are there any computations using variables having the same data type but different lengths? This can be a problem in IBM FORTRAN.

4. Is the target variable of an assignment smaller than the right—hand expression?

5. Is an overflow or underflow exception possible during the compution of an expression? That is, the end result may appear to have a valid value, but an intermediate result might be too big or too small for the machine's data representations.

6. Is it possible for the divisor in a division operation to be zero?

7. If the underlying machine represents variables in base—2 form, are there any consequences of the resulting inaccuracy? That is, 10 x 0.1 is rarely equal to 1.0 on a binary machine.

8. Where applicable, can the value of a variable go outside its meaningful range?

9. For expressions containing more than one operator, are the assumptions about the order of evaluation and precedence of operators correct?

10. Are there any invalid uses of integer arithmetic, particularly divisions? For instance, if I is an integer variable, whether the expression I/2*2 is equal to I depends on whether I has an odd or even value and whether the multiplication or division is performed first.

COMPARISON ERRORS

1. Are there any comparisons between variables having inconsistent data types (eg comparing a character string to an address)?

2. Are there any mixed—mode comparisons or comparisons between variables of different lengths? If so, ensure that the conversion rules are well understood.

3. Are the comparison operators correct? Programmers frequently confuse such relationships as at most, at least, greater than, not less than or equal.

4. Does each Boolean expression state what it is supposed to state? Programmers often make mistakes when writing logical expressions involving "and", "or" and "not".

5. Are the operands of a Boolean operator Boolean? Have comparison and Boolean operators been erroneously mixed together? This represents another frequent class of mistakes.

6. Are there any comparisons between fractional or floating point numbers that are represented in base—2 by the underlying machine?

7. For expressions containing more than one Boolean operator, are the assumptions about the order of evaluation and the precedence of operators correct?

8. Does the way in which your compiler evaluates Boolean expression affect the program?

CONTROL—FLOW ERRORS

1. If the program contains a multiway branch (eg a computed GOTO in FORTRAN), can the index variable ever exceed the number of branch possibilities? For example, in the FORTRAN statement

$$\text{GOTO } (200,300,400),\ I$$

will I always have the value 1, 2 or 3?

2. Will every loop eventually terminate? Devise an informal proof or argument showing that each loop will terminate.

3. Will the program, module or subroutine eventually terminate?

4. Is it possible that, because of the conditions upon entry, a loop will never execute? If so, does this represent an oversight?

5. For a loop controlled by both iteration and Boolean condition (eg a searching loop), what are the consequences of "loop fallthrough"? for example, for a loop headed by

$$\text{DO } I=1 \text{ TO TALESIZE WHILE (NOTFOUND)}$$

what happens if NOTFOUND never becomes false?

6. Are there any "off by one" errors (eg one too many or too few iterations)?

7. If the language contains a concept of statement groups (eg DO/END groups in PL/I), is there an explicit END for each group and do the ENDs correspond to their appropriate groups?

8. Are there any non—exhaustive decisions? For instance, if an input parameter's expected values are 1, 2 or 3, does the logic assume that it must be 3 if it is not 1 or 2? If so, is the assumption valid?

INTERFACE ERRORS

1. Does the number of parameters received by this module equal the number of arguments set by each of the calling modules? Also is the order correct?

2. Do the attributes (eg type and size) of each parameter match the attributes of each corresponding argument?

3. Does the units system of each parameter match the units system of each corresponding argument? For example, is the parameter expressed in degrees by the argument expressed in radians?

4. Does the number of arguments transmitted by this module to another module equal the number of parameters expected by that module?

5. Do the attributes of each argument transmitted to another module match the attributes of the corresponding parameter in that module?

6. Does the units system of each argument transmitted to another module match the units system of the corresponding parameter in that module?

7. If built—in functions are invoked, are the number, attributes, and order of the arguments correct?

8. If a module has multiple entry points, is a parameter ever referenced that is not associated with the current point of entry?

9. Does a subroutine alter a parameter that is intended to be only an input value? Side effects in FORTRAN are well known.

10. If global variables are present (eg PL/I variables having the EXTERNAL attribute, variables listed in a FORTRAN COMMON statement), do they have the same definition and attributes in all modules that reference them?

11. Are constants ever passed as arguments? In some FORTRAN implementations a statement such as

CALL SUBX(J,3)

is dangerous, since if the subroutine SUBX assigns a value to its second parameter, the value of the constant 3 will be altered.

INPUT/OUTPUT ERRORS

1. If files are explicitly declared, are their attributes correct?

2. Are the attributes on the OPEN statement correct?

3. Does the format specification agree with the information in the I/O statement? For instance, in FORTRAN, does each FORMAT statement agree (in terms of the number and attributes of the items) with the corresponding READ or WRITE statement?

4. Is the size of the I/O area in storage equal to the record size?

5. Have all files been opened before use? Are all files closed correctly?

6. Are end–of–file conditions detected and handled correctly?

7. Are I/0 error conditions handled correctly?

8. Are there spelling or grammatical errors in any text that is printed or displayed by the program?

OTHER CHECKS

1. If the compiler produces a cross–reference listing of identifiers, examine it for variables that are never referenced or referenced only once.

2. If the compiler produces an attribute listing, check the attributes of each variable to ensure that no unexpected default attributes have been assigned.

3. If the program compiled successfully, but the compiler produced one or more "warning" or "informational" messages, check each one carefully. Warning messages are indications that the compiler suspects that you are doing something of questionable validity; all these suspicions should be reviewed. Informational messages may list undeclared variables or languages uses that impede code optimization.

4. Is the program or module sufficiently robust? That is, does it check its input for validity?

REFERENCES

G M Weinberg, 'The Psychology of Computer Programming', (van Nostrand).

G J Myers, 'The Art of Software Testing', (Wiley).

PARALLEL PROCESSING ON SHARED MEMORY MULTI–USER SYSTEMS

V.R. Saunders

SERC Daresbury Laboratory, Daresbury, Warrington
Cheshire, WA4 4AD

INTRODUCTION

The present notes attempt to give a feeling for the techniques available to the programmer when using shared memory parallel processing systems, such as the CRAY–XMP,–YMP,–2, CONVEX C–2, IBM 3090, SEQUENT Balance and Symmetry, or the ENCORE Multimax series of systems. We hope to present:

(*a*) A style of parallel programming (within the context of FORTRAN77) which is portable over this range of machines, although unfortunately the lack of language standardization precludes the portability of parallel syntax at the present time. It is intended that the style give rise to efficient use of such systems taking into account both the existence of shared memory and the fact that each computing node may be given over to multi–user operation; by way of contrast, in distributed memory systems, such as the Intel iPSC/2 hypercube or the Meiko transputer based series, it is normal for each node to be dedicated to a single user. We assert that whilst multi–user nodes should be inherently the more efficient and flexible, it is necessary to take account of the effects of the multi–user environment when evolving a programming style.

(*b*) An explanation of much of the jargon of the subject

(*c*) An indication of the range of applicability of parallel concepts in the calculation of molecular electronic structure by the usual methods of quantum chemistry.

The purist may argue that the existence of a single shared memory precludes the existence of a massive amount of parallelism, and it is certainly true that one cannot connect a very large number of processors to a single memory at a cost which is linear in the number of processors. (The architecture is said to be not *scaleable*). However, in the present state of the art perhaps 10 to 100 processors may be coupled to a shared memory, so given that the processors are of reasonably high power, a very useful computing engine nonetheless becomes available. The existence of a shared memory solves at a stroke the communication problems associated with distributed memory architectures, considerably simplifying programming problems. In a subject such as quantum chemistry, where the fundamental theories and algorithms are rather involved, and present day codes often even messier and certainly very large, ease of programming is of prime concern.

Supercomputational Science
Edited by R.G. Evans and S. Wilson
Plenum Press, New York, 1990

The question may be asked as to why it is necessary to multi–process a job when each node is operating in multi–user (*multi–programming*) mode. Multi–programming can be expected to keep all the processors busy given that there is sufficient memory to maintain a sufficiently large number of active jobs. Suppose one job occupies all or most of the memory. It is then clearly impossible for normal multi–programming to keep all processors busy. The memory greedy job must multi–process if one is not to waste machine cycles. There is however a more subtle reason. Let us assume that the overall aim is to reduce the number of idle cycles to a minimum. Obviously the presence of a number of small memory multi–processing jobs in the general job–mix, which may include large memory (perhaps heavily I/O bound as well) jobs is a great help in acheiving our overall aim. Or perhaps the system is relatively low in work sometimes, so that only a few jobs can be found to run. Again, if these jobs are multi–processed, the risk of idle cycles is much reduced. I beleive that such considerations should be reflected in the charging formula for the use of such machines. Suppose in a given time frame:

MEM = Memory used by a given job

TMEM = Total memory of all jobs concurrently scheduled for execution

CYCLE = Number of cycles consumed by the given job

IDLE = Total number of idle cycles in the time frame

Then I would suggest that the charge for the given job should be proportional to:

IDLE*MEM/TMEM + CYCLE

which would apportion most of the blame for idle cycles to the large memory jobs, yet still give an incentive for smaller memory jobs to multi–process. For an article detailing the impact of multi–processing small memory jobs in the context of a CRAY multi–user environment see M. Bieterman, Cray Channels (Summer 1989) page 10.

THE ARCHITECTURE OF A SHARED MEMORY PARALLEL SYSTEM

A schematic diagram of a shared memory parallel system (a dual processor system) is shown in Fig. 1. We note that each processor is symmetrically connected to the shared memory and may read or write to any word of that memory. Each processor is normally connected to a local memory, to which the other processors have no access. These local memories will constitute the fast registers (for example on a CRAY or IBM system the vector, scalar and addressing registers) which may perhaps be supplemented by conventional local memory banks. Probably the least familiar feature of the Fig. 1 is the item marked *'locks'*. These provide a synchronization mechanism for the various processes of a parallel job, and have the following characteristics:

(*a*) Any lock can be accessed by any processor (and hence *process*; a process is a software construct eventually mapped onto the processors). The locks are therefore a shared memory, and can be a separate set of registers, as on CRAY machines, or can be any word in the central shared memory, as in ENCORE Multimax systems.

(*b*) A lock can be represented as a 1–bit data structure with values of 0 (when it is said to be *unlocked* or *disabled*) or 1 (*locked* or *enabled*).

(*c*) To enable (or *aquire*) a lock, a process simply reads the lock–bit, using a special order. There are two possible outcomes:

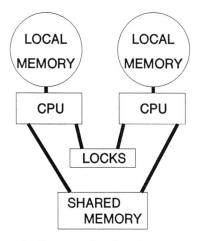

Fig. 1. A schematic diagram of a shared memory parallel system

(i) A value of 0 is returned.

> This means that the lock was unlocked, the usual interpretation being that it is safe for the process to continue. During the read operation the lock will have been set to 1, indicating a locked status to any other process which may subsequently read the lock. The reading and setting of the lock occurs in one indivisible step — said to be *atomic*. Thus it is impossible for two process to enable the lock simultaneously.

(ii) A value of 1 is returned.

> Some other process has enabled the lock, and it is not safe for the present process to continue. The present process must execute a tight loop continuosly checking the lock, until a 0 is returned. This is known as *spinning* and the lock is sometimes referred to as a *spinlock* because of this. Obviously spinning involves an unproductive use of machine cycles; procedures to minimize or eradicate the spinning overhead will be discussed below.

(d) To enable (or *release*) a lock, a process need only write a 0 to it. If there are other processes spinning on the lock, one of them will be allowed to aquire the lock, and to proceed.

The primary purpose of the locks is to provide protection for data structures which are shared between processes, for example to ensure that a given data structure is being updated by only one process at any given time. Typical coding for processing such a protected data structure might look like:

CALL LOCKON(LOCKNO)

Process protected data structure

CALL LOCKOFF(LOCKNO)

where LOCKNO identifies the particular lock, whilst the subroutine names LOCKON, LOCKOFF may vary from system to system. A full description of the type of protection needed requires a formal description of processing dependencies of data structures, a matter to which we now turn our attention.

DATA STRUCTURES

It is now convenient to define the characteristics of a number of data structures, the classification being sufficiently fine for the purposes of shared memory parallel processing of such structures.

1. Local Data Structures

A local (also known as *private*) data structure has the following attributes:

(*a*) It is created before being used by a given process.

(*b*) It is not needed by another parallel process.

It may exist in local memory, or on the *heap* (an area of memory which expands from low to high address values) or the *stack* (an area of memory which expands from high to low address values).

2. Shared Data Structures

These are characterized by being read before written within a given process. In FORTRAN programs, shared data structures are invariably stored in COMMON blocks. On some systems (CRAY for example) a COMMON block is assumed to be shared unless the user directs that it be local while on other systems (SEQUENT for example) the user must declare the COMMON block to be shared, the default being local. It is necessary to sub—classify shared data structures as follows:

2.1 Shared Independent Data Structures

Either:

(*a*)   All processes use the data structure in read only mode,

or

(*b*)   Each shared variable within the data structure can be read/written by only one process. For example, consider the matrix addition:

$$A = A + B$$

partitioned as:

$$(A_1 / A_2) = (A_1 / A_2) + (B_1 / B_2)$$

where we produces A_1 and A_2 in two separate processes. The B—matrix is clearly shared independent since it is processed in read—only mode. The A—matrix is also shared independent since any given element is read/written by only one process.

2.2 Shared Locked Data Structures

(*a*)   A shared locked data structure can be read/written by more than one process.

(b)   If the processes were executed serially but in random order, the operations involving the data structure would produce the same result.

Some typical examples are:

$$B = MAX(\ B\ ,\ R_i)$$

$$B = B + R_i \qquad \text{(scalar or matrix arithmetic)}$$

$$B = B * R_i \qquad \text{(scalar arithmetic only)}$$

where R_i is a result from the ith process, while B denotes the shared locked data structure. A shared locked data structure needs protection from multiple access from the point where it is first read to the point where it is last written within a given process. Such protection can be provided with lock. Most commonly, associative/commutative arithmetic is used in the construction of a shared locked data structure. Given the finite precision of floating point arithmetic it is usually true that a shared locked data structure is not strictly bit—wise invariant to the order in which it was produced, since different orderings produce different roundings and affect the low order bits of the result. In quantum chemistry this is not normally a serious problem, since the algorithms are rather numerically stable. On the contrary, the trajectories computed by the methods of molecular dynamics are often very numerically unstable, and it is not uncommon for such trajectories to vary greatly depending on the ordering of the processes whereby they are computed.

A direct access data set which requires that transactions be carried out by only one process at a time (but in any order) may also be regarded as a locked data structure.

2.3 Shared Ordered Data Structures

(a)   A shared ordered data structure may be read/written by more than one process.

(b)   If the processes were executed serially but in random order, the operations involving the data structure would not produce the correct results.

As an example we quote the construction of a matrix by means of a sequence of matrix multiplications:

$$R = A_1 A_2 A_3 A_4.......$$

where the matrix multiplication processes must be carried out in the correct order because they are non—commutative. so the matrix **R** is a shared ordered data structure.

Another example concerns the processing of a sequential data set, which may require ordering protection to ensure that it is processed serially.

It is not possible to provide ordering protection directly via a lock; it is necessary to create data structures known as *semaphores* to provide this level of protection.

SEMAPHORES

A semaphore is a shared locked data structure (which can and must be protected by a lock) which is introduced to provide more sophisticated control mechanisms than possible through a spinlock. Examples of the use of semaphores are:

(a) To provide protection for a shared ordered data structure.

(b) To provide buffered or queued access to a data structure.

We discuss some aspects of the use of semaphores.

1. Global Index

The updating algorithm within a parallel process for a global index is:

$I = I + 1$

where I is usually initialized to zero before parallel working commences. The global index is usually used to indicate how far through a calculation being carried out in parallel has got. Imagine for example that the following serial code:

DO 1 I=1,N

Multiply matrix A_i with matrix B_i to give result matrix R_i

1   CONTINUE

is to be prepared for M—way parallel execution. The coding might look like:

```
EXTERNAL PROCESS
COMMON /GLOBAL/ I, LOCKI, N
I=0
CALL FORK (PROCESS , M)
CALL BARRIER
```

where the system supplied routine FORK creates M identical copies of the subroutine PROCESS to be executed in parallel, whilst BARRIER (system supplied) causes a return to serial processing after waiting for all parallel processes to complete. I is the global index while LOCKI denotes the lock to be used to protect I from simultaneous updates. Of course the FORK/LOCK syntax may vary widely between different machines (for example on the CRAY one may use the TSKSTART/TSKWAIT routines). The user supplied parallel routine PROCESS might look like:

```
        SUBROUTINE PROCESS
        COMMON /GLOBAL/ I , LOCKI, N
        COMMON /MATRIX/ R(), A(), B()
999     CALL LOCKON(LOCKI)
        IF(I.EQ.N)THEN
        CALL LOCKOFF(LOCKI)
        RETURN
        ENDIF
        I=I+1
        J=I
        CALL LOCKOFF(LOCKI)
            Multiply A_j by B_j to give R_j
        GOTO 999
        END
```

Notice that when I equals N all work is complete, so all processes return to the calling routine which is waiting at the barrier. Note also that a local copy of I is placed in J to ensure that that if the global index is subsequently updated by another copy of PROCESS, the logic of the present copy of PROCESS when multiplying the matrices is not disturbed. Locks are not required to protect **A**, **B** or **R** as these are shared independent structures. Note the distinction between a *task* (in this case a matrix multiplication) and a process. A process in general carries out many tasks.

The above represents a case based on the sharing of work out amongst the processes using *data partitioning* (also known as *homogeneous multitasking*) where one performs the same task on different sets of data.

Function partitioning (*hetereogeneous multitasking*), where one performs different tasks on the same data structures is less common in scientific work (except perhaps in data–base management systems), but can easily be driven by allowing the global index, possibly supplemented by a task list, to select the required function.

On a dedicated machine, and given a sufficiently large number of tasks, every process will carry out an almost identical amount of work, even if the dimensions of the matrices are variable, and the job is said to be in *dynamic balance*. On a non–dedicated machine, each processor supplies to its assigned process as many cycles as it is able to, bearing in mind that the "effective power" of a given processor depends on the behaviour of the other user jobs it is dealing with. In the case that all the matrices are of the same dimension it would be possible to assign N/M of the tasks to each of the M processes and acheive "*static balance*", where each process by design performed an equal amount of work, with perhaps somewhat simpler coding (indeed on single user node distributed memory systems this is often the aim of algorithm design). On a multi–user system this programming style is far from ideal, since it loads each processor equally, without regard to how busy the processors are with other work. The processes terminate in considerably different elapsed times, with a consequent degradation in the degree of parallelism of the job, particularly in its latter stages.

2. Counting/Queuing Semaphores

This is an example of a software engineering device to reduce or eradicate the time spinning in locks while protecting shared locked data structures. The semaphore (which is itself a shared locked data structure) consists of a queue list together with an integer, N. The interpretation of N is as follows:

N > 0   Number of copies (or *images*) of the shared locked data structure available.

N $\leq$ 0   No copy of the data structure available. $-$N equals the length of the queue for the data structure.

Also part of the semaphore is an array, denoted INF(), such that when INF(i)=0, the I*th* image of the shared locked data structure is available, whilst if INF(i)=1, the I*th* image is in use by a process and unavailable to other processes. To aquire the semaphore (under control of a lock):

(*a*)   N = N $-$ 1

(*b*)   If N $\geq$ 0 then
An image of the data structure is available to the process. Find an INF(I)=0. Set INF(i)=1. Release the lock and then process the I*th* image of the data structure

(c)   If N < 0 then
         Put process ID (*Pid*) on the −N*th* slot of the queue. Release the
         lock, and then *Block* the process.

The Pid simply corresponds to some tag (often simply an integer) to uniquely identify
the process. The action of blocking consists of yielding the processor to some other
job. The process is suspended until woken up later by some other process.

       To release the semaphore (under control of a lock), after processing the shared
locked data structure:

(a)   If N < 0 then
         Wake–up the process at the head of the queue, and remove it from
         the queue. Tell it which image of the data structure to use (the one
         being released).

(b)   If N ≥ 0 then
         Set INF(I) = 0.

(c)   N = N + 1
         Release the lock.

       Obviously two system routines are required, which we will generically denote
by the names BLOCK and WAKEUP. Of course, the names of these routines will be
different, for example, on a CRAY these functions can be provided by means of the
EVWAIT and EVPOST routines.

       On many systems the user does not directly spin on the hardware locks, the
LOCKON/LOCKOFF functions being provided by a queuing semaphore, which is a
simplification of the counting/queuing semaphore such that the number of images of
the shared ordered data structure is one. On such a system one does not need to
construct a counting/queuing semaphore unless one wishes to use multiple images of
the shared locked data structure.

       The principle of the semaphore should be clear. One spins on the lock only
when there is contention for access to the semaphore, rather than for the data
structure being protected by the semaphore. The time taken to either aquire or
release the semaphore is very short, so that the chances for contention for access to
the semaphore are slight.

3. An Example of the Use of Multiple Images

       Suppose the shared locked data structure, a matrix $\mathbf{R}$, is updated in the i'th
task by:

$$\mathbf{R} = \mathbf{R} + \mathbf{A_i}$$

commencing from $\mathbf{R}=\underline{0}$. Initially we create a number of images of $\mathbf{R}$ so that $\mathbf{R_1}=\underline{0}$,
$\mathbf{R_2}=\underline{0}$, $\mathbf{R_3}=\underline{0}$ etc. Updates now proceed via either $\mathbf{R_1}=\mathbf{R_1}+\mathbf{A_i}$ or $\mathbf{R_2}=\mathbf{R_2}+\mathbf{A_i}$ *etc.* After
the barrier we form:

$$\mathbf{R} = \mathbf{R_1} + \mathbf{R_2} + \mathbf{R_3} \ etc$$

which of course defines the full $\mathbf{R}$–matrix. The creation of the multiple images of $\underline{\mathbf{R}}$
reduces contention for $\mathbf{R}$ during the parallel processing phases. In the direct CI
method the σ–vector is updated as envisaged above (see V.R. Saunders and J.H. van
Lenthe, Molecular Physics, **48**, 923 (1983)) and is thus an obvious candidate for
multiple imaging.

If we create as many images as there are parallel processes, there is no need for a semaphore at all, since we can assign one image to each process. In this form the method can be used in the construction of Fock matrices from two–electron integrals (or supermatrices) or in the construction of the gradient vector (with respect to geometrical variations) from the gradient integrals in analytic gradient SCF theory.

4. Ordering/Queuing Semaphore

This semaphore (which is itself a shared locked data structure) is designed to provide ordering protection for a shared ordered data structure. It consists of a queue list and an integer, N, initialized to zero, which will be used to count the number of iterations carried out on the ordered data structure.

To aquire the semaphore (under control of a lock):

(a)   Work out how many iterations on the shared ordered data structure must have occurred before the current task can proceed, probably using a global index, K.

(b)   If $N \geq K$ Release the lock. Operate on ordered structure.

(c)   If $N < K$ It is too early to process the ordered data structure. Put process ID and K on the queue list, release the lock and then block.

To release the semaphore after processing the shared ordered data structure:

(a) $N = N + 1$

(b)   Check the queue for a process with $N \geq K$. If such a process exists, wakeup the process, and adjust the queue list.

(c)   Release the lock.

CONCLUSION

We have discussed a style of programming (dynamic balance) which we consider to be very suitable for application on shared–memory multi–user systems. The programming style requires three pairs of routines, which have been generically denoted:

> LOCKON/LOCKOFF
> FORK/BARRIER
> BLOCK/WAKEUP

Given these three constructs (which are available on all the systems we have investigated) it has been shown how to define global indices and appropriate queuing semaphores to enable the protection of shared locked and shared ordered data structures in an economic way (for example, the use of multiple images of shared locked data structures). In summary, locks protect semaphores which in turn protect data structures.

RUNNING FORTRAN PROGRAMMES IN AN OCCAM ENVIRONMENT

Lydia Heck

Physics Department, The University, Durham DH1 3LE

INTRODUCTION

Concurrency is not a new concept. It is practised widely in every branch of the industry and our daily life. The most prominent example is probably the conveyor belt in a factory. Every worker on the belt is dedicated to one assembly phase in the manufacturing of a product. Worker (i) receives the product in its prestate (i–1) from worker (i–1), performs his task and hands the product in its state (i) to worker (i+1). While worker (i) is busy performing his task on the nth product, worker (i–1) is working on product (n+1) and worker (i+1) on product (n–1). Each worker's task in this example is assumed to be different. The conveyor belt is the communication line between the workers. To make this production scheme cost effective and optimal there must be excellent load balancing in the tasks every worker performs. To achieve this load balancing different methods can be applied which might be more or less sensitive to each worker's capability.

In studying this example of concurrency it is emphasised that its main feature is that different workers act *simultaneously* in a well defined way to achieve a final product. Furthermore it also shows that to achieve optimal output the *communication* between the different product stages has to be organised systematically. Concurrency is, in general, a group of "workers" acting in parallel with well established intercommunication lines.

To reproduce concurrency in the world of computing two stages in the development have to be considered. Firstly the technical one. The assembly of 'workers' is represented by a number of processors and the communication between the workers is established via real hardware connections between the processors. Naturally this requires a fair amount of technology as the communication lines must transmit data almost unrestrictedly at high speed to guarantee the optimal effect.

Secondly the organisational side of it, which is expressed primarily in the computing language dealing with parallelism and communication, but also in the ability of the programmer to recognise parallel features and to explore them optimally; this requires a somewhat new way of thinking.

In the next section I will introduce the basic features of one parallel programming language, OCCAM, and show how it differs from standard languages. I will then introduce the transputer. In the final sections I will discuss a piece of software called Fortnet which makes it possible to run FORTRAN code on an array

Supercomputational Science
Edited by R.G. Evans and S. Wilson
Plenum Press, New York, 1990

of transputers. Much of the information given in the last section will be required only by potential users of Fortnet.

THE OCCAM PROGRAMMING LANGUAGE

Languages like standard FORTRAN 77, Pascal or C assume implicitly that the computation of a numerical problem is done sequentially. This is the default and no explicit mentioning of it is necessary. Also because there is only one processor working on the problem with its own memory, there is no question of interprocess–data–communication either. The only data–passing is to and from files.

The OCCAM programming language is designed to write codes for interacting parallel processes which can be performed on a set of interconnected processors with local memory (distributed memory machine). Both interaction–communication and parallelism are introduced at the programming level. The basics of the language are (Inmos Ltd., 1988b):

An OCCAM programme is built from three primitive processes:

(1) assignment
     variable: = expression
(2) communication
     input from channel
     channel ? variable
     output to channel
     channel ! expression
(3) SKIP and STOP
     The primitive process SKIP starts, performs *no* action and terminates.
     The primitive process STOP starts, performs *no* action and never terminates.

Primitive processes are combined in a construct. There are three main constructs:

(1) SEQ – sequential
(2) PAR – parallel
(3) ALT – alternation.

A process in general is a construct of constructs. Processes belonging to the same construct are indented relative to the construct name by two mandatory blanks (replacing "begin" and "end").

All quantities have to be declared. There are two forms:

data type	f.i.	channel type	f.i.
INT	integer	CHAN OF	INT
REAL	real		REAL
BYTE	byte		ANY
and others			and others, also user defined protocols

The elements of the OCCAM language are written in capital letters and are reserved words.

The processes in a SEQ construct are performed in the order in which they are listed which is equivalent to normal sequential programming; only when a process within the construct is terminated will the next start. The processes in a

PAR—construct are performed in parallel, irrespective of the order in which they appear. Generally, "in parallel" means "simultaneously". The third construct is ALT. An ALT construct contains two or more processes. The first process to become ready, and only this one, is executed. If two processes become ready at the same time only one of them is executed but which one is decided at machine level. The ALT construct is often used to guard a set of channels for data input.

THE TRANSPUTER

The processor which belongs intrinsically to the OCCAM programming language is the transputer. It was designed by Inmos together with the Inmos OCCAM language; an OCCAM process simulates the working of a transputer (Barron et al., 1983).

The transputer is constructed from a family of very large scale integrated (VLSI) components. Figure 1 shows the setup of the Inmos T800. It comprises

> 64 bit floating point unit
>
> 32 bit processor (CPU)
>
> 4 kbyte RAM
>
> Timer
>
> external memory interface
>
> link services and 4 links.

The floating point unit works concurrently with the CPU.

Every link is bidirectional. The two directions are distinct. The mapping of OCCAM channels on links is done at programme level and the direction has to be preserved.

Transputers can be connected into variable topologies either manually using pieces of wire with a little plug on each side or by means of an electronic configuration chip. Examples of topologies are given in figure 2. The only restriction to different hardware topologies are that the transputer has only 4 links.

The transputer is designed to process a great number of instructions; a performance comparison of the T800–20 Mhz with other processors is given by White et al. (1988). They measured for the IMS T800–20 a top performance of 4600 K Whetstones/sec whereas other processors ranked significantly below.

Processes can be run concurrently on different transputers; or they can be run in parallel on one transputer. The latter is done in time sharing. Each process gets an equal slice of time. When the allocated time has passed the current process is placed at the bottom of the waiting queue of processes and the following process is run. Channels which communicate between processes run in parallel on one transputer are called soft channels and are represented by a word in memory, OCCAM channels communicating between transputers are called hard and are mapped on the physical links between the microchips. Soft and hard channels are distinguished by their address in memory, otherwise they are not treated differently. Therefore the form of the processes does not depend on whether they are run in time—sharing parallel on a single processor or truly parallel on a *distributed* system (Inmos Ltd., 1988c). This is most advantageous in designing a concurrent programme, which can be done on a single transputer and after successful debugging can be transferred to the array of transputers available. Message passing is truly synchronous.

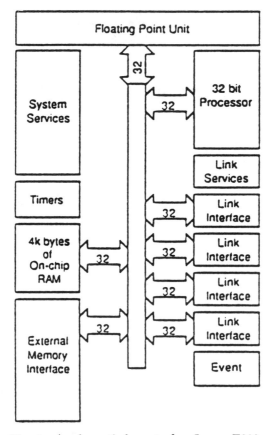

Fig. 1. A schematic layout of an Inmos T800.

The transputer is not a multi−user device. If one programme is performed on it, it will be locked to other user programmes until that programme is finished.

The transputer gives great computing power for a very reasonable amount of money. For about $150,000 it is possible to acquire a dedicated computer system which is comparable in its computing power to the CRAY−XMP in scalar operation.

In this way small research groups can afford their own mini–supercomputers (subject to grants) making feasible research which requires more and more computing time.

A NEW COMPUTER DESIGN, NEW COMPUTER LANGUAGE AND OLD FORTRAN PROGRAMMES

OCCAM is a high level computing language and the language of the transputer and thus the most natural to use in programming code destined to be run on this processor. Furthermore the OCCAM implementations by Inmos and Meiko (Inmos, 1988a and Meiko Ltd., 1988) provide standard functions like sin, cos, exp, tanh, etc. as well as input/output routines making data handling easily manageable. Why then does not everyone with access to a transputer array want to jump at the opportunity of learning something new and exciting, and start programming everything in OCCAM? There is at least one very good reason: the extensive investment in existing codes, some of which are in the format of commercial libraries like the NAG, CPC libraries, and others freely available to the scientific community. To rewrite these libraries would be a waste of time and manpower and is quite unnecessary. Meiko's implementation of OCCAM (and Inmos's, I believe) allow in an OCCAM programme for the call of alien language routines written in FORTRAN, Pascal, or C. The Fortnet harness (Allan et al., 1989), which I will discuss in greater detail in later sections, is based on the OCCAM and FORTRAN software provided by Meiko (Meiko Ltd., 1988, 1989). Therefore I will restrict myself to discussing the procedure for preparing a FORTRAN programme to run as an 'OCCAM' process, using Meiko software.

Meiko's implementation of FORTRAN includes one important extension of standard FORTRAN which makes it possible to communicate data to the outside world other than through a variable list and files. A set of data passing routines are

IO$XBLI (user,message,length)

and

IO$XBLO (user,message,length)

where the arguments

user	is a number 1,2,3,... representing an OCCAM channel in the FORTRAN programme.
message	is a data array
length	is the actual length of the data array,

and X represents one of the following symbols

C for complex,

D for double precision,

I for integer

R for real

reflecting the nature of the array 'message'.

To input data of type X from channel 'user' to the FORTRAN routine the routine IO$XBLI is called and to output data of type X to channel 'user' the routine IO$XBLO is called.

When a FORTRAN programme called 'worker' is written including these extensions it is compiled using the Topexpress f77–compiler distributed by Meiko. In a linking process the channels which are referred to as the numbers 1,2, etc. are established as type CHAN OF ANY and in the call of the FORTRAN process are listed as arguments, e.g.

worker (fromF,toF,keyboard,screen,user1,user2,user3).

The first four entries are reserved. fromF, toF represent the access to the filing system and are replaced in the FORTRAN part of the programme by logical unit numbers of files which are opened for reading (fromF) or writing (toF). The channels keyboard and screen are by default coupled to the logical units for keyboard (5) and screen (6). Thus the FORTRAN command

WRITE(6,*) 'word'

will send the string 'word' along channel screen into the OCCAM message– passing environment, and if this channel is properly connected the message 'word' will appear on the terminal screen.

The numbers 1,2,3, etc. in the calls of the subroutines IO$XLBI(O) refer to the 'user' channels user1,user2,user3, etc. respectively, i.e. a message array received in FORTRAN with the call of

CALL IO$IBLI (1,message,length)

has been sent along the channel user1. These numbers do *not* correspond to logical unit numbers of files.

MODELS OF PARALLELISM

As the examples of transputer configurations show (see figure 2) there are different ways of realising parallel solutions of a problem and one recognises immediately that a given problem will not be optimally solved by every possible configuration. Certain criteria have to be considered carefully before settling on one or other method of parallelisation and transputer configuration. To get optimal results from a computing surface of transputers an algorithm should lead to a well–balanced use of all processors, which means that the computations on each of them should be well synchronised and that they should not have to wait for data. Secondly, message passing does take time and although transputer links are fast it is still time which cannot be spent on computation. Only well–balanced CPU–intensive algorithms with few data exchanges will lead to an optimal speed up on a computing surface.

Considering these criteria, the first parallel application which springs to mind is the so–called *data farming*. The same code is loaded on to all the transputers on the surface, but every process works on a different data set. There is no communication between the slave processes and only if there is a master task sending out the data and collecting the results will there be considerations of message passing and, to some extent, of load balancing. However even in such a case there is data flow as input and output data have to be transported between the individual slaves and the filing system.

Another approach is that of the conveyor belt, in which worker n relies on the output of n–1 etc. In this case it is most important to consider the CPU requirements of each task, as it is easily possible to suffer great losses in time through processors waiting for each other. The grid is used in calculations depending on nearest neighbours. Other applications like the binary tree are very specialised and model – dependent. Scott et al. (1988) investigate the performance of a parallel

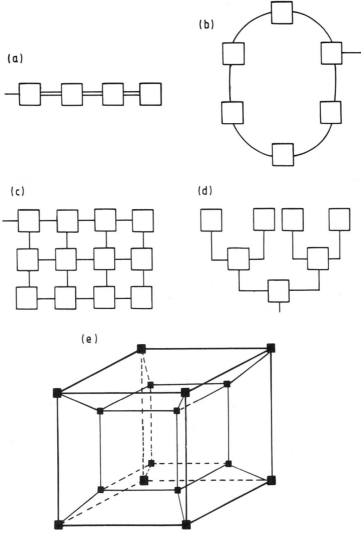

Fig. 2. Examples of multi–processor topologies
(a) daisy chain, (b) a ring, (c) 2–dimensional grid,
(d) a binary tree, (e) a hypercube.

programme to compute Racah coefficients on dependence of input data and processor topology; one of their topologies is a ring of transputers, the other is a simple tree.

One more model which does not depend too specifically on the topology of the computer array is *task farming*. In this case a compiled code is loaded on to a transputer, the task is run, and when it terminates the next code is loaded. In this way completely independent codes can make use of a computing surface. The resulting achievement in load balancing depends on the tasks to a certain extent but also on the number of tasks. If there are many more tasks than there are transputers, the array can be occupied for a long time and a final load imbalance between the last tasks only (moderately) affects the ideal speed–up. Task farming can also be performed in highly interactive systems. However in this case great care is needed at the basic programming level to ensure message routing and synchronisation between the different programme parts.

DESCRIPTION OF THE FORTNET HARNESS

The Fortnet harness is an OCCAM programme for running FORTRAN codes on the Meiko computing surface (Allan et al., 1989; Allan and Heck, 1989). Adaptation of the Meiko system–specific routines should ensure portability to an Inmos computing surface.

The harness is designed to be loaded down on a daisy chain of transputers (see Figure 3). Every transputer hosts one FORTRAN user programme hidden in SLAVE and which will be called 'worker', which is run in parallel (time sharing) with the message routing processes. The general setup is such that the first transputer runs the driver process and the master FORTRAN process and all the other transputers run identical slave FORTRAN processes in data farming. Every process knows its process number. The driver process has number 0, the master is number 1 and the slaves are number 2 to number of transputers. The process number is the address of the process.

The OCCAM programme allows for message passing in two ways. The first is direct access to the host filing system, and the channels dedicated to this job will be called filing system streams. These channels are accessed from the FORTRAN process by addressing files in the usual FORTRAN way. The management of the filing system streams is performed by Meiko software processes (Meiko Ltd., 1988) which are run in priority parallel to the FORTRAN and interprocess communications processes on the same transputer. Two hard links per transputer are dedicated to the filing system streams (see figure 3).

The other possibility is the interprocess (interFORTRAN) communication. These channels are accessed from within the FORTRAN routine using the FORTRAN–OCCAM routines IO$IBLI/O described above and henceforth they will be referred to as 'interprocess' channels. The interprocess message passing is dealt with through a set of OCCAM processes which receive and direct the messages. All channels are of the type CHAN OF INT¦¦[]INT which means (for input from a channel, for instance): expect one integer which is the total length of a following array of integers; then expect the integer array itself. Every message has the form given in figure 4 (Allan et al., 1989).

For the message routing processes, only the first array element is relevant, as they only evaluate the message according to its destination. The message directing is done centrally on every transputer by the process message.controller (figure 5) (Allan et al., 1989; Allan and Heck, 1989). Three different channels enter the process and 3 leave it. The channel array 'in' carries messages from the neighbouring transputers to either side whereas 'data' is the channel passing data from the FORTRAN process into the stream of interprocess communication. The channel array 'out' passes messages from the transputer under consideration to its two nearest neighbours and channel 'comm' passes data received from one of the neighbouring processes into the FORTRAN process.

To connect to the neighbouring transputer on the interprocess channels, two free links per transputer are again necessary as there is one in and one out channel to either side of 'mynode' (see figure 3). Together with the two hard links per transputer for the filing system streams, this makes a total of four. This requirement restricts the application of the harness to a closed chain, where only the last transputer and the first one have two and one free link respectively.

Let me refer back to the considerations of transputer configurations. The Fortnet harness is an example of how service requirements impose directly the topology of a transputer array. We recall that only four links per transputer are available.

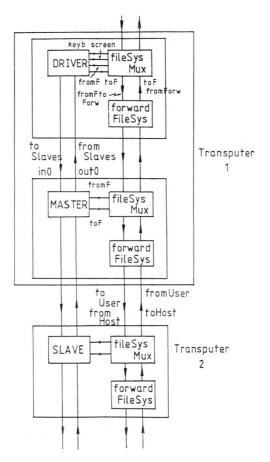

Fig 3. Placement of the driver, master and slave processes of the Fortnet harness on a dual daisy–chain configuration of transputers. The Meiko filing system procedures and filing system streams are shown on the right; the interprocess channels on the left (Allan and Heck, 1989; Allan et al., 1989)

$$\boxed{\text{isiz}} \;::\; \boxed{\text{TADDR}}\;\boxed{\text{FADDR}}\;\boxed{\text{TAG}}\;\boxed{A[\imath\!>\!3]}$$
$$\quad\quad\quad A[1]\quad\quad A[2]\quad\quad A[3]$$

Fig. 4. Message protocol for interprocess data communication where A[i] is an integer array and A[1] = TADDR is the address node, A[2] = FADDR is the sender node and A[3] = TAG is the tag describing the nature of the message; the array elements A[3+n], n $\geq$ 1 carry the real data (Allan et al., 1989).

73

EXPLANATION OF INDIVIDUAL FORTRAN PROGRAM PARTS OF FORTNET

In the driver process (figure 3) all services connecting the computing surface to the host are established and process server which is a FORTRAN programme is started. Process 'server' is standing by, to handle read and write requests to the filing system from the worker processes via the interprocess channels. Each worker starts by sending a startup message to server. The workers must send this startup message, otherwise following messages from the worker will not be handled. The potential user has to interact with the server programme to a small degree. Firstly files accessed by the workers via server have to be opened in server and secondly the files' logical unit numbers have to be entered into an array which is part of programme server in order to identify the files according to the requests. These changes are not frequent and entries in server should not change for an established FORTRAN programme. As the file **server.f** is partly user dependent it is not taken up in a library. The user has to have access to it.

The Fortnet FORTRAN library **iosub.f** contains message passing routines and other services; their descriptions can be found in Allan et al. (1989). I propose to explain the message passing routines in detail, as their understanding will promote efficient use.

SUBROUTINES READ AND WRITE

Two routines have been developed which allow access to files via the server program run by PROC driver. In relation to their function they are called subroutines READ and WRITE and are always called in conjunction with their FORTRAN counterparts, as in

CALL READ (LU,ISIZE,BUFFER)
READ (BUFFER, FORTRAN format) variable list.

The two subroutines READ and WRITE work in similar ways where the former performs the reading from and the latter the writing to a file via the interprocess channels. The discussion of one will serve to explain the working of both.

CALL READ (LU,ISIZE,BUFFER) sends a request to server (which has address 0) to read data from a 'logical unit LU' and send the data array to the requesting worker. The local 'logical unit LU' is translated to an actual logical unit number in server. Programme server then reads one character string of length 132 (the maximal length of a line) from this logical unit (file), encodes it as an integer array and sends it off to the requesting worker where the first 3 array elements contain the worker address, the server's address and the type description of the message (see figure 4). The requesting worker process is in the meantime waiting for a reply from server. When the message arrives it is equivalenced into a character array of length 132. The character string is treated as an internal FORTRAN file and read by a FORTRAN READ in a user–chosen format.

IDEAS ON FILE SHARING

This method of accessing files leads to an effective way of sharing files amongst different slaves. However, it has to be remembered that individual lines in the file have to be closed data sets. In order to read two lines from a file, two 'Read' requests have to be sent to the server programme. As other workers are wholly or partly independent in their work from the requesting worker programme, a 'Read'

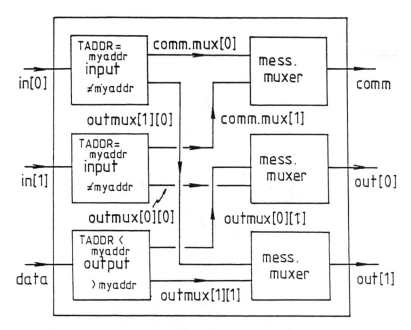

Fig. 5.   PROC message.controller ([]CHAN OF INT::[]int in, out, comm, data, VAL INT my.addr). Internal channels of the message controller and procedures which redirect messages between transputers and the FORTRAN code. Messages received from in[0] are tested for their address TADDR. If TADDR = my.addr the message is passed to the FORTRAN code via comm, otherwise it is forwarded down the chain via out[1]. Likewise messages coming up the chain are received on in[1], and passed to either comm or out[0]. A message from the FORTRAN code on channel data is sent to out[0] or out[1] depending on its direction on the chain determined from TADDR (Allan et al., 1989; Allan and Heck, 1989).

request from one of these could precede the second 'Read' request. The result would be a mix—up of data and the running of at least two of the worker programmes would be worthless.

Furthermore in sharing a file in this way the line—by—line entries in the file must not depend on the worker address requesting to read, as there is no guarantee that an entry assigned to worker i is not requested by worker j. Thus, the sharing of files has to be planned carefully and can even then contain only 'simple' sets of data; for instance do—loop variables or data file names. Although this seems a severe restriction, the latter in particular can be used to great advantage in data and task—farming of FORTRAN code and provides a very simple and effective means of load balancing.

Another means of file sharing can be via the filing system streams and depends on the way the host handles its filing system. In Unix it is possible to access the same file simultaneously from different programmes, each programme working on it independently and not 'knowing' about the other operating programmes. Thus the same file can be input to several programmes, each programme setting its own file marks, and if several processors run the same programme with one data set common to each copy of the programme, this data set can be read via the filing system streams by each worker from just one file.

Writing to the same *sequential* data file by different programmes via the filing system streams however will lead to (in view of the above properties of file handling) total confusion and data loss.

If an input/output file is a direct access file and if records are uniquely determined as a function of the worker programmes this file can be shared properly and to great advantage considering the way that Unix handles files.

INTERPROCESS COMMUNICATION

The harness has a secure way of handling interprocess communication. Several routines are involved in this and the way they work will now be discussed in detail.

The routines for sending data from one process to another process are

SEND(M,ISIZ,ARRAY)
which sends the ISIZ bytes from ARRAY to processor M
SENDS(M,ISIZ,SARRAY)
to send a string SARRAY of ISIZ bytes to processor M.

The routines for receiving data from another process are

RECEVE(M,ISIZ,ARRAY)
to receive ISIZ bytes from processor M and store them in the array ARRAY
RECEVS(M,ISIZ,SARRAY)
to receive a string SARRAY of ISIZ bytes from processor M.

A large amount of data may be sent and received during a numerical concurrent calculation on a transputer array, and the calculations of a process may depend on data provided by several processes which need not be nearest neighbours. The calculations of each process will depend on individual data sets and initial conditions and the times used on the different processes between message passing will vary accordingly. Although we talk about concurrent programming, individual processes are sequential and should be CPU intensive. For example, let us assume that worker m relies consecutively on data from process k and process ℓ, where the data of process k are required first. To make sure that the data of process k are indeed received first, message blocking and handshaking before message passing can be achieved by careful use of the routines WAIT and CHECK. Routines WAIT and CHECK must be used in conjunction with each other. The two routines will now be explained.

CALL WAIT(N) : wait for 'CHECK' message from process N. Before WAIT expects a message from process N it checks its list of pending processes. If process N is entered into this list, WAIT will send the pending resolve message -4 (see Table 1). It then returns control to the calling routine. If process N is not in the pending list routine WAIT is awaiting a message. The message it receives is checked if

(a) the sender is process N
(b) the message is sent by routine CHECK (tag -2).

If both are true routine WAIT replies to process N with -3 and returns control to calling routine.

If the sender is not the desired process N routine MESERR is called which puts the message in the pending queue and returns the message to the sending process. The sending process is then blocked until its message is needed.

If the message is not sent by routine CHECK, WAIT will wait for the next message. The message will be lost and the programme might even deadlock.

Table 1.

Message Tags (Allan et al., 1989; Allan and Heck, 1989)

TAG	reply from source
0	SEND
-1	MESERR
-2	response from CHECK
-3	normal response from WAIT
-4	WAIT responding from pending state
integer >0	local 'logical' unit number for READ and WRITE

CALL CHECK(M) : check if process M is ready for sending data. Routine CHECK sends a message tag $= -2$ to process M; it then waits for a reply message. CHECK receives a message and checks it if

(a) the sender is process M

(b) it is the normal reply (tag $= -3$).

If *(a)* and *(b)* are true control is returned to the calling routine. If the reply message is tagged -1 the message is returned and pending. Routine CHECK then waits for the activation signal (tag $= -4$).

If the reply message is not a normal reply and not a pending message signal, the message is reported as lost and routine MESERR takes over. A programme which leads to lost messages may be faulty and could deadlock eventually. Every lost message report should be noticed and the programme reconsidered.

The routines CHECK and WAIT are used in connection with the routines RECEIVE (RECEVS) and SEND(S) in the form (for example see Allan et al., 1989)

process M	process N
CALL CHECK(N)	CALL WAIT(M)
CALL RECEVE(N,ISIZ,ARRAY)	CALL SEND(M,ISIZ,ARRAY)

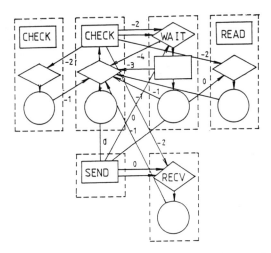

Fig. 6. Data paths used in Fortnet for error—correcting protocol of messages. The negative integers are tags defined in table 2. Independent routines are shown in dashed boxes. Their internal parts are shown in shaped boxes depending on the functions as follows: [ ] send message or request; <> receive reply or message; O handle errors, update pending list and send message (usually by calling the routine MESERR) (Allan et al., 1989, Allan and Heck, 1989).

In a balanced and correct programme CHECK and WAIT should interact properly.

However imbalancing and faulty programming can lead to an involved pattern of message passing as fig. 6 shows (Allan et al., 1989; Allan and Heck, 1989). I would like to discuss this, as it illustrates an agony which a concurrent programmer occasionally meets.

In a well balanced and correct programme (for the TAG explanations see table 2)

> CHECK sends a message to a WAIT (−2)
> WAIT replies normally with 'ready' (−3), at most with 'resolve pending state' (−4)
> then SEND and RECEVE can proceed.

However CHECK could also send its message to a waiting routine READ, RECEVE or another CHECK. These routines react via MESERR sending replies (−1) back to CHECK. If the programming is very unbalanced or faulty, it will deadlock eventually.

SEND should meet RECEVE in the waiting process. Both then perform normally and the programme continues. However in unbalanced and faulty programming the SEND signal (0) could be received by a CHECK or a WAIT or a READ on the other process handing its message over to MESERR; the whole might then lead to deadlock.

Although data transport is, in principle, straightforward within OCCAM and also with the Fortnet harness programming, planning is more than ever necessary to achieve data synchronisation of your programme.

A detailed description of all the aspects of the Fortnet harness can be found in Allan et al. (1989) and Allan and Heck (1989).

ACKNOWLEDGEMENTS

The author would like to thank Dr. J. Welford for discussions on the functional aspects of the transputer and Dr. D.R. Flower for carefully reading the manuscript.

REFERENCES

Allan, R. J. and Heck, L., 1989, Fortnet: A parallel FORTRAN harness for porting application codes to Transputer arrays, Proc. Int. Conf. on Applications of Transputers, Liverpool, 23–25 August 1989.

Allan, R. J., Heck, L. and Zureck, S., 1989, Parallel FORTRAN in Scientific Computing: a new OCCAM harness called Fortnet, submitted for publication in Computer Physics Communications.

Barron, I., Cavill, P., May, D. and Wilson, P., 1983, Transputer does 5 or more MIPS even when not used in parallel, Electronics, Nov. 17, 109.

Hutson, J. M., 1989, private communication.

Inmos Limited, 1988a, "Transputer Development System", Prentice Hall, New York.

Inmos Limited, 1988b, "OCCAM 2 Reference Manual", Prentice Hall, New York.

Inmos Limited, 1988c, "Transputer Reference Manual", page 54, Prentice Hall, New York.

Meiko Limited, 1988, "Software Reference Manual", Meiko Ltd., Bristol.

Meiko Ltd., 1989, "FORTRAN Reference Manual for the Computing Surface", Meiko Ltd., Bristol.

Scott, N. S., Milligan, P. and Riley, H. W. C., 1987, The Parallel Computation of Racah coefficients using Transputers, Computer Physics Communications 46, 83.

White, D. N. J., Ruddock, J. N. and Edgington, P. R., 1988, Molecular Design with Transparallel Supercomputers in Molecular Simulation, Vol. 3, 71–100, Gordan and Breach.

NUMERICAL RECIPES FOR SUPERCOMPUTERS

S. Wilson

Rutherford Appleton Laboratory, Chilton, Oxfordshire, OX11 0QX

INTRODUCTION

From the earliest days of the computer era, state–of–the–art scientific calculations have almost always demanded efficient computer programs. But in the present decade we have seen the advent of general purpose computing machines which perform parts of a calculation concurrently.

What has changed with the advent of the parallel computer is the ratio between the performance of a good and a bad computer program. This ratio is not likely to exceed a factor of two or three on a serial computer, whereas factors of ten or more are not uncommon on parallel computers. Quite simply the stakes in the programming game have been substantially raised.

(Hockney and Jesshope, 1981)

As we approach the end of the decade, the "*factors of ten*" can often be replaced by factors of one hundred or even more. This, in turn, can critically affect the research that we can undertake. Given the intricate connection between algorithms and the theory upon which they are based, it is clear that huge factors can emerge when the same quantity is calculated by different methods just because of the suitability of the methods to parallel computation. It is clearly of central importance to establish the extent to which parts of a computation can proceed concurrently, if at all.

This lecture is concerned with the synthesis of parallel numerical algorithms and the analysis of their complexity. We all have our favourite recipes, and favourite recipe books (*e.g.* the excellent book by Press *et. al.* (1986)), for achieving a given computational task but frequently these recipes do not perform well when implemented directly on supercomputers. The creation of parallel algorithms and programs is often intimately related to the architecture of the target machine and so cannot be examined completely in isolation. This is not a lecture on how to adapt code for a particular machine, a vectorizing compiler or a multiprocessing environment. Neither is it a lecture about particular numerical techniques for that would require much more space than we have available here. It is rather a lecture about the general principles of parallel algorithm design and the construction of numerical recipes for supercomputers.

Supercomputational Science
Edited by R.G. Evans and S. Wilson
Plenum Press, New York, 1990

PARALLEL COMPUTATION AND CONTROL FLOW GRAPHS

It is clearly important to establish the extent to which a particular calculation can be subdivided into parts which can be carried out concurrently. There appear to be some computations which cannot be performed more rapidly on N processors than on a single processor. A simple example, due to Kung (1979), is provided by the evaluation of

$$y = x^{2^k}$$

by successive squaring; that is, by putting

$$y := x$$

and using the recursion

$$y := y * y.$$

Thus after one cycle we have x^2, after two cycles x^4, *etc.* and the required result can be obtained in k cycles on a single processor. Using N processors no power higher than 2^m can be achieved in m cycles and thus the time required for the whole computation is seen immediately to be independent of the number of processors available.

Following Dongarra and his coworkers (1988) in their SCHEDULE tool for portable parallel algorithms in FORTRAN, we find it useful to represent parallel computations graphically. A parallel program can be derived by breaking up the computation into discrete units and then constructing a *control flow graph* which exhibits the execution dependences between these units. The idea is probably best described by example. Let us suppose that we have ten subroutines, designated A, B, ... , J. A typical control flow graph is shown in Figure 1. In this Figure, we show a scheme for subroutines A, B, ... , I in which we start by executing subroutines B, E, G, H and I simultaneously since they appear as leaves in the control flow graph. Note that there are three "copies" of subroutine B and four copies of subroutine I operating on different data. As soon as each of the routines I have been completed, the

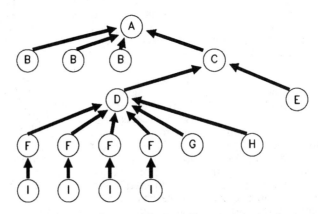

Fig. 1. A control flow graph. Details are given in the text.

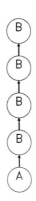

Fig. 2. A control graph for the evaluation of x^{2^k}. A represents the first step, that is putting $y := x$ and B represents the successive squaring step $y := y * y$. Each execution of step B is dependent on the completion of the previous step.

corresponding "copies" of F may execute. When execution of each of the F subroutines has been completed, execution of subroutine D can commence provided that both G and H have been completed. When D and E have been completed execution, C may start. Finally, when the three "copies" of the subroutine B have been completed together with C, C may start. When A is completed the entire computation is finished.

A control flow graph for the evaluation of x^{2^k} is given in Figure 2. Here A represents the first step, that is putting $y := x$ and B represents the successive squaring step $y := y * y$. Each execution of step B is dependent on the completion of the previous step. None of the steps in the computation can be executed concurrently. It is also clear from Fig. 2 that only one of the available processors is active at any one time.

There are broadly two methods for partitioning a given task between the available processors :

a) partitioning of the computation

b) partitioning of the data.

The two approaches, which are not mutually exclusive, are considered in the following sections.

COMPUTATION PARTITIONING.

A parallel algorithm can be devised by distributing a computation amongst the available processors.

Let us illustrate the concept of computational partitioning by means of a simple example, the evaluation of a polynomial, which is one of the most ubiquitous operations in computing. For example, polynomials have to be evaluated in the computation of transcendental and more complex algebraic expressions, and in the approximation of logarithmic and trigonometric expressions.

Consider the problem of evaluating a polynomial expression

$$f_n(x) = \sum_{i=0}^{n} c_i x^i$$

It is well known that the direct evaluation of this expression

$$f_n(x) = c_0 + c_1 x + c_2 x^2 + c_3 x^3 + c_4 x^4 + \ldots + c_n x^n$$

is less efficient than the Horner scheme

$$f_n(x) = c_0 + x(c_1 + x(c_2 + x(c_3 + x(c_4 + \ldots))))$$

which can be written as the recursion

$$y_n = c_n$$

$$y_j = y_{j+1} x + c_j, \quad j = n-1, n-2, \ldots, 1, 0$$

$$f_n(x) = y_0$$

Let us analyse the computational complexity of these schemes. The evaluation of the polynomial term by term requires $(2n-1)$ multiplications and n additions whereas the Horner scheme involves n multiplications and n additions. The time required by the Horner scheme is, therefore, $2n\tau$, where τ is the time for a floating point operation, compared with a time of $(3n-1)\tau$ for the term by term evaluation.

On a single processor of the CRAY X–MP/48, which is itself a vector processor, the evaluation of a polynomial of order 99 using the term by term expansion for 1000 values of x was found to execute at a rate of 86 MFLOPS (Million of FLoating–point OPerations per Second) requiring 32.9 milliseconds of central processor unit time. The same task can be carried in 23.0 milliseconds using the Horner scheme; the rate of execution in this case being only 9 MFLOPS. (The maximum rate of execution on a single processor of the CRAY X–MP/48 is about 235 MFLOPS). The Horner scheme is faster, requiring about 70% of the time for the term by term evaluation. However, the rate of execution observed for the Horner scheme is only 10% of that for the term by term algorithm. *A high rate of execution does not necessarily indicate an efficient program.*

However, as described above, the Horner scheme is not suitable for parallel computation since it involves the computation of n sums and n products in strictly sequential order.

Can we modify the Horner algorithm to partition the computation between two or more processors ? Let us, for the moment, restrict our attention to the case of two processors and write the polynomial in the form

$$f_n(x) = (c_0 + c_2 x^2 + c_4 x^4 + \ldots + c_{n-1} x^{n-1})$$

$$+ (c_1 + c_3 x^2 + c_5 x^4 + \ldots + c_n x^{n-1}) x$$

We can evaluate the first parenthesis on processor 0 by performing the recursion

$$y_n = c_{n-1}$$

$$y_{n-j} = y_{n-j+2} \, x^2 + c_{n-j}, \qquad\qquad j = 2,4, \ldots, n-1, \; (n)$$

whilst on processor 1 we evaluate the second parenthesis

$$y_{n-1} = c_n$$

$$y_{n-j} = y_{n-j+2} \, x^2 + c_{n-j}, \qquad\qquad j = 3,5, \ldots, n-1, \; (n)$$

Finally, the value of the polynomial is given by

$$f_n(x) = y_0 + y_1 x$$

This algorithm requires that n additions be performed on processor 0 and concurrently n additions on processor 1. One multiplication is required to evaluate x^2 and one further addition is required to obtain the final result. Thus the time required by this two–processor algorithm is $(n+2)\tau$, where τ is the time required for a single floating point operation.

This algorithm can be generalized to a p processor computer provided that $p < n/2$. On processor 0 we compute

$$g_0(x) = \sum_{j=0}^{[n/p]} c_{pj} \, x^{pj}$$

on processor 1 we compute

$$g_1(x) = \sum_{j=0}^{[(n-1)/p]} c_{pj+1} \, x^{pj}$$

and on processor q we compute

$$g_q(x) = \sum_{j=0}^{[(n-q)/p]} c_{pj+q} \, x^{pj}$$

The value of the polynomial is then given by

$$f_n(x) = \sum_{q=0}^{p-1} g_q(x) \, x^q$$

The Horner scheme is used to evaluate each of the polynomials which arise in this p processor algorithm. An analysis of the computational complexity of this algorithm reveals that the time required by the p–processor algorithm is $(2n/p + 2 \log p)\tau$.

Consider again the practical problem of evaluating a polynomial of order 99 for 1000 values of x on a single processor of the CRAY X—MP/48. Partitioning the calculation into four parts, we can code this as follows:—

```
DO 1 I=1,1000
    X=XX(I)
    X2=X*X
    X4=X2*X2
    DO 2 K=1,4
        FTMP(K)=A(101-K)
2   CONTINUE
    DO 3 J=97,5,-4
        DO 4 K=1,4
            FTMP(K)=FTMP(K)*X4+A(J-K)
4       CONTINUE
3   CONTINUE
    F(I)=FTMP(1)+X*(FTMP(2)+X*(FTMP(3)+X*FTMP(4)))
1 CONTINUE
```

Execution of this code required 13.7 milliseconds of central processing unit time on a single processor of the CRAY X—MP/48.

Let us now briefly return to the problem of calculating $y=x^{2^k}$ by successive squaring. There are, in fact, cases in which a degree of parallel computation can be incorporated into this calculation by means of computational partitioning. For any x>1, the value of y will increase rapidly as k increases. It may be required, therefore, that y be evaluated to multiword precision. Multiword precision is usually implemented by software operations rather than hardware operations. It is then obviously possible for different words to be processed in parallel and, thus, some concurrent computation can be introduced. However, more spectacular results can be obtained by the data partitioning technique to which we now turn our attention.

DATA PARTITIONING

It is frequently the case in practical computations that we require a number of sets of data to be processed. By partitioning the data we can devise a parallel algorithm in which the same calculation is carried out on different processors using different data.

Consider, again the evaluation of a polynomial. We required the value of a function, f(x), not for just one value of the argument x but for a number of values x_i, i=1,2,... N. The computation of $f(x_i)$ for each x_i can proceed concurrently. Note that data partitioning can be

(i)   either static or dynamic — that is, we can divide the data between the available processors before the computation is commenced or we can assign new data to the processors as the tasks previously given to them are completed;

(ii)   use in conjunction with computation partitioning.

Data partitioning can be introduced into the problem of evaluating a 99th order polynomial for 1000 values of x using the following code:—

```
DO 1 I=1,1000
    F(I)=A(100)
```

```
      1  CONTINUE
         DO 2 J=99,1,-1
            DO 3 I=1,1000
               F(I)=F(I)*X(I)+A(J)
      3     CONTINUE
      2  CONTINUE
```

This code requires 2.7 milliseconds to execute on a single processor of the CRAY X–MP/48 and achieves an execution rate of 124 MFLOPS. The time required is xx% of the 32.9 milliseconds used in the term by term evaluation described at the beginning of the preceding section.

We leave it as an exercise for the reader to devise an algorithm to evaluate a polynomial of order 99 for 1000 values of x using both computational partitioning and data partitioning.

A control graph for the evaluation of $x_i^{2^k}$, i=1,2,...,N is displayed in Figure 3, from which the fact that the most of the computation can proceed concurrently is immediately apparent. The computation which appears to be totally sequential when only one value of x is considered is in fact amenable to concurrent computation when more than one value of x is to be considered. Consider the case when, say, k=15 and 1000 values of x_i. "Scalar code" can be constructed by considering a particular value of x_i which is then squared fifteen times. Executing the following FORTRAN code on a single processor of the CRAY X–MP/48

```
      *
      *     Scalar code
      *
         KMAX=15
         DO 1 I=1,1000
            DO 2 K=1,KMAX
               X(I)=X(I)*X(I)
      2     CONTINUE
      1  CONTINUE
```

a rate of execution approaching 5 MFLOPS was obtained. On the other hand, executing the following "vector code" on a single processor of the CRAY X–MP/48

```
      *
      *     Vector code
      *
         KMAX=15
         DO 2 K=1,KMAX
            DO 1 I=1,1000
               X(I)=X(I)*X(I)
      1     CONTINUE
      2  CONTINUE
```

resulted in an execution rate approaching 75 MFLOPS — 15 times that of the scalar code.

THE ERROR FUNCTION

Having introduced some general principles of parallel algorithm design and the construction of numerical recipes for supercomputers, we turn now to some specific examples. In this sections, we consider the evaluation of the error function and, in the following section, we turn our attention to matrix multiplication.

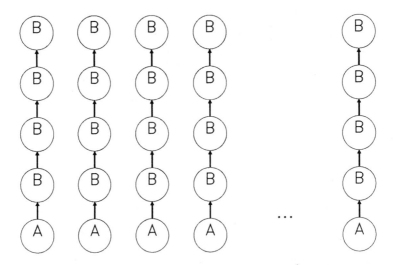

Fig. 3. A control graph for the evaluation of $x_i^{2^k}$, i = 1, 2, ...

The error function arises in many scientific computations. It is defined by

$$\text{erf}(x) = \int_0^x dt \, \exp(-t^2)$$

It can be accurately and efficiently evaluated using expansions in terms of Tchebyshev polynomials. Different expansions are employed for three different ranges of values of x. For $|x| \leq 2$ the expansion

$$\text{erf}(x) = x \sum_r a_r T_r(t)$$

is employed where

$$t = \tfrac{1}{2} x^2 - 1$$

For $2 < |x| \leq x_h$ we put

$$\text{erf}(x) = \text{sign}(x) \left[1 - \frac{\exp(-x^2)}{|x| \sqrt{\pi}} \sum_r b_r T_r(t) \right]$$

where

$$t = (x-7)/(x+3)$$

Finally, for $|x| \geq x_h$ the expression

$$\text{erf}(x) = \text{sign}(x)$$

is used where x_h is the value of x above which $|\text{erf}(x)| = 1$ within the rounding error of the machine being used.

In Figure 4 FORTRAN code suitable for evaluating the error function on a scalar processor is presented. The scalar FUNCTION ERF(X) returns the value of the error function for the scalar argument X.

FORTRAN code suitable for implementation on a vector processor is shown in Figure 5. Data partitioning is employed to obtain a suitable algorithm. The FUNCTION VERF(X) returns a vector each element of which contains the error function for the corresponding element of the vector argument X. The conditional statements in the code given in Figure 4 inhibit efficient implementation on vector processing computers. By replacing the scalar argument X by a vector argument much improved efficiency can be achieved.

The code shown in Figure 5 is written in FORTRAN 200, the dialect of FORTRAN which is employed on the Cyber 205 and ETA 10 machines. The use of the WHERE block in this code and the FORTRAN 200 vector notation should be noted. To illustrate the FORTRAN 200 vector syntax, which closely resembles the proposed FORTRAN 8X syntax (Metcalf and Reid, 1988), consider the following simple DO loop

```
      DO 1 I= 1,N
           A(I+NA) = C + B(I+NB)
  1   CONTINUE
```

```
      REAL FUNCTION ERF(X)
C
C     Evaluation of the error function, erf(x)
C
C     .. Scalar Arguments ..
      REAL            X
C     .. Local Scalars ..
      REAL            CJ, CJP1, CJP2, HALF, ONE, SQRTPI, THREE,
     *                TWENTY, TWO, X2, XUP, XV, ZERO
      INTEGER         J, NA, NB
C     .. Local Arrays ..
      REAL            A(15), B(15)
C     .. Intrinsic Functions ..
      INTRINSIC       ABS, EXP, SIGN
C     .. Data statements ..
      DATA NA,NB/15,15/,XUP/5.75E0/,SQRTPI/1.7724538509055/
     A,A(1),A(2),A(3),A(4),A(5),A(6),A(7),A(8),A(9),A(10)
     A,A(11),A(12),A(13),A(14),A(15)
     A/1.9449071068179,4.20186582324E-2,-1.86866103977E-2
     A,5.1281061839E-3,-1.0683107462E-3,1.744737872E-4
     A,-2.15642056E-5,1.7282658E-6,-2.00479E-8,-1.64782E-8
     A,2.0008E-9,2.58E-11,-3.06E-11,1.9E-12,4.0E-13/
     A,B(1),B(2),B(3),B(4),B(5),B(6),B(7),B(8),B(9),B(10)
     A,B(11),B(12),B(13),B(14),B(15)
     A/1.4831105640848,-3.010710733866E-1,6.89948306898E-2
     A,-1.39162712647E-2,2.4207995224E-3,-3.658639686E-4
     A,4.86209844E-5,-5.7492565E-6,6.113243E-7,-5.89910E-8
     A,5.2070E-9,-4.233E-10,3.19E-11,-2.2E-12,1.0E-13/
      DATA ZERO, ONE, TWO, THREE, TWENTY, HALF /0.0,1.0,2.0,3.0,20.0,
     * 0.5/
C     .. Executable Statements ..
      XV = ABS(X)
      IF (XV.GE.XUP) GO TO 600
      IF (XV.LE.TWO) GO TO 300
      X2 = TWO - TWENTY/(XV+THREE)
```

Fig. 4. FORTRAN code suitable for the evaluation of the error function on a scalar processor. For a given value of the scalar x this function returns the value of erf(x). Expansions in terms of Tchebyshev polynomials are employed as described in the text.

```
C
      CJP2 = ZERO
      CJP1 = A(NA)
      J = NA - 1
100   CONTINUE
      CJ = X2*CJP1 - CJP2 + A(J)
      IF (J.EQ.1) GO TO 200
      CJP2 = CJP1
      CJP1 = CJ
      J = J - 1
      GO TO 100
200   CONTINUE
      X2 = HALF*(CJ-CJP2)/XV*EXP(-X*X)/SQRTPI
      ERF = (ONE-X2)*SIGN(ONE,X)
      GO TO 700
C
300   CONTINUE
      X2 = X*X - TWO
      CJP2 = ZERO
      CJP1 = B(NB)
      J = NB - 1
400   CONTINUE
      CJ = X2*CJP1 - CJP2 + B(J)
      IF (J.EQ.1) GO TO 500
      CJP2 = CJP1
      CJP1 = CJ
      J = J - 1
      GO TO 400
500   CONTINUE
      ERF = HALF*(CJ-CJP2)*X
      GO TO 700
C
600   CONTINUE
      ERF = SIGN(ONE,X)
700   RETURN
      END
```

Fig. 4. (continued)

```
          REAL FUNCTION VERF(X;*)
C
C    Evaluation of the error function, erf(x)
C
C    FORTRAN 200 version for CYBER 205 and ETA 10 machines
C
C    .. Array arguments ..
     REAL X(100)
C    .. Local Scalars ..
     REAL            HALF, ONE, SQRTPI, THREE,
    *                TWENTY, TWO, XUP, ZERO
     INTEGER         J, NA, NB
C    .. Local Arrays ..
     REAL X2(100),XV(100),CJ(100),CJP1(100),CJP2(100),V(100),
    *        A(15), B(15)
C    .. Intrinsic Functions ..
     INTRINSIC       ABS, EXP, SIGN
     DESCRIPTOR      VERF
C    .. Data statements ..
     DATA NA,NB/15,15/,XUP/5.75E0/,SQRTPI/1.7724538509055/
    A,A(1),A(2),A(3),A(4),A(5),A(6),A(7),A(8),A(9),A(10)
    A,A(11),A(12),A(13),A(14),A(15)
    A/1.9449071068179,4.20186582324E-2,-1.86866103977E-2
    A,5.1281061839E-3,-1.0683107462E-3,1.744737872E-4
    A,-2.15642056E-5,1.7282658E-6,-2.00479E-8,-1.64782E-8
    A,2.0008E-9,2.58E-11,-3.06E-11,1.9E-12,4.0E-13/
    A,B(1),B(2),B(3),B(4),B(5),B(6),B(7),B(8),B(9),B(10)
    A,B(11),B(12),B(13),B(14),B(15)
    A/1.4831105640848,-3.010710733866E-1,6.89948306898E-2
    A,-1.39162712647E-2,2.4207995224E-3,-3.658639686E-4
    A,4.86209844E-5,-5.7492565E-6,6.113243E-7,-5.89910E-8
    A,5.2070E-9,-4.233E-10,3.19E-11,-2.2E-12,1.0E-13/
C
C
     DATA ZERO, ONE, TWO, THREE, TWENTY, HALF /0.0,1.0,2.0,3.0,20.0,
    * 0.5/
C    .. Executable Statements ..
     N=100
C
     CJ(1:N)=1.0
     XV(1;N)=VABS(X(1;N);XV(1;N))
     V(1;N)=VSIGN(CJ(1;N),X(1;N);V(1;N))
```

Fig. 5. FORTRAN 200 code suitable for the evaluation of the error function on the Cyber 205 and ETA–10 computers using the vector processing facility. Given a vector containing 100 elements x_i this vector function returns a vector containing $erf(x_i)$.

```
C
      X2(1;N)=X(1;N)*X(1;N)-2.0
      CJP2(1:N)=0.0
      CJP1(1:N)=B(NB)
      DO 100, J=NB-1,2,-1
      CJ(1;N)=X2(1;N)*CJP1(1;N)-CJP2(1;N)+B(J)
      CJP2(1;N)=CJP1(1;N)
      CJP1(1;N)=CJ(1;N)
100   CONTINUE
      CJ(1;N)=X2(1;N)*CJP1(1;N)-CJP2(1;N)+B(1)
      WHERE (XV(1;N).LE.2.0)
      V(1;N)=HALF*(CJ(1;N)-CJP2(1;N))*X(1;N)
      ENDWHERE
      X2(1;N)=2.0-20.0/(XV(1;N)+3.0)
      CJP2(1:N)=0.0
      CJP1(1:N)=A(NA)
      DO 200, J=NA-1,2,-1
      CJ(1;N)=X2(1;N)*CJP1(1;N)-CJP2(1;N)+A(J)
      CJP2(1;N)=CJP1(1;N)
      CJP1(1;N)=CJ(1;N)
200   CONTINUE
      CJ(1;N)=X2(1;N)*CJP1(1;N)-CJP2(1;N)+A(1)
      X2(1;N)=-X(1;N)*X(1;N)
      X2(1;N)=VEXP(X2(1;N);X2(1;N))
      X2(1;N)=0.5*(CJ(1;N)-CJP2(1;N))/XV(1;N)*X2(1;N)/SQRTPI
      CJP1(1;N)=1.0
      CJ(1;N)=VSIGN(CJP1(1;N),X(1;N);CJ(1;N))
      WHERE (.NOT.((XV(1;N).GE.XUP).OR.(XV(1;N).LE.TWO)))
      V(1;N)=(CJP1(1;N)-X2(1;N))*CJ(1;N)
      ENDWHERE
      VERF=V(1;N)
      RETURN
      END
```

Fig. 5. (continued)

In FORTRAN 200 vector syntax this becomes

$$A(NA;N) = C + B(NB;N)$$

where NA and NB are the starting addresses for A and B, respectively, and the length of the vector is given after the semicolon. Intrinsic functions such as ABS are available in vector form. For example, the statement

$$Y(1;N) = VABS(X(1;N);Y(1;N))$$

results in each element of the vector Y(1;N) containing the absolute value of the corresponding element of the vector X(1;N).

The WHERE block is a particularly power feature of FORTRAN 200. In its simplest form it has the form

```
WHERE (LBIT(1;N))
     A(1:N) = B(1;N)
ENDWHERE
```

in which LBIT(1;N) is a BIT vector whose elements are either .TRUE. or .FALSE. and the elements of the vector B(1;N) are assigned to the corresponding elements of A(1;N) according to the elements of LBIT(1;N). In Figure 6, the code which is equivalent to that given in Figure 5 is presented using the DESCRIPTOR notation of FORTRAN 200. In this notation, the about simple WHERE block would take the form

```
WHERE (LBIT)
     A = B
ENDWHERE
```

LBIT, A and B are declared DESCRIPTORS. The code given in Figure 6 has an advantage over that given in Figure 5 in that the work arrays that are required are assigned dynamically. The intrinsic function Q8SLEN returns the length of the argument vector X. The ASSIGN statements then allocate memory to the various work arrays. The DESCRIPTOR syntax is used throughout and thus X(1;N) is replaced by X where X is declared a DESCRIPTOR.

In Table 1, a comparison is made of the time required on the Cyber 205 vector processor (2 pipelines) using the "scalar" code given in Figure 4 and the code given in Figure 6. these timing test were performed on the Cyber 205 installation at the University of Manchester Regional Computer Centre.

A similar approach can be employed in the evaluation of any function which can be approximated by a polynomial. For example, given a vector x, $0 \leq x_i \leq \pi/2$, the reader may consider the design a program to approximate the vector f, where

$$f_i = (\sin x_i)/x_i$$

using the polynomial approximation (Abramowitz and Stegun, 1965)

$$\frac{\sin x}{x} = 1 + a_2 x^2 + a_4 x^4 + \epsilon(x)$$

Table 1

Central processing time required to evaluate the error function, $\text{erf}(x_i)$, $i=1,...,N$ on a Cyber 205 (two pipeline) computers using scalar instructions and vector instructions.

N	scalar code time/milliseconds τ_s	vector code time/milliseconds τ_v	ratio τ_s/τ_v
500	9.4	1.6	5.9
1000	18.6	2.4	7.8
1500	27.8	3.4	8.2
2000	37.7	4.5	8.4
2500	46.4	5.6	8.3
3000	55.4	6.6	8.4
3500	64.1	7.7	8.3
4000	73.2	8.8	8.3
4500	82.8	9.9	8.4
5000	92.5	11.0	8.4

```
      REAL FUNCTION VERF(X;*)
C
C     Evaluation of the error function, erf(x)
C
C     FORTRAN 200 version for the CYBER 205 and ETA 10 using descriptors
C     .. Array arguments ..
C     REAL X(100)
C     .. Local Scalars ..
      REAL            HALF, ONE, SQRTPI, THREE,
     *                TWENTY, TWO, XUP, ZERO
      INTEGER         J, NA, NB
C     .. Local Arrays ..
C     REAL X2(100),XV(100),CJ(100),CJP1(100),CJP2(100),V(100)
     *                A(15), B(15)
C     .. Descriptors ..
      DESCRIPTOR      VERF,X,XV,X2,CJ,CJP1,CJP2,V
C     .. Data statements ..
C
      DATA NA,NB/15,15/,XUP/5.75E0/,SQRTPI/1.7724538509055/
 A,A(1),A(2),A(3),A(4),A(5),A(6),A(7),A(8),A(9),A(10)
     A,A(11),A(12),A(13),A(14),A(15)
     A/1.9449071068179,4.20186582324E-2,-1.86866103977E-2
     A,5.1281061839E-3,-1.0683107462E-3,1.744737872E-4
     A,-2.15642056E-5,1.7282658E-6,-2.00479E-8,-1.64782E-8
     A,2.0008E-9,2.58E-11,-3.06E-11,1.9E-12,4.0E-13/
     A,B(1),B(2),B(3),B(4),B(5),B(6),B(7),B(8),B(9),B(10)
     A,B(11),B(12),B(13),B(14),B(15)
     A/1.4831105640848,-3.010710733866E-1,6.89948306898E-2
     A,-1.39162712647E-2,2.4207995224E-3,-3.658639686E-4
     A,4.86209844E-5,-5.7492565E-6,6.113243E-7,-5.89910E-8
     A,5.2070E-9,-4.233E-10,3.19E-11,-2.2E-12,1.0E-13/
C
C
C         .. Executable Statements ..
      N=Q8SLEN(X)
      ASSIGN XV,.DYN.N
      ASSIGN X2,.DYN.N
      ASSIGN CJ,.DYN.N
      ASSIGN CJP1,.DYN.N
      ASSIGN CJP2,.DYN.N
      ASSIGN V,.DYN.N
C
      XV=VABS(X;XV)
```

Fig. 6. Alternative FORTRAN 200 code, uses the DESCRIPTOR language element, suitable for the evaluation of the error function on the Cyber 205 and ETA–10 computers using the vector processing facility.

```
C
      X2=X*X-2.0
      CJP1=X2*B(NB)+B(NB-1)
      CJP2=B(NB)
      DO 100, J=NB-2,2,-1
      CJ=X2*CJP1-CJP2+B(J)
      CJP2=CJP1
      CJP1=CJ
100   CONTINUE
      CJ=X2*CJP1-CJP2+B(1)
      WHERE (XV.LE.2.0)
      V=0.5*(CJ-CJP2)*X
      ENDWHERE
      X2=2.0-20.0/(XV+3.0)
      CJP1=X2*A(NA)+A(NA-1)
      CJP2=A(NA)
      DO 200, J=NA-2,2,-1
      CJ=X2*CJP1-CJP2+A(J)
      CJP2=CJP1
      CJP1=CJ
200   CONTINUE
      CJ=X2*CJP1-CJP2+A(1)
      X2=-X*X
      X2=VEXP(X2;X2)
      X2=0.5*(CJ-CJP2)/XV*X2/SQRTPI
      CJP1=1.0-X2
      CJ=VSIGN(CJP1,X;CJ)
      WHERE (XV.GT.2.0)
      V=CJ
      ENDWHERE
      VERF=V
      FREE
      RETURN
      END
```

Fig. 6. (continued)

where $a_2 = -0.16605$ and $a_4 = 0.00761$. The performance of the code should be monitored as a function of the length of the vector $\mathbf{x}$.

MATRIX MULTIPLICATION

Many scientific calculations involve extensive linear algebra. Such calculations can be efficiently executed on modern supercomputers by exploiting a set of Basic Linear Algebra Subroutines (BLAS) (see, for example, Lawson, Hanson, Kincaid, and Krogh, 1979; Lawson, Hanson, Kincaid, and Krogh, 1979; Dongarra, Du Croz, Hammarling, and Hanson, 1986; Dongarra, Du Croz, Hammarling, and Hanson, 1986; Dongarra, Du Croz, Duff, and Hammarling, 1987; Du Croz, Mayes, Wasniewski, and Wilson, 1988) tailored to the particular target machine. These subroutines are sometimes divided into three types:—

1) Level 1 BLAS – vector operations

2) Level 2 BLAS – matrix–vector operations

3) Level 3 BLAS – matrix operations

By structuring programs around these BLAS, not only can very efficient code be obtained but also a degree of portability results which is important for general purpose numerical software libraries (Du Croz and Mayes, 1990).

In this section, we consider as an example one of the most fundamental operations of linear algebra, namely matrix multiplication. Consider the product of two square matrices $\mathbf{A}=\mathbf{B}\,\mathbf{C}$, which can be written in terms of the matrix elements as

$$A_{ij} = \sum_{k}^{n} B_{ik}\,C_{kj}$$

FORTRAN code for evaluating this product can be written in at least three distinct ways. In each of the following cases we assume that the elements of the array A have been set to zero. First, we have what might be termed the inner product method which is clearly sequential, since it has the form of a scalar summation :

```
*
*       Matrix multiplication using a scalar loop
*       structure.
*
        DO 1 I = 1,N
            DO 2 J = 1,N
                DO 3 K = 1,N
                    A(I,J) = A(I,J) + B(I,K) * C(K,J)
3               CONTINUE
2           CONTINUE
1       CONTINUE
```

In this code, the inner DO loop runs over k and thus $A(I,J)$ is effectively a scalar quantity. Next we have the middle product method which has a loop structure suitable for vector processing computers :—

```
*
*      Matrix multiplication using a loop
*      structure suitable for vector processors.
*
       DO 1 J = 1,N
           DO 2 K = 1,N
               DO 3 I = 1,N
                   A(I,J) = A(I,J) + B(I,K) * C(K,J)
3              CONTINUE
2          CONTINUE
1      CONTINUE
```

Here the inner DO loop is over I and thus $A(I,J)$ is effectively a vector quantity. The inner loop in this construction can be executed in vector mode. Finally, we have the outer product method, which has the following form :

```
*
*      Matrix multiplication using a loop
*      structure suitable for array processors.
*
       DO 1 K = 1,N
           DO 2 I = 1,N
               DO 3 J = 1,N
                   A(I,J) = A(I,J) + B(I,K) * C(K,J)
3              CONTINUE
2          CONTINUE
1      CONTINUE
```

in which the inner two DO loops are over I and J and $A(I,J)$ is treated as a array. Whereas the middle product method can be said to have a degree of parallelism n, the outer product method can be seen to have a degree of parallelism n^2, since the inner two loops are independent.

In Table 2 we present the results of timing tests for the inner product, middle product and outer product matrix multiplication schemes performed on a single processor of the CRAY X–MP/48. Both the middle product scheme and the outer product scheme are able to exploit the vector processing capabilities of this machine and this is reflected in the times quoted.

When performing matrix multiplication on machines with more than one processor two approaches suggest themselves :

a)   partitioning the computation of a single matrix product

b)   partitioning the data by performing a number of matrix multiplications simultaneously

We consider each of these cases in turn.

a)   partitioning the computation of a single matrix product

Table 2

Results of timing tests for the inner product, middle product and outer product matrix multiplication schemes performed on a single processor of the CRAY X–MP/48. The matrices are taken to be square and have dimension N.

Dimension N	Inner product	CPU time/seconds Middle product	Outer product
20	0.001	0.000	0.000
40	0.007	0.002	0.002
60	0.019	0.005	0.005
80	0.036	0.012	0.011
100	0.060	0.021	0.021
120	0.093	0.034	0.033
140	0.139	0.054	0.055
160	0.187	0.075	0.074
180	0.245	0.106	0.105
200	0.324	0.146	0.144
300	0.875	0.454	0.458
400	1.852	1.059	1.060
500	3.321	1.946	1.964

Figure 7 illustrates the partitioning of the matrices **A**, **B** and **C** for the multitasking of a single matrix multiplication. Given matrices **A** and **B** of dimension $n_1 \times m$ and $m \times n_2$, respectively, we wish to compute the matrix product $C = A B$ in which **C** is of dimension $n_1 \times n_2$. The partitions of the matrices **A**, **B** and **C** shown in Figure 7 are of dimension $p_1 \times p_2$, $p_2 \times n_2$, and $p_1 \times n_2$, respectively. The matrix C is initially set to be a null matrix. One block row of the matrix **C** is updated according to

$$C_{i,k} <- C_{i,k} + A_{i,j} B_{j,k}$$

$$k = 1, 2, ..., n_2$$

for

$$i = i_1, i_2, ..., i_{p_1}$$

and

$$j = j_1, j_2, ..., j_{p_2}$$

b)   partitioning   the   data   by   performing   a   number   of   matrix multiplications simultaneously

FORTRAN code for the simultaneous multiplication of several distinct matrices on a multitasking computer, again the CRAY X–MP/48, is given in Figure 8. This code is applicable to an arbitrary number of processors, although in the present discussion we are, of course, limited to four physical processors and we shall assume this limit for both the number of physical processors and the number of logical processors in the immediate discussion of the code. The code in Figure 8 employs Cray macrotasking facilities to calculate each of the matrix products as a separate task. Clearly, we only wish to initialize four tasks at any one time since otherwise the tasks will be competing for resources. TASK(*,*) is the task control array. The vector TASK(1,n), TASK(2,n), TASK(3,n), n=1,2,3,4, corresponds to each of the tasks being performed at a given time. TSKTUNE modifies tuning parameters in the library scheduler and is called during initialization to establish the number of processors to be used. Each call to TSKSTART initializes a task. The arguments of TSKSTART are the task control array, the external entry and a list of arguments. TSKWAIT monitors the completion of the tasks. It should be noted that the Cray macrotasking feature allows control over the number of logical processors and not the number of physical processors. Timing data for the code presented in Figure 8 is shown in Figure 9. This program uses the Cray provided matrix multiplication routine MXMA which is coded in assembler language (CAL) and achieves a rate of execution approaching 220 MFLOPS.

We conclude this section by briefly discussing the algebraic complexity of matrix multiplication. In 1968, Winograd suggested that the matrix product

$$C_{ij} = \sum_{k=1}^{n} A_{ik} B_{kj}$$

```
          PROGRAM MULTIMAT
          PARAMETER(N=256, NCPUS= 4, MTSK=100, NTSK=8)
          INTEGER TASK
          DIMENSION DUMP(200)
          COMMON /A/ A(N,N),B(N,N),C(N,N)
          COMMON /TSK / TASK (3,NCPUS)
          EXTERNAL MXMA
          N1=1
          NN=N
          DO 1 I=1,NCPUS-1
              TASK(1,I)=3
              TASK(3,I)=I
   1      CONTINUE
          IF (NCPUS.GT.1) THEN
          CALL TSKTUNE('MAXCPU',NCPUS)
          CALL TSKTUNE('DBRELEAS',NCPUS)
          ENDIF
C
          DO 2 I=1,N
              DO 2 J=1,N
   2              A(I,J)=0.987654321
C
          I=0
          DO 3 K=1,MTSK
              I=I+1
              IF(I.NE.NTSK) THEN
                  CALL TSKSTART(TASK(1,I),MXMA ,
   1              A(1,1),N1,NN,B(1,1),N1,NN,C(1,1),N1,NN,NN,NN,NN)
              ELSE
                  CALL MXMA (
   1              A(1,1),N1,NN,B(1,1),N1,NN,C(1,1),N1,NN,NN,NN,NN)
                  DO 4 J=1,NCPUS-1
   4                  CALL TSKWAIT(TASK(1,J))
                      I=0
              ENDIF
   3      CONTINUE
          DO 6 J=1,I
   6          CALL TSKWAIT(TASK(1,J))
          STOP
          END
```

Fig. 8. Matrix multiplication code for the CRAY X–MP/48.

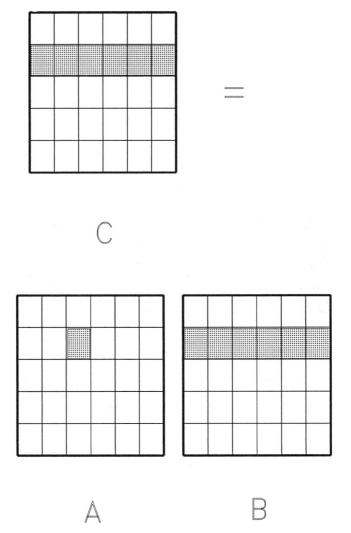

Fig. 7. Partition of matrices for matrix multiplication on multiprocessing computers. (See text for details).

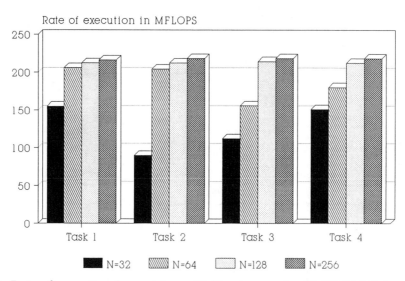

Fig: 9. Rate of execution for matrix multiplication on the CRAY X–MP/48. Four tasks, that is matrix multiplications, are carried out concurrently on the four processors of the CRAY X–MP/48. The rate of execution is given for matrices of dimension, N = 32, 64, 128, 256.

be rewritten as

$$C_{ij} = \sum_{k=2,4,..}^{n} (A_{i\,k-1} + B_{k\,j})(A_{i\,k} + B_{k-1\,j})$$

$$- \sum_{k=2,4,...}^{n} A_{i\,k-1}\,A_{i\,k} - \sum_{k=2,4,...}^{n} B_{k-1\,j}\,B_{kj}$$

where, for simplicity, we have taken n to be even. It can be demonstrated that these two equations are identical and furthermore that the Winograd matrix multiplication involves $1/2\,n^3 + n^2$ multiplications compared with n^3 for the standard scheme. Work by Strassen has shown that the number of scalar multiplications involved in a matrix multiplication scales as n^s where $s = \log_2 7 = 2.807$. However, both the Winograd and the Strassen scheme involve more floating point additions than the standard scheme. For instance, the total number of floating point additions involved in the Winograd scheme is of the order $3n^3/2$ compared with only $n^2(n-1)$ for the standard approach. Thus on a machine like the CRAY X–MP for which all floating point operations take the same time the standard scheme is preferred. For a machine with more addition units than multiplication units the Winograd and Strassen algorithms deserve attention.

MEMORY MANAGEMENT

So far we have limited our discussion to the utilization of the central processing units. In this final section, it is emphasized that we should not be solely concerned with central processing unit activity in designing efficient algorithms for supercomputers. Dongarra claims that

> *The key to using a high–performance computer effectively is to avoid unnecessary memory references. In most computers, data flows from memory into and out of registers and from registers into and out of functional units, which perform the given instructions on the data. Algorithm performance can be dominated by the amount of memory traffic rather than by the number of floating point operations involved. The movement of data between memory and registers can be as costly as arithmetic operations on data.*

In the implementation of numerical techniques on parallel machines it is vital to organize the use of not only the processing units but also the memory and the input–output channels. The performance of an algorithm can be dominated by the amount of memory traffic rather than the number of floating–point operations.

To illustrate the effect of memory management on the performance of a piece of FORTRAN code consider again matrix multiply using the middle product DO loop structure which was given previously as

```
*
*       Matrix multiplication using a loop
*       structure suitable for vector processors.
*
```

```
          DO 1 J = 1,N
             DO 2 K = 1,N
                DO 3 I = 1,N
                   A(I,J) = A(I,J) + B(I,K) * C(K,J)
      3            CONTINUE
      2         CONTINUE
      1      CONTINUE
```

and let us modify this whilst maintaining the "vector nature" of the inner DO loop as follows

```
          DO 1 I = 1,N
             DO 2 K = 1,N
                DO 3 J = 1,N
                   A(I,J) = A(I,J) + B(I,K) * C(K,J)
      3            CONTINUE
      2         CONTINUE
      1      CONTINUE
```

As in the original structure $A(I,J)$ is effectively a vector. However, it is the second array subscript J which is increasing most rapidly in this modified code. The elements of the array A are actually stored in memory in the order $A(1,1)$, $A(2,1)$, $A(3,1)$, ..., $A(1,2)$, $A(2,2)$, $A(3,2)$, ..., $A(1,3)$, $A(2,3)$, $A(3,3)$, ... and thus whereas the original code involved a unit "stride" the modified code requires a stride of n, where n is the matrix dimension. This is reflected in the computer time observed for the original and the modified middle product codes. For n=200, the original code uses 0.137 milliseconds whereas the modified code requires 0.251 milliseconds. Increasing the dimension to 500, we find that 1.887 milliseconds are required by the original code compared with 3.420 milliseconds for the modified middle product code. The last time quoted should be compared with that given for the scalar code given in Table 2 (3.321 milliseconds) — poor memory management used in conjunction with a DO loop structure apparently suited to vector processing has thus resulted in a degradation of performance to levels below that observed for scalar code !

The most efficient matrix multiplication routines coded in FORTRAN achieved rates of execution of around 130 − 140 MFLOPS. The assembler language routine MXMA, which was used to generate the results displayed in Figure 9 leads to execution rates approaching 220 MFLOPS. Memory management is one of the main contributing factors to this speed in that by using CAL (Cray Assembler Language) it is possible to write intermediates which arise in the matrix multiplication to vector register rather than memory.

REFERENCES

Abramowitz, M., and Stegun, I, 1965, Handbook of Mathematical Functions, Dover, New York.

Dongarra, J.J., Sarensen, D.C., Connolly, K., and Patterson, J., 1988, Parallel Computing **8** 41

Dongarra, J.J., Du Croz J.J., Hammarling, S., and Hanson, R., 1986, *An Extended Set of Fortran Basic Linear Algebra Subprograms: Model Implementation and Test programs*, Argonne National Laboratory Report ANL−MCS−TM−81.

Dongarra, J.J., Du Croz, J.J., Hammarling, S., and Hanson, R., 1986, *An Extended Set of Fortran Basic Linear Algebra Subprograms*, Argonne National Laboratory Report ANL–MCS–TM–41.

Dongarra, J.J., Du Croz J.J., Duff, I.S., and Hammarling, S., 1987, *A Proposal for a Set of Level 3 Basic Linear Algebra Subprograms*, Argonne National Laboratory Report ANL–MCS–TM–88.

Du Croz, J.J., Mayes, P.J.D., Wasniewski, J., and Wilson, S., 1988, Parallel Computing **8** 345

Du Croz, J.J., Mayes, P.J.D., 1990, this volume

Hockney, R.W., and Jesshope, C.J., 1981, *Parallel computers*, Adam Hilger, Bristol.

Kung, H.T., 1979, J. ACM **23** 252

Lawson, C, Hanson, R., Kincaid, D., and Krogh, F., 1979, ACM Trans. Math. Software **5**

Lawson, C, Hanson R.,, Kincaid, D., and Krogh, F., 1979, Algorithm 539, ACM Trans. Math. Software **5**

Metcalfe, M., and Reid, J, 1988, *FORTRAN 8X*, MacMillan

Press, W., Flannery, B., Teukolsky, S., and Vetterling, W., 1986, Numerical Recipes, Cambridge Univesity Press.

Strassen, V., 1969, Num. Math **13** 354

Winograd, S., 1968, IEEE Trans. Computers C–17 693.

THE NAG LIBRARY IN A SUPERCOMPUTING ENVIRONMENT

J.J. Du Croz and P.J.D. Mayes

The Numerical Algorithms Group Ltd.,
Wilkinson House, Jordan Hill Road, Oxford OX2 8DR

Parts of this paper are reproduced with permission from two articles published in the NAG Newsletter, issues 1/89 and 2/89.

INTRODUCTION

In a supercomputing environment the role of a numerical subroutine library is even more important than in a more conventional computing environment. Not only should the library provide accuracy, reliability and robustness in performing standard numerical computations, but it should also — as far as possible — offer the high levels of performance which users of supercomputers may expect. Indeed, users may reasonably look to a subroutine library to relieve them of some of the burden of acquiring the specialised expertise — for example, knowledge of architectural details or of the capabilities of a vectorizing compiler — that may be necessary to use a supercomputer efficiently.

The aim of this paper is twofold: first, to describe what levels of performance the NAG library can offer; and second, to explain how this performance is achieved, in the hope that the techniques will be of help to readers in improving the efficiency of their own codes.

The NAG Fortran Library is a library of Fortran 77 subroutines for standard numerical and statistical computations. At the time of writing, Mark 13 of the Library, containing 735 documented routines, is generally available; and Mark 14, containing almost 900 routines, is at an advanced stage of preparation. The Library has been implemented on a wide range of machines, including the following which may in some sense be classified as supercomputers: the Alliant FX series; the Amdahl/Fujitsu/Siemens VP series; the CDC Cyber 205; the CDC Cyber 990; the Convex C1 and C2; the Cray 1; the Cray X–MP; the Cray 2; the Cray Y–MP; the FPS M64 series; the Gould NP1; the IBM 3090 VF; the NAS 9160 and XL (see Luecke, 1988); the NEC SX series; the Stellar GS1000; and the Unisys ISP (see Du Croz and Wasniewski, 1988).

On almost all these machines, the NAG library runs at present in uniprocessor mode (the Alliant is the only exception). So far our work has concentrated on exploiting the vector–processing capabilities of supercomputers; exploitation of parallelism will come in the next phase.

Supercomputational Science
Edited by R.G. Evans and S. Wilson
Plenum Press, New York, 1990

STRATEGY

The following aims were stated at the start of our work on adapting the NAG library to supercomputers:

(a) to provide the user of the NAG Library on a supercomputer with access to computational power which comes reasonably close to the full power of the machine.

(b) to preserve the existing specifications of the Library routines, so that no changes need be made to documentation or users' programs;

(c) to preserve as much generality in the code as possible, ideally to develop a single version of the code which performs satisfactorily on both conventional and vector machines − this simplifies management and maintenance of the Library.

In practice the aims (a) and (c) are incompatible; some basic computations may need to be coded in different ways for different vector machines. Our policy has been to confine any machine–specific coding to a small number of simple kernel routines.

The second aim (b) is important, since a supercomputing environment in the broadest sense includes also the workstations and minicomputers on which programs may be developed before being sent via a network to run on a supercomputer.

Initially we concentrated our attention on routines for dense linear algebra, and our work in this area is described in the next section.

The following three sections discuss random number generation, quadrature and FFT's. To provide efficient routines for these computations, we added a fourth principle to our strategy:

(d) to design new routines with a vectorisable user interface, so that the design of the interface does not become an obstacle to vectorization.

LINEAR ALGEBRA

In linear algebra, we have been able to re–structure the code of many existing routines without disturbing the user–interface, and thus have achieved very satisfactory levels of performance, as will be illustrated in subsection 3. Our guiding principle has been to organise the code so that as much as possible of the computation is performed by lower–level kernel routines, which can then be tuned for maximum efficiency on different vector–processors. However, implementing even a small number of kernel routines efficiently on each new vector–processing machine could have imposed a large burden on NAG in terms of specialised programming effort.

Therefore we adopted a policy of collaborating in the specification of standard sets of kernel routines, in the hope that optimised implementations of those routines would be developed for particular machines, by manufacturers or others. In practice this meant that we became actively involved in the specification of the Level 2 and Level 3 BLAS.

1. The Level 2 BLAS

By 1984 a number of people concerned with the development of numerical software had recognized the potential benefits of defining a standard set of kernel routines, in the same spirit as the original set of BLAS, defined by Lawson *et al*

(1979). (BLAS is an acronym for Basic Linear Algebra Subprograms.) The original BLAS — now known as Level 1 BLAS — perform simple vector operations, but are of too small a granularity to be efficient on most vector machines. It was clear that operations of larger granularity were needed. They would allow greater flexibility in adapting the code to the architecture of the machine; and on machines with vector registers they would allow a reduction in the ratio of memory references to arithmetic operations.

NAG took part in an international collaborative project to define an extended set of BLAS for matrix–vector operations. These became known as the Level 2 BLAS.

The Level 2 BLAS perform the following types of matrix–vector operation in real arithmetic:

(a) matrix–vector products of the forms:

$$y \longleftarrow \alpha\, A x + \beta\, y$$

and

$$y \longleftarrow \alpha\, A^T x + \beta\, y$$

where α and β are scalars, **x** and **y** are vectors, and **A** is a rectangular matrix, and:

$$x \longleftarrow T x$$

and

$$x \longleftarrow T^T x$$

where **T** is an upper or lower triangular matrix;

(b) rank–one and rank–two updates of the forms:

$$A \longleftarrow \alpha\, x y^T + A$$

and:

$$H \longleftarrow \alpha\, x x^T + H$$

and

$$H \longleftarrow \alpha\, x y^T + \alpha\, y x^T + H$$

where **H** is a symmetric matrix;

(c) solution of triangular equations of the form:

$$x \longleftarrow T^{-1} x$$

and

$$x \longleftarrow T^{-T} x$$

Analogues of these operations in complex arithmetic are also provided, and routines are specified which cater for various storage schemes, including band matrices and packed storage for symmetric or triangular matrices.

Many numerical algorithms in dense linear algebra can be programmed so that the bulk of the computation is performed by calls to Level 2 BLAS, and this results in concise and elegant code.

2. The Level 2 BLAS in the NAG Library

The Level 2 BLAS were introduced into the NAG Fortran Library at Mark 12. At the same time some refinements were made to the infrastructure of the Library software.

A new chapter was created: F06 — Linear Algebra Support Routines. It includes all the Level 2 BLAS, as well as the original Level 1 BLAS. (It also contains many other routines for scalar, vector and matrix operations.) Standard Fortran code for all the BLAS is provided for use when no specialised implementation is available.

The BLAS routines have been given NAG—type names (for example, F06PAF), but they can also be called by their more familiar BLAS names (for example, SGEMV in single precision or DGEMV in double precision). Routines in the NAG Library always refer to the BLAS by their BLAS names, so that Library routines can easily be linked to machine—specific implementations of the BLAS as and when they are available.

Some manufacturers — for example Cray, Convex and Alliant — already provide efficient implementations in their run—time libraries. IBM have included a few of the routines in their ESSL library for the 3090 VF. An implementation of the real Level 2 BLAS for the CDC Cyber 205 has been developed by Lioen *et al* (1987) and for the Siemens VP series by Geers (1989). All such specialised implementations of the BLAS are rigorously tested by NAG before they are used in conjunction with the Library.

In addition NAG has prepared alternative Fortran versions of the code for some of the Level 2 BLAS, for use on vector machines where no other specialised implementation is available. The alternative code may, for example, make use of compiler directives or the technique of unrolling vector loops due to Dongarra and Eisenstat (1984).

Calls to Level 2 BLAS have been introduced into many of the older linear algebra routines in the Library, and are used in new routines included at Mark 13, for real and complex singular value decomposition, and for solution of almost block diagonal systems of equations (1989). Level 2 BLAS are also used in other chapters: for example, linear, quadratic and nonlinear programming; nonlinear equations; nonlinear least—squares; and curve and surface fitting. Altogether 117 documented routines in the Mark 13 Library call Level 2 BLAS either directly or indirectly. Some details of the performance of these routines are given in subsections 3 and 4.

3. Performance of linear algebra routines

Table 1 presents performance measurements of selected NAG Linear Algebra routines on a variety of vector processing machines. The routines selected perform various factorizations or transformations of matrices which are required for the solution of systems of linear equations or matrix eigenvalue problems. They are the following:

F01AEF: reduction of a real symmetric–definite eigenproblem to standard form

F01AGF: reduction of a real symmetric matrix to tridiagonal form

F01AKF: reduction of a real matrix to upper Hessenberg form

F01AMF: reduction of a complex matrix to upper Hessenberg form

F01AXF: QR factorization of a real matrix, with column pivoting

F01BCF: reduction of a complex Hermitian matrix to tridiagonal form

F01CKF: matrix multiplication

F03AEF: Cholesky factorization of a real symmetric positive–definite matrix

F03AFF: LU factorization of a real matrix, with partial pivoting

F03AHF: LU factorization of a complex matrix, with partial pivoting

Table 1 shows current performance measurements from the Amdahl VP 1200, Cray 1, Cray X–MP, Cray 2 and IBM 3090E VF.

Table 1

Speed of NAG Library routines in megaflops for square matrices of order 500.

	Amdahl VP1200	Cray 1	Cray X–MP	Cray 2	IBM 3090E V
Precision	double	single	single	single	double
Max speed	571	150	235	488	114
F01AEF	179	86	193	287	34
F01AGF	156	52	201	289	32
F01AKF	253	95	199	271	38
F01AMF	303	72	182	165	33
F01AXF	386	60	186	210	27
F01BCF	274	72	165	161	35
F01CKF	519	137	219	376	46
F03AEF	299	103	188	272	39
F03AFF	262	67	172	244	55
F03AHF	173	62	193	212	29

4. Routines for nonlinear problems

The Level 2 BLAS have also proved useful in improving the performance of routines for nonlinear problems. This should not be surprising, since many algorithms for nonlinear problems work by solving a sequence of linear subproblems.

We have studied in particular the NAG Library routines for solving systems of nonlinear equations (C05NBF, –NCF, –PBF and –PCF), which perform a sequence of QR factorizations, and those for nonlinear least squares problems (E04FCF, –FDF, –GBF, –GCF, –GDF, –GEF, –HEF and –HFF), which perform a sequence of singular value decompositions (Du Croz et al (1988)).

It is more difficult to present meaningful performance measurements for such routines than it is in the field of linear algebra. The path taken by the algorithm is problem–dependent, and a significant proportion of the computing time may be spent in the user–supplied code which defines the problem. However Table 2 illustrates clearly the improvement in performance between Mark 12 and Mark 13, as a result of modifying the code to call the Level 2 BLAS.

Table 2 refers to the solution of a particular system of nonlinear equations of order 129 on a Cray 1. The Mark 12 Library code and the user–supplied code was vectorizable — it ran about 4 times faster than when compiled in scalar mode. However incorporating calls to the Level 2 BLAS — and using the best available implementation of them — allowed the Library code to be speeded up by over 40%. The effect on the total time taken to solve the problem depends on the time spent in the user–supplied code — which varies enormously in this example depending on whether the Jacobian is computed analytically or by finite differences.

Table 2

Time taken to solve a system of nonlinear equations on a Cray 1

(a) using C05NCF (computes a finite–difference Jacobian)

	Mark 12	Mark 13
time taken by NAG Library code	0.352	0.202
time taken by user–supplied code	0.510	0.510
total time	0.862	0.712

(b) using C05PCF (uses a user–supplied analytic Jacobian)

	Mark 12	Mark 13
time taken by NAG Library code	0.350	0.201
time taken by user–supplied code	0.026	0.026
total time	0.376	0.227

Comparable improvements were observed for the routines in the E04 chapter which solve nonlinear least squares problems. On large problems the bulk of the work is done by routines which compute the singular value decomposition (SVD) of the Jacobian matrix J. There is scope for using Level 2 BLAS in the first stage of the SVD, which consists of forming the QR factorization of J, but in the remaining stages plane rotations must be used, and so we were led to focus attention on improving the efficiency of applying plane rotations.

5. Applying sequences of plane rotations

The design of the Level 2 BLAS involved a certain amount of compromise. We wanted to make their scope broad enough to implement a large range of linear algebraic computations, without making the set of routines so complex as to reduce the chances of having them implemented efficiently on a wide range of machines. To quote from Dongarra et al. (1988) "The hard decision was to restrict the scope only to these operations [that is, those listed in Section 3], since there are many other potential candidates, such as matrix scaling and sequences of plane rotations."

The last—mentioned type of operation has the same level of granularity as the Level 2 BLAS, and offers similar scope for performance improvements from machine—specific coding, including a reduction in the ratio of memory references to arithmetic operations. The most important instance is the application of a sequence of plane rotations to the rows or columns of a rectangular matrix. It is implemented by the NAG Library routine F06QXF (in real arithmetic), and, as for the Level 2 BLAS, we have developed alternative code for this routine in order to achieve greater efficiency on certain vector machines.

Applying sequences of plane rotations is important in the computation of eigenvectors, singular vectors, Schur and generalized Schur factorizations, and also in updating QR or Cholesky factorizations, especially in methods for linearly constrained optimization.

For example, when all the eigenvectors of a symmetric tridiagonal matrix are computed by the QL algorithm (as in NAG Library routine F02AMF), each iteration of the QL algorithm generates a sequence of plane rotations which must be applied to the columns of a matrix $\mathbf{Q}$; at the end of the algorithm, $\mathbf{Q}$ is the matrix of eigenvectors. Thus the work of computing the eigenvectors consists entirely of applying sequences of plane rotations.

We have modified F02AMF to call F06QXF to apply the rotations, and when using tuned machine—specific code for F06QXF, have observed a 25% reduction in the time taken on an IBM 3090 VF. The modified code has been included in the 3090 VF implementation at Mark 13, and will be adopted generally at Mark 14.

For the Cray 1 and Cray X—MP, F06QXF has been coded in CAL (Cray Assembly Language), achieving 110 megaflops on the Cray 1 and 155 megaflops on the Cray X—MP. This enables the modified version of F02AMF to run 40% faster on a Cray 1 and 20% faster on a Cray X—MP.

The routine F02WEF which computes the SVD of a real matrix, benefits from the CAL—coded F06QXF when singular vectors are to be computed. For example, on a Cray X—MP the last stage in the computation — the SVD of a bidiagonal matrix — runs about 2.5 times faster than when the standard Fortran version of F06QXF is used.

6. The Level 3 BLAS

Section 3 showed that the level of performance achieved by NAG linear algebra routines on some machines — Cray 2 and IBM 3090 VF — is still disappointing even when good implementations of the relevant Level 2 BLAS are available.

Linear algebra algorithms which call Level 2 BLAS usually compute their results one vector (row or column) at a time. Unfortunately this approach to software construction is often not well—suited to computers with a hierarchy of memory (global memory, local memory, cache, vector—registers) and restricted bandwidth for data–transfer between the different levels. The Cray 2 and IBM 3090 VF both fall into this category. On these machines it is more effective to partition matrices into blocks, and to compute the results one block at a time, in order to reduce the volume of data traffic and to provide for maximum re–use of data while it is held in cache or local memory.

Hence, no sooner had the specification of the Level 2 BLAS been finalised than NAG joined a similar project to specify a set of Level 3 BLAS (see Dongarra *et al*), to provide the necessary modules for constructing block algorithms and implementing them efficiently.

The Level 3 BLAS perform the following types of matrix–matrix operation in real arithmetic:

(a) matrix–matrix products of the forms:

$$C \longleftarrow \alpha \, AB + \beta \, C,$$

$$C \longleftarrow \alpha \, A^T B + \beta \, C,$$

$$C \longleftarrow \alpha \, AB^T + \beta \, C$$

and

$$C \longleftarrow \alpha \, A^T B^T + \beta \, C$$

where α and β are scalars, and A, B and C are rectangular matrices, and:

$$B \longleftarrow \alpha \, TB,$$

$$B \longleftarrow \alpha \, T^T B,$$

$$B \longleftarrow \alpha \, BT$$

and

$$B \longleftarrow \alpha \, BT^T$$

where T is an upper or lower triangular matrix;

(b) rank–k updates of a symmetric matrix of the forms:

$$C \longleftarrow \alpha \, AA^T + \beta \, C,$$

$$C \longleftarrow \alpha \, A^T A + \beta \, C,$$

$$C \longleftarrow \alpha \, AB^T + \alpha \, BA^T + \beta \, C$$

and

$$C \longleftarrow \alpha \, A^T B + \alpha \, B^T A + \beta \, C$$

(c) solution of triangular equations with multiple right hand sides of the form:

$$B \longleftarrow \alpha\, T^{-1} B,$$

$$B \longleftarrow \alpha\, T^{-T} B,$$

$$B \longleftarrow \alpha\, B T^{-1}$$

and

$$B \longleftarrow \alpha\, B T^{-T}$$

Analogues of these operations in complex arithmetic are also provided.

The Level 3 BLAS achieve a higher ratio of arithmetic operations to data movement than the Level 2 BLAS, and also offer more scope for parallel processing.

7. Exploiting the Level 3 BLAS

The Level 3 BLAS will be included in the NAG Fortran Library at Mark 14.

However, two of the Level 3 BLAS are already provided in release 3 of the ESSL Library on the IBM 3090 VF; and by making use of them we have already improved the performance of the routine F03AFF for ULU⁻ factorization from 26 to 56 megaflops. Figure 1 shows the performance of the routine *(a)* calling Level 2 BLAS; *(b)* calling Level 3 BLAS. We plan to make more extensive use of the Level 3 BLAS at Mark 14 (see Mayes and Radicati di Brozolo. 1989).

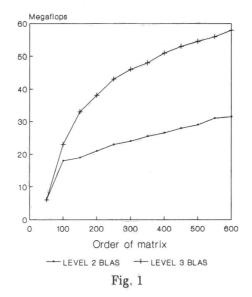

Fig. 1

Speed of *LU* factorization on an IBM 3090E VF

In general, exploiting Level 3 BLAS is not as simple as exploiting Level 2 BLAS. It is necessary to re–formulate the algorithms of linear algebra so that they work on "blocks" (that is, submatrices) of the original matrix, rather than on individual elements or rows or columns. For some algorithms, the re–formulation is straightforward; for others, some research has been or will be needed.

Developing software for block algorithms in linear algebra is the goal of the LAPACK project (Demmel *et al*, 1987). Our aim is to include LAPACK routines in the NAG Library so that we can further improve the level of performance of our linear algebra routines over an ever wider range of supercomputers, including many machines with parallel processing capability as well as vector facilities.

RANDOM NUMBER GENERATORS

Large–scale simulations may require the generation of many millions of random numbers. All practical algorithms for generating random numbers – strictly speaking, pseudo–random numbers – repeat themselves eventually with a fixed period. A good rule of thumb is that, in order to maintain good statistical properties in the simulation, the total number of numbers generated should not exceed the square–root of the period.

Many generators in common use have periods of at most 2^{32} (as a consequence of relying on 32–bit integer arithmetic), and hence the statistical properties of a simulation may deteriorate if more than 2^{16} ($\simeq 10^5$) random numbers are used. On very many modern computers 10^5 random numbers can be generated in less than a second, so such generators are clearly inadequate. Since 1977 (Mark 6), the NAG Fortran Library has relied on a generator with a period of 2^{57}, and this is satisfactory for simulations involving up to about 10^9 random numbers.

The basic generator in the NAG Library returns the same sequence of random numbers on all machines, up to the accuracy of real variables – that is, from a user's point of view, it is completely portable. The routine G05CAF returns at each call the next random number in the sequence. It uses a multiplicative congruential algorithm, which can easily be vectorized, with any desired vector length l. Random numbers can be generated in batches of length l, stored in a buffer, and drawn on as needed.

The code for G05CAF is complicated by the fact that the algorithm requires 59–bit integers; so multi–length integer arithmetic is used in all current implementations of the library. For most machines Fortran code is provided, with variants tailored for different wordlengths (that is, for different ranges of integer variables). Assembler code is provided for a few implementations.

Vectorized code for generating random numbers was introduced into some implementations of the Library at Mark 13. But the total time required to call G05CAF is dominated by the overhead of a function call, especially on the more powerful vector–processors. Therefore at Mark 14 we are introducing a new routine G05FAF – a subroutine which in a single call can return an array of n random numbers, identical to those that would be obtained by n successive calls of G05CAF. The first column of Table 3 shows the speed–up between G05CAF at Mark 13 and G05FAF at Mark 14.

G05CAF returns random numbers from a uniform distribution over $(0,1)$. The G05 chapter of the NAG Library also contains a large number of routines for generating random numbers from other distributions, in each case performing some transformation on the results of one or more calls of G05CAF – and thus incurring at least double the overhead of a function call. Routines which return a vector of random numbers from different distributions can provide further gains in efficiency, in two ways:

> by using vectorized code to apply the transformations;

> by applying the transformations directly to the basic sequence of random numbers stored in the buffer, and avoiding a hierarchy of function or subroutine calls.

At Mark 14, G05FAF can return numbers uniformly distributed over a general interval $[a,b]$, at very little extra cost compared with a uniform $(0, 1)$ distribution. G05FBF returns a vector of numbers from an exponential distribution, and G05FDF from a normal distribution. For the uniform and exponential distributions, the new routines return the same numbers as would successive calls of the old routines (at least to within rounding error). For the normal distribution, the new routine uses the Box–Muller method rather than Brent's algorithm used by the old routine G05DDF: Brent's algorithm is somewhat faster on scalar machines, but is not vectorizable, whereas the Box–Muller transformations can be vectorized.

Table 3 shows the speed–up between the routines at Mark 13 which return a single random number, and the new Mark 14 routines which return a vector of random numbers. Even on a scalar machine (DEC VAX 8700) there is a slight speed–up (except for the normal distribution).

Table 3

Average time in microseconds required to generate a random number from different distributions using:

a) routines which return a single random number, as implemented at Mark 13

b) new Mark 14 routines which return a vector of random numbers.

		uniform (0,1)	Distribution uniform (a,b)	exponential	normal
Routine	a)	G05CAF	G05DAF	G05DBF	G05DDF
	b)	G05FAF	G05FAF	G05FBF	G05FDF
Amdahl	a)	2.7	4.8	6.5	11.5
VP 1200	b)	0.23	0.25	0.39	0.76
Cray X–MP	a)	1.7	3.5	5.8	7.4
	b)	0.32	0.37	0.51	0.87
Convex C1	a)	13.0	24.0	43.0	55.0
	b)	5.5	6.4	9.8	14.6
DEC	a)	13.0	24.0	46.0	50.0
VAX 8700[a]	b)	12.0	16.0	37.0	54.0

[a] on the VAX 8700 both sets of timings used assembly language for the basic generator.

QUADRATURE

There are a number of areas of numerical computing where a user is required to provide a function or subroutine in order to specify the problem to be solved. For quadrature a user must usually provide code to calculate the value of the integrand at a point requested by the routine. Gladwell (1986) pointed out that the existing interfaces to most NAG quadrature routines inhibit the possibilities for vectorization, and here we describe ways in which a redesign of the interface has greatly improved the performance of some NAG quadrature algorithms on vector–processing machines. As with routines for random number generation, the new routines can outperform the earlier routines on conventional scalar machines as well.

1. One–dimensional quadrature

We have concentrated on the two routines D01AJF and D01AKF, which are based respectively on the QUADPACK routines QAGS and QAG (Piessens *et al*, 1980). D01AJF uses an adaptive integration method, based on the Gauss 10–point and Kronrod 21–point rules, and is designed as a general–purpose integrator over a finite interval, able to handle integrands which have certain types of singularities. D01AKF, which is based on the Gauss 30–point and Kronrod 61–point rules, is designed particularly for oscillating, non–singular integrands.

Both these routines require the user to supply a function to evaluate the integrand at a single point. Inside the NAG routines, most of the calls to the user–supplied function occur within the innermost DO–loop, which cannot therefore be vectorized. Also, since the user is only required to evaluate the integrand at a *single* point, for problems with very simple integrands there is unlikely to be sufficient work in a single function call to permit any vectorization within the user's code. There can also be a penalty on those machines where the overhead of a subprogram call is high, since the user's function can be called a large number of times.

The call of the user's function can be moved out of the innermost loop of the integrator, at the cost of some extra workspace to store the function values. There may then be some gain from vectorization within the integrator, but in fact the vector lengths are quite short, and little time is spent in vectorizable code. To achieve greater speed–ups, it is also necessary to allow the user to vectorize the evaluation of the integrand. In other words, n calls to a user–supplied function F within the innermost loop

```
      DO 10 I = 1, N
            FVAL(I) = F(X(I))
10    CONTINUE
```

must be replaced with a single call to a user–supplied subroutine FCN

    CALL FCN(N,X,FVAL)

At Mark 13, two new routines, D01ATF and D01AUF were introduced into the library implementing this design. D01ATF uses an identical algorithm to D01AJF, and D01AUF is very similar to D01AKF, but extends the functionality by including a number of different Gauss–Kronrod rules.

Table 4 shows the time taken to compute the following integral

$$\int_0^1 \cos(2^a \sin x)\, dx$$

$$\text{for } a = 8$$

on a range of machines. The table shows that even on a conventional scalar machine, such as the VAX 8700, reducing the number of subprogram calls can be beneficial.

2. Multi–dimensional Quadrature

With multi–dimensional quadrature, the gain from vectorizing the user interface is potentially much greater, because the number of integrand evaluations is usually very much higher. We have examined the routine D01GCF, which calculates a definite integral in up to 20 dimensions, using the Korobov–Conroy number–theoretic method. D01GCF will integrate over an arbitrary n–dimensional region by first transforming the region of integration to the n–cube. The user must supply a subroutine REGION which evaluates the limits c_i, d_i in the ith dimension, where in general c_i and d_i may be functions of $x_1, x_2, ..., x_{i-1}$.

For Mark 14 we have developed an alternative routine D01GDF implementing the same algorithm, but with the user–supplied routines re–designed so that they return a vector of function values or integration limits at each call. The Korobov–Conroy method is particularly simple in that all the points at which the integrand value is required are known in advance. However in order to limit the amount of internally declared workspace, the points are passed to the user–supplied code in segments of 128.

Table 5 shows the time taken to compute the integral

$$\int_0^1 dx_1 \ldots \int_0^1 dx \prod a_i \exp(-a_i x_i), \text{ where the } a_i \text{ are constants,}$$

with n = 10, using both the existing routine D01GCF and the new routine D01GDF. In each case 80,021 points are used.

For Mark 15 we plan to extend this approach to other algorithms for multi–dimensional quadrature.

Table 4

Time in milliseconds to evaluate a single integral.

	D01AJF (old)	D01ATF (new)	D01AKF (old)	D01AUF (new)
Amdahl VP 1200	33	8.5	13	1.5
Convex C1	282	78	120	17
Cray X–MP	33	7.2	15	1.7
IBM 3090/VF	60	23	28	6.8
VAX 8700	409	390	194	188

Table 5

Time in seconds to calculate a 10–dimensional integral.

	Time for D01GCF	Time for D01GDF	Speedup
Amdahl VP 1200	22.5	0.8	27.4
Convex C1	102.4	20.6	5.0
Cray X–MP	11.3	1.2	9.6
IBM 3090/VF	41.1	5.5	7.5
VAX 8700	149.8	82.2	1.8

An alternative strategy has been applied in the routine D01EAF, introduced at Mark 12. D01EAF implements the same adaptive algorithm for multi–dimensional quadrature as D01FCF (see Genz and Malik (1980)), but allows several integrands to be treated simultaneously. This strategy only makes sense if the integrands have similar behaviour — for example, functions differing only in the value of one or two parameters — because the adaptive strategy will be governed by the worst case, and more function evaluations may be used than if each integral had been computed individually. However the overall computing time can be significantly reduced, firstly by vectorization of the user's code to evaluate the vector of integrands, and secondly by taking advantage of common terms in the integrands (which can also be beneficial on scalar machines).

FAST FOURIER TRANSFORMS

1. Complex Transforms

The fast Fourier transform, or FFT, is an algorithm for computing the discrete Fourier transform $\{\hat{x}_k\}$ of a sequence $\{x_j\}$ of complex numbers

$$\hat{x}_k = (\sqrt{n})^{-1} \sum_0^{n-1} x_j \exp(ijk\pi/n), \quad k=0,1,...,n-1$$

If n can be factorized as the product of small integers $n = n_1 \, n_2... \, n_q$, then the computation can be decomposed into q passes over the data, each pass corresponding to one of the factors n_i, in such a way that the total amount of work is proportional to $n \, (\, n_1 + n_2 + \, ... \, + n_q)$, or $n \log n$, rather than n^2. This is the nub of the FFT algorithm. It is the fact that the ratio $n/\log n$ becomes large as n becomes large that has made the FFT such a powerful computational tool.

There are a number of variants of the basic FFT algorithm, which differ only in the way the computations are organised internally. They are reviewed (especially from the point of view of vectorization) by Swarztrauber (1982, 1984)and Temperton (1983).

The earlier NAG routines for complex FFT's — C06ECF and C06FCF, introduced at Mark 8 — use an *in–place* variant, usually known as the Gentleman–Sande form. This has the advantage that all the arithmetic operations required to compute the transform, can be performed without any extra workspace — that is, the transform can overwrite the original sequence — but the transform is produced in scrambled order; it must then be rearranged into the correct order. The arithmetic phase of the computation can be vectorized, but the re–ordering phase cannot be vectorized, at least not efficiently, and certainly not if no extra workspace is available. Hence the re–ordering phase consumes a disproportionately large amount of time. (The re–ordering phase is often referred to as "bit–reversal", because when n is a power of 2, it involves reversing the bits in the indices of the computed quantities $\hat{x}_k$.)

The need for a re–ordering phase can be avoided altogether by using a *self–sorting variant* of the FFT, as in the newer NAG routine C06FRF, which was introduced at Mark 12. There is, however, a price to be paid: the computation requires a separate work–array which is used alternately as an input or output array in successive passes of the computation.

Each pass, corresponding to one of the factors n_i is performed by a call to an auxiliary kernel routine. These kernels play the same kind of role in FFT computations as the BLAS do in linear algebra, although there has as yet been no effort to specify standardised calling sequences. In the NAG Library specialised kernel routines are provided for factors 2, 3, 4, 5 and 6, and it is here that efforts to speed up the code need to be concentrated. (The Library also includes a kernel routine for odd factors > 6, so that there is no constraint on the value of n, but this is much less efficient.)

The kernels consist, in their simplest form, of two nested DO–loops. They can be nested in either order, and in both cases the inner loop can be vectorized (on some machines compiler directives must be inserted). However, the vector length varies between 1 and at most $n/2$. This is unsatisfactory, since for at least part of the calculation the vector lengths will be very short. It is possible to do better by reversing the order of the two DO–loops midway through the calculation, with the result that the minimum vector length is approximately $\sqrt{n}$. Another point to be considered is that at some stages of the computation, the arrays are being accessed with large stride, which can cause memory bank conflicts on machines with interleaved memory, and inefficient memory usage on machines which use a cache, or some other form of intermediate storage between the main memory and CPU.

This is much less satisfactory than, say, matrix multiplication, where we can use vectors with stride 1 and constant length n. Also, on most vector–processors, the maximum speed of the machine is achieved only if floating–point additions can be paired with multiplications; but in the FFT kernels there are always more additions than multiplications (the actual ratio varies between the different kernels). Nevertheless, speeds of 244 megaflops on an Amdahl VP1200, and 100 megaflops on a Cray X–MP have been measured for a single transform of length $14{,}400 = 4^2 \text{x} 5^2 \text{x} 6^2$; on both machines this is almost half the maximum speed. For comparison, the earlier routine C06FCF performed the same computation at 11 and 12 megaflops on the two machines respectively.

2. Multiple Complex Transforms

In many applications – for example, 2–dimensional transforms and solving P.D.E.'s, as discussed in Sections 6.3 and 6.6 – several transforms of the same length are required. The new routine C06FRF has the additional feature that it can compute all m transforms in a single call, in such a way that the minimum vector length in the kernels is approximately $m\sqrt{n}$ rather than just $\sqrt{n}$. In addition, the trigonometric function values which are required, are computed just once (and can be re–used in subsequent calls). This is more efficient on scalar machines as well, as is the reduction in subprogram calls from m to 1.

Figure 2 shows the speed of C06FRF performing several complex transforms on a Cray X–MP, for different values of m and n. The figure shows the considerable improvement in performance as m increases. (It also shows the detrimental effects of memory–bank conflicts for some values of n, when, as in this example, both m and n are powers of 2.)

3. Two–Dimensional Complex Transforms

At Mark 13 a new routine C06FUF was introduced to calculate a two–dimensional transform of an m by n array of complex data. C06FUF calls C06FRF once to perform a one–dimensional transform of each of the rows of the array, transposes the array, calls C06FRF again, and transposes the array once more to leave the transform in the correct location. Thus the efficiency of C06FRF in performing multiple one–dimensional transforms is fully exploited; in fact, a significant proportion of the time is spent in the transpositions of the array, especially when the values of m and n lead to memory–bank conflicts or on machines with a cache or paged memory. Table 6 illustrates the speed of C06FUF compared with that of the earlier routine C06FJF.

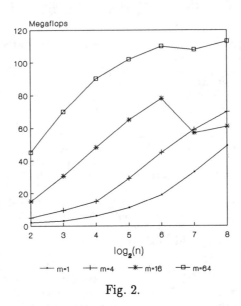

Fig. 2.

Speed of multiple complex FFT's using C06FRF on a Cray X–MP

Table 6

Speed in megaflops for a 512 x 512 2–dimensional complex FFT

	C06FJF (old)	C06FUF (new)
Amdahl VP 1200	5.0	322.0
Convex C1	0.3	5.7
CRAY X–MP	7.0	109.0
IBM 3090/VF	0.6	15.8

4. Real Transforms

So far we have considered only transforms of complex data. In many practical problems the data is in fact real. The transform of a purely real sequence is complex, but has an internal symmetry. It is called a "conjugate symmetric", "hermitian" or "half–complex" sequence; it can be represented by the same number of real values as the input sequence, and it is possible to exploit this fact to cut both the storage and arithmetic by half, as described by Swarztrauber (1982, 1986) and Temperton (1983).

The remarks above, about the design of the kernel routines and about the advantages of performing multiple transforms, apply with little change to the design of software for real transforms. These features are implemented in the routines:

C06FPF which transforms real sequences to Hermitian sequences, and
C06FQF which transforms Hermitian sequences to real sequences.

In order to show the full mixed–radix capability of our codes, Table 7 presents the speeds of multiple transforms, both real and complex, of various lengths involving different combinations of the factors 2, 3, 4, 5 and 6.

5. Real Symmetric Transforms

Further savings in computation and storage can be made if the sequence to be transformed has additional internal symmetry. For example, the transform of a real even sequence $(x_j = x_{n-j})$ is again a real even sequence, and the transform is a Fourier cosine transform.

Table 7

Speed in megaflops for 128 transforms of various lengths.

		Transform Length					
		180	192	200	216	240	256
Amdahl VP1200	real	303	265	309	298	296	274
	complex	376	360	370	371	381	351
Convex C1	real	6.4	5.9	6.8	6.3	6.9	6.7
	complex	5.6	5.7	6.6	5.1	6.0	6.2
Cray X–MP	real	114	101	115	114	111	102
	complex	121	121	115	128	119	120
IBM 3090/VF	real	21	18	21	20	21	18
	complex	24	22	24	23	23	22

At Mark 13 four new routines were introduced into the Library for performing the following transforms with additional symmetry:

C06HAF performs transforms of odd sequences ($x_j = -x_{n-j}$, sine transforms)

C06HBF performs transforms of even sequences ($x_j = x_{n-j}$, cosine transforms)

C06HCF performs transforms of quarter–wave odd sequences ($x_j = -x_{n-1-j}$, quarter–wave sine transforms)

C06HDF performs transforms of quarter–wave even sequences ($x_j = x_{n-1-j}$, quarter–wave cosine transforms)

All these routines can perform multiple transforms in a single call. The method is described in Section 5 of (Swarztrauber, 1986), the problem is reduced by pre– and post–processing phases to the computation of general real transforms, which is performed by calls to C06FPF, and thus takes advantage of the efficient vectorization of that routine.

The efficiency of the NAG routines for symmetric FFT's are illustrated indirectly in the next section.

6. Applications to Solving P.D.E.'s

The FFT can be used to solve Poisson's equation

$$u_{xx} + u_{yy} = f(x,y), \quad (x,y) \in [a,b] \times [c,d]$$

where either the solution or its derivative are prescribed on the boundaries – full details may be found in Swarztrauber (1984). When Poisson's equation is discretized using central differences, the approximate solution u_{ij} may be obtained as the solution of a system of linear equations. As described in Swarztrauber (1984), if the Fourier transform in the i–index is computed, then the Fourier coefficients u_{kj} are easier to compute than the original u_{ij}, being the solution of independent tridiagonal systems of linear equations.

In fact, the Fourier transform (1) of a real sequence can only be used to simplify the difference equations in this way when the boundary conditions are periodic, i.e. $u(a,y) = u(b,y)$. When either the solution or its derivative are prescribed on $x = a$ or $x = b$, then the symmetric transforms described in Section 3 have to be used:

the sine transform when $u(a,y)$ and $u(b,y)$ are prescribed.

the cosine transform when $u_x(a,y)$ and $u_x(b,y)$ are prescribed.

the quarter–wave sine transform when $u(a,y)$ and $u_x(b,y)$ are prescribed.

the quarter–wave cosine transform when $u_x(a,y)$ and $u(b,y)$ are prescribed.

At Mark 14, a new routine D03FAF will be introduced which computes a solution to the three–dimensional Helmholtz equation

$$u_{xx} + u_{yy} + u_{zz} - \lambda u = f(x,y,z)$$

The routine is derived from the routine HW3CRT in Fishpack (Swarztrauber and Sweet, 1984). The FFT is applied to the $i-$ and $j-$indices of the approximate solution u_{ijk}, resulting in multiple tridiagonal systems of equations to be solved. The original FFT code has been replaced by calls to the NAG FFT routines described above, and this change has speeded up the solution time by factors between 5 and 10 on various vector–processors. Table 8 shows the time taken by HW3CRT and D03FAF to solve Poisson's equation ($\lambda = 0$) when the solution is prescribed on the boundaries in the x and z directions, and is periodic in the y direction.

Table 8

Time in seconds to solve Poisson's equation on a 64x64x64 grid

	HW3CRT	D03FAF
Amdahl VP 1200	2.4	0.2
Convex C1	19.3	3.7
Cray X–MP	1.7	0.2
IBM 3090/VF	6.2	2.3

CONCLUSIONS

This article has described advances in vectorization of NAG routines in certain fundamental areas of numerical computing. The routines which have been described are used by many other routines in the NAG Library, for solving nonlinear equations, O.D.E.'s, P.D.E.'s, integral equations, for nonlinear optimization, regression and time series analysis; thus the benefits of the improvements in performance are available, through those higher–level routines, to a wide range of users' applications.

ACKNOWLEDGEMENTS

The work of implementing the NAG Library on supercomputers has been shared among many people. Margaret Day, Karl Knapp, Kevin Schrier and Jerzy Wasniewski deserve special mention; they also provided the timing measurements quoted in this paper.

REFERENCES

Brankin, R.W., and Gladwell, I., 1989
Codes for Almost Block Diagonal Systems.
NAG Technical Report TR1/89, (to be published in Comp. and Math. with Applics.).

Demmel, J., Dongarra, J.J., Du Croz, J.J., Greenbaum, A., Hammarling , S.J., and Sorensen, D.C., 1987
Prospectus for the Development of Linear Algebra Library for High Performance Computers.
Argonne National Laboratory, Mathematics and Computer Science Division, Technical Memorandum No. 97.

Dongarra, J.J., Du Croz, J.J., Duff, I.S. and Hammarling, S.J., 1989
A Set of Level 3 Basic Linear Algebra Subprograms.
to be published in ACM Trans. Math. Software.

Dongarra, J.J., Du Croz, J.J., Hammarling, S.J., and Hanson, R.J., 1988
An Extended Set of Fortran Basic Linear Algebra Subprograms.
ACM Trans. Math. Software, 14, pp. 1–17.

Dongarra, J.J., Du Croz, J.J., Hammarling, S.J., and Hanson, R.J., 1988
Algorithm 656: An Extended Set of Basic Linear Algebra Subprograms: Model
Implementation and Test Programs.
ACM Trans. Math. Software, 14, pp. 18–32.

Dongarra, J.J., and Eisenstat, S.C., 1984
Squeezing the Most out of an Algorithm in Cray Fortran.
ACM Trans. Math. Software, 10, pp. 221–230.

Du Croz, J.J.,Mayes, P.J.D., Wasniewski, J., and Wilson, S., 1988
Applications of Level 2 BLAS in the NAG Library.
Parallel Comput., 8, pp. 345–350.

Du Croz, J.J., and Wasniewski, J., 1988
Basic Linear Algebra Computations on the Sperry ISP.
Lecture Notes in Computer Science, 297, pp. 629–638.

Geers, N, 1989
Optimization of Level 2 BLAS for Siemens VP systems, University of Karlsruhe,
Computer Centre, Report No. 37.89.

Genz, A.C., and Malik, A.A., 1980
An adaptive algorithm for numerical integration over an Un~@THdimensional
rectangular region
J. Comput. Appl. Math., 6, pp. 295–302.

Gladwell, I., 1986
Vectorization of one–dimensional quadrature codes
NAG Technical Report TR 7/86, December
Lawson, C., Hanson, R.J., Kincaid, D., and Krogh, F.T., 1979
Basic Linear Algebra Subprograms for Fortran Usage.
ACM Trans. Math. Software, 5, pp. 308–323.

Lioen W.M., Louter–Nool, M., and te Riele, H.J.J., 1987
Optimization of the Real Level 2 BLAS on the Cyber 205.
In: Algorithms and Applications on Vector and Parallel Computers.
Elsevier Science Publishers.

Luecke, G.R., 1988
Performance of the Numerical Algorithms Group (NAG) Mark 12 Library
on National Advanced Systems Vector Computers.
In: Proceedings of 3rd International Conference on Supercomputing,
Volume II, pp. 354–359.
International Supercomputing Institute, Inc.

Mayes, P.J.D., and Radicati di Brozolo, G., 1989
Portable and Efficient Factorization Algorithms on the IBM 3090/VF.
Proceedings of the 3rd International Conference on Supercomputing, Crete,
pp. 263–270 ACM, New York.

Piessens R.,, E. de Doncker–Kapenga, E., Uberhuber, C.W., and Kahaner, D.K., 1980
QUADPACK – A Subroutine Package for Automatic Integration,
Springer–Verlag, Berlin.

Swarztrauber, P.N., 1982
Vectorizing the FFTs.
In, Parallel Computations, G. Rodrigue (Ed.).
Academic Press.

Swarztrauber, P.N., 1984
FFT algorithms for vector computers.
Parallel Comput., 1, pp. 45–63.

Swarztrauber, P.N., 1984
Fast Poisson Solvers
In, Studies in Numerical Analysis, G. H. Golub (Ed.).
Mathematical Association of America.

Swarztrauber, P.N., 1986
Symmetric FFT's
Math. Comp., 47, pp. 323–346.

Swarztrauber, P.N., and Sweet, R.A., 1979
Efficient Fortran subprograms for the solution of elliptic partial
differential equations.
ACM Trans. Math. Software, 5, pp. 352–364

Temperton, C. 1983
Self–sorting mixed–radix fast Fourier transforms.
J. Comput. Phys., 52, pp. 1–23.

Temperton, C. 1983
Fast mixed–radix real Fourier transforms.
J. Comput. Phys., 52, pp. 340–350.

COMPUTER SIMULATION OF PLASMAS

A.R. Bell

Physics Department, Imperial College, London SW7 2BZ.

A) INTRODUCTION

A plasma consists of charged particles moving relatively freely, but interacting through the electric and magnetic fields produced by each particle. It is well known that all except a very small (but nevertheless important) fraction of the detectable universe is a plasma. Most plasma physics can be expressed in terms of five fairly straightforward equations, the four Maxwell equations for electromagnetism and the equation of motion for charged particles in electromagnetic fields. Why then is plasma physics such a mathematically difficult subject and why is numerical simulation so important? The most basic reason is that any experimental plasma contains a very large number of particles, $10^{18}-10^{20}$ in a typical fusion experiment. Moreover, particles in plasmas have a tendancy to act independently of each other. In conventional hydrodynamics, large numbers of particles can be described by a few simple numbers such as their temperature, density and mean velocity. Sometimes we can do this with a plasma but even then we have a few more numbers to include such as current and charge density, along with the electromagnetic fields. More usually, plasmas are not so simply described. Plasmas are not usually Maxwellian and we have to think in terms of distribution functions in phase space. Whenever we can, we model the non−Maxwellian nature of the plasma by transport models, e.g. for heat flow, but this is a specialised skill in itself. When one considers that conventional hydrodynamics is very complex and involves advanced numerical simulation, it is hardly surprising that simulation plays such an important role in plasma physics.

In plasma physics, numerical methods are important for theoretical work since the equations are often too difficult to solve analytically, but simulation is just as important for experimentalists. As an example, consider a typical laser plasma experiment. A high power laser, $\sim 10^{12}$ Watt, is focussed onto a small area on the surface of a solid target. The temperature immediately rises to around 1 keV and the atoms of the solid ionise to form a plasma. The plasma is ~ 0.1mm across, it moves at around 5×10^5 m sec^{-1}, it exists for $\sim 10^{-9}$ sec, and it is optically thick to probing at visible wavelengths. Quite clearly, experimental diagnostics are a major problem. The only way to understand such experiments is to make as many measurements as possible, and then run a computer simulation to see how well it agrees. If the simulation does not reproduce the measurements, then alter the simulation model to see whether the agreement improves. When simulation and measurements agree then it is possible that the physics in the code is correct. Of course there is the danger that agreement between simulation and experiment is coincidental but, on the whole, this methodology works well, and interaction between experiment and simulation has produced a reasonable understanding of laser−produced plasmas.

Supercomputational Science
Edited by R.G. Evans and S. Wilson
Plenum Press, New York, 1990

B) CLASSIFICATION OF SIMULATION MODELS

Not all plasmas are the same, and different simulation models are used in different cases. For example, plasmas can be collisionless or collision−dominated, magnetised or unmagnetised. Even the same plasma can be dominated by different effects depending on which phenomena you are interested in. Broadly speaking, plasmas can be divided into two classes, plasmas in which particles intially close to each other remain close to each other, and plasmas in which particles wander well away from their initial neighbours. Particles can be localised by collisions with other particles or because they are unable to cross magnetic field lines. If particles are localised then a collection of neighbouring particles can be treated as a fluid element and a hydrodynamic treatment may be possible. If particles are not localised then a full phase space model is probably necessary.

If particles are not localised then a very appealing and successful simulation model is the particle code. The motions of a representative selection of particles are followed in their self−consistent electromagnetic fields. This has the immense advantage of making very few assumptions and approximations. It is close to reality. Its weakness is that very large numbers of particles (~10^5) may have to be followed for the results to be statistically valid. Long code runs may therefore be necessary, and it is not unknown for one run to take ~100 Cray hours.

If the particles are localised, the plasma can be modelled hydrodynamically. Although fluid models are often of doubtful validity for plasmas because of their non−Maxwellian nature, fluid simulation has the advantage of computational speed. All quantities are a function of position and time only, not requiring solution in phase space. With fluid models it is possible to model complete experiments in more than one dimension. Hence its importance for experiments. In contrast, particle codes can only model idealised problems or small parts of experiments. When the plasma is magnetised then the fluid model becomes a magnetohydrodynamic (MHD) model in which electromagnetic fields are added to the conventional fluid equations. In the MHD model, magnetic forces are often comparable to or exceed the thermal pressure forces. The MHD model is very important for magnetic confinement, e.g. tokamaks such as JET in Oxfordshire.

Sometimes, a plasma is too collisional to be modelled by a particle code but not sufficiently localised for the use of a fluid code. Then it is usual to use solve the Boltzmann or Fokker−Planck equation for a collisional plasma in phase space.

There are a large number of numerical models used in plasma physics which I will not have room to discuss here, e.g. codes to model wave propagation and codes to perform stability analyses. The algorithms discussed here are chosen because they are a) having a major impact on the development of basic plasma physics, b) likely to be relevant outside plasma physics, c) being actively developed by the Collaborative Computing Project in Plasma Physics (CCP10).

C) PARTICLE CODES

C.1 Introduction

A particle code follows the motions of N particles (N~10^2-10^6) in their self−consistent fields. The equations solved are

$$dv_i/dt = (q_i/m_i)(E(x_i)+v_i \times B(x_i)) \quad (1), \qquad dx_i/dt = v_i \quad (2),$$

$$\nabla \cdot E = \rho/\epsilon_0 \quad (3), \quad \nabla \times E = -\partial B/\partial t \quad (4), \quad \nabla \cdot B = 0 \quad (5), \quad \nabla \times B = \mu_0 j + \mu_0 \epsilon_0 \partial E/\partial t \quad (6),$$

$$\rho(x) = \sum_i q_i \delta(x-x_i) \quad (7), \qquad j(x) = \sum_i q_i v_i \delta(x-x_i) \quad (8),$$

where m_i, q_i, x_i and v_i are the mass, charge, position and velocity of the ith particle.

$\rho(x)$ and $j(x)$ are the charge and current density. E and B are the electric and magnetic fields. Particle codes have been immensely successful, and they are well described by Birdsall & Langdon (1985) and Hockney & Eastwood (1981).

C.2 Particle motions

Equations (1) and (2) describe the motion of each particle in given electromagnetic fields. The equations can easily be solved by the leap−frog method with good stability and accuracy $O(\Delta t^2)$.

At each timestep:
a) starting from the particle positions at time $(n - \frac{1}{2})\Delta t$, integrate equation (2) using the velocities at time $n\Delta t$ to find the particle positions at time $(n + \frac{1}{2})\Delta t$.
b) starting from the particle velocities at time $n\Delta t$, integrate equation (1) using the forces at time $(n + \frac{1}{2})\Delta t$ to find the particle velocities at time $(n + 1)\Delta t$.

Step a) is differenced in the obvious way. Step b) is not so obvious, but can straightforwardly be solved by splitting the step into an acceleration due to E and a rotation in velocity space due to B. The fields are varying in time, but 2nd order accuracy is preserved if they are evaluated (as described below) after step a), i.e. the field values are held, along with the particle positions, at the half timesteps.

The complete 3−dimensional algorithm (Birdsall & Langdon, 1985) is

$$x^{n+\frac{1}{2}} = x^{n-\frac{1}{2}} + v^n \Delta t$$

$$v_\alpha = v^n + \tfrac{1}{2}(q/m)E^{n+\frac{1}{2}}\Delta t, \quad v_\beta = v_\alpha + v_\alpha x t, \quad v_\gamma = v_\alpha + v_\beta x s, \quad v^{n+1} = v_\gamma + \tfrac{1}{2}(q/m)E^{n+\frac{1}{2}}\Delta t$$

where $t = \frac{1}{2}(qB/m)\Delta t$ and $s = 2t/(1+t^2)$.

E and B are the electric and magentic fields; q and m are the particle's charge and mass.

The particle mover is ideal for vectorisation. The equations for each particle are independent and the calculation for each can proceed in parallel.

C.3 The Field−Solver

The function of the field−solver is to calculate the electric and magnetic fields experienced by each particle and determined by the motion of all the other particles. This is not so straightforward. The principles involved can be illustrated by considering the purely electrostatic case in which particles only interact through the Coulomb potential, and the magnetic fields arising from particle currents are neglected. This is equivalent to the limit in which the speed of light is infinite. Equation (8) is not needed, and equation (7) can be replaced by:

$$E(x_j) = \frac{1}{4\pi\epsilon_0} \sum_{i \neq j}^{N} q_i \frac{x_j - x_i}{|x_j - x_i|^3} \qquad \text{in 3-dimensions}$$

with equivalent expressions for E due to charge slabs or charge rods if only one or two dimensions respectively are considered.

The electric field has to be evaluated for each of N particles, and each evaluation involves a sum of contributions from the $(N-1)$ other particles. The number of operations is $\sim N^2$. Since N can be 10^5 or larger, a straight summation is too slow. Fortunately, there are ways of speeding up the calculation so that the number of operations is $\sim N\log N$. There is necessarily a loss in accuracy, but the loss is of a form which is acceptable as indicated by the physics.

C.3.1 Cell methods

Cell methods provide one means of speeding up the field−solver. Instead of calculating the electric field at the position occupied by each of N particles, it is initially calculated on a grid and then interpolated from the grid to the particle positions. The calculation of the field at the grid−points is also simplified by firstly associating the charge of particle with the nearest grid−point(s). After accumulating all charges at the grid−points, the field at each grid−point is calculated from equation (3) using a Fast Fourier Transform (FFT). Care has to be taken with the charge accumulation and interpolation to avoid spurious effects. For example, if an incorrect rule for accumulation and interpolation is chosen, particles can find themselves repelled from the nearest grid−point.

The errors arising from incorrect choice of accumulation and interpolation methods can be seen in the following 1−dimensional example. Let there be M grid−points with the mth grid−point at $m\Delta x$, and calculate the field using the following steps:

i) Let the accumulated charge at each grid−point be

$$\sigma_m = \sum_i q_i \, W_{ngp}(x_i - m\Delta x) \qquad \text{where } W_{ngp}(z) = \begin{cases} 1 \text{ if } |z| < \tfrac{1}{2}\Delta x \\ 0 \text{ otherwise} \end{cases}$$

This associates the charge of each particle with the grid−point nearest to it.

ii) The potential φ_m at each grid−point is calculated from the difference form of $\partial^2 \varphi / \partial x^2 = -\rho / \epsilon_0$:

$$\frac{\varphi_{m-1} - 2\varphi_m + \varphi_{m+1}}{\Delta x^2} = \frac{-\sigma_m}{\epsilon_0 \Delta x}$$

iii) The electric field E_m at each grid−point is calculated from the difference form of $E = -\partial \varphi / \partial x$:

$$E_m = -\frac{\varphi_{m+1} - \varphi_{m-1}}{2\Delta x}$$

iv) Calculate the electric field at x_j, the position of the jth particle:

$$E(x_j) = \sum_m E_m \, W_{cic}(x_j - m\Delta x) \qquad \text{where } W_{cic}(z) = \begin{cases} 1 - |z|/\Delta x \text{ if } |z| < \Delta x \\ 0 \text{ otherwise} \end{cases}$$

N.B. This is incorrect!

Step iv) looks as though it ought to give good accuracy since it calculates $E(x_j)$ by taking a weighted average of E_m at the two nearest grid−points, whereas use of the weighting function W_{ngp} instead of W_{cic} would set it equal to the value at the nearest grid−point. However, the error becomes clear if we calculate the force exerted by a particle on itself, i.e. set N=1 and i=j=1. Without loss of generality, let $q_1 = 1$ and $0 < x_1 < \tfrac{1}{2}\Delta x$, making m=0 the nearest grid−point, and m=1 the next nearest.

For this example, step i) gives $\sigma_0 = 1$ and all other $\sigma_m = 0$. Step ii) has the solution $\varphi_0 = 0$, and $\varphi_m = -|m|\Delta x/2\epsilon_0$ all $m \neq 0$. Step iii) gives $E_m = -\tfrac{1}{2}/\epsilon_0$ for $m \leqslant -1$, $E_0 = 0$, and $E_m = \tfrac{1}{2}/\epsilon_0$ for $m \geqslant 1$. Step iv) then gives

$$E(x_1) = E_0 W_{cic}(x_1) + E_1 W_{cic}(x_1 - \Delta x) = \tfrac{1}{2}x_1 / \epsilon_0 \Delta x$$

Our single isolated particle is therefore subject to a force which pushes it away from the nearest grid−point when in reality a single isolated charge cannot exert a force on itself. Steps i) to iv) given above are not acceptable, but the situation is easily remedied. If we replace step iv) by

$$E(x_j) = \sum_m E_m \, W_{ngp}(x_j - m\Delta x)$$

where W_{ngp} is defined in step i) above, then $E(x_1)= 0$ and the problem is avoided.

The general condition that a particle should not suffer a self force is that the weighting functions W should be the same in steps i) and iv). Equally well the function could be W_{cic} in both cases. In fact this would be preferable since it is more accurate, and it is indeed the usual choice in particle simulations.

Use of W_{ngp} is referred to as the NEAREST−GRID−POINT method. W_{cic} is the CLOUD−IN−CELL (CIC) or PARTICLE−IN−CELL (PIC) method.

A physical interpretation of the CIC or PIC method is easily given. It is equivalent to spreading the charge of a particle uniformly over a distance $\pm\frac{1}{2}\Delta x$ on each side of the particle position. Instead of each charge being a point charge, it is simulated as a cloud of charge. Hence the CIC name, although it is more usually referred to as the PIC method.

Cell methods are clearly an approximation. The method cannot simulate close interactions between individual particles. In other words, binary particle collisions are not correctly treated. However, collisions are not important in many aspects of plasma physics. Plasmas exhibit a rich variety of collective effects, meaning that the plasmas can be viewed in terms of large collections of particles interacting with other collection of particles. For example, an electron plasma wave can be viewed as consisting of a large collection of particles being displaced from their equilibrium position, setting up an electric field which exerts a force on them which pulls them back towards the equilibrium position. The physics of this and many other kinds of waves are often unaffected by collisions and appropriate for simulation with PIC codes.

The inability of PIC codes to model collisions has a major advantage. PIC codes model large numbers of particles acting collectively. All particles in one region of space follow very similar trajectories as determined by spatially smooth fields. We do not need to follow each particle separately. It is possible to lump together large numbers of particles into one macro−particle. Hence a PIC code does not need to simulate the very large number of particles present in a real plasma. This would be prohibitively slow and expensive. Instead, only a limited number of macro−particles need to be simulated. In effect, each particle modelled in a PIC simulation has the charge and mass of many electrons or ions, but its trajectory correctly represents individual electrons or ions provided the charge to mass ratio of the macro−particle is the same as that of the electrons or ions.

The electric field on the grid is calculated from the charges on the grid with a Fast Fourier Transform. If there are M grid−points, this involves ~MlogM operations. Since M is usually an order of magnitude smaller than the number of particles, N, and library FFTs are available which use the full power of a vector machine, this part of the code runs quickly. Charge assignment to the grid and field interpolation from the grid require ~N operations. Unfortunately, this does not easily vectorise since the nearest grid−point to particle depends on its position. If naively programmed, this would require calculation of an array index within the central loop over all the particles.

Figure 1 shows some typical output from a 1−D PIC code. In 'Beat−wave' experiments, two laser beams are injected into a plasma. The beams have slightly different frequencies such that the beat between the laser beams resonantly drives up electron oscillations (electron plasma waves). Figure 1a shows a clean well−behaved plasma wave, but the experiment (Dangor et al, 1989) did not see a wave of the expected amplitude. However, only the ions, not the electrons, were allowed to move in Fig. 1a. Recent analytical work (e.g. Pesme et al, 1988) has shown that despite the relatively large mass, and hence slow response, of the ions, ion motion can disrupt a plasma wave through the modulational instability. Fig. 1b shows what happens when the ions are allowed to move. The plasma wave breaks up and the amplitude reaches a value in good agreement with that seen in experiments.

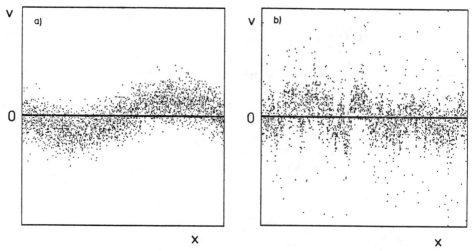

Fig. 1. Particle plots in phase space (x,v). Each point represents the position of a simulation particle. a) ions not allowed to move. b) ions allowed to move. The plasma wave in b) is broken up by the modulational instability.

C.3.2 Linked–List and Tree methods

Cell methods have been extraordinarily successful in modelling collective effects in plasmas, and it is difficult to see them being replaced. However, they cannot model collisions directly. There have been particle codes written which include collisions by randomising particle velocities (e.g. Mason, 1980) in accordance with the Fokker–Planck model of collisions. Instead of adapting a particle code, it is more usual to solve the Fokker–Planck equation in finite difference form. In either case, this is satisfactory provided that the collision model is adequate, which it is in most cases. Generally speaking, the Fokker–Planck model is adequate at low densities, high temperatures and for low Z plasmas where collisions are mainly small angle deflections. But as the density is increased or the temperature decreased, large angle collisions become progressively more important. Eventually the motion of each particle becomes dominated by strong interaction with its few nearest neighbours. The plasma is then said to be strongly coupled. The problem becomes similar to the Molecular Dynamics problems of interest in the theory of solids and liquids. A favourite model is the one component plasma (OCP) in which the electrons are treated as a smeared out background. More recently, two component plasmas (TCP) have been studied (e.g. Clerouin & Hansen, 1987), and this field will probably develop further in the next few years.

The actual modelling of the collisions themselves needs a particle code which correctly models binary interactions between nearby particles. One way of doing this is to calculate all $N(N-1)$ binary interactions, but this is unnecessary since binary interactions between individual particles are only important between close neighbours. If r_0 is the typical distance between nearest neighbours, then at an interparticle separation of many times r_0 it is not the individual position of each particle that matters, but the nett charge imbalance, positive or negative, averaged over large numbers of particles.

The calculation of electric field at a point can in effect be split into two parts a) the field exerted by nearby particles and depending on the exact positions of each of those particles, and b) the field exerted by collections of particles at large distances, which depends on overall charge densities rather than the detailed position of each particle. The number of operations to calculate contribution a) to the field is $\sim N_c N$ where N_c is the number of nearby particles which make an individual contribution to the field. Contribution b) from large collections of more distant particles can be calculated by the cell method described above with the (relatively) small number of operations appropriate to that method. If the calculation is separated in this way, the number of operations is far less than the $\sim N^2$ operations required to calculate all individual binary inertactions. This approach is used in the P^{3}M method decribed by Hockney and Eastwood. Conceptually the most difficult part of the method is identifying the particles which need to be considered as being nearby. Since initially nearby particles can subsequently drift apart, and vice versa, the identification of nearby particles has to be performed frequently in the calculation. In practice, lists linking particles with all nearby particles can be generated quite easily at each timestep. The method given by Hockney and Eastwood generates a Linked−List by associating each particle with a mesh grid−point. The electric field at any point due to nearby interactions is then found by reference to the list of particles close to the nearby grid−points.

The principle of modelling nearby interactions exactly but distant interactions as an average can be applied in many ways. A more recent method is the Tree Method which comes in a variety of forms. This has been applied mainly in the astrophysical community where it has been used for the similar problem of calculating the motion of large numbers of stars interacting gravitationally (Hernquist, 1987). One of the seminal papers on tree algorithms was the short paper by Barnes and Hutt (1986). Their method divides space into a series of boxes of different sizes. The largest box contains the whole system. In three dimensions this is then subdivided into 8 boxes of half the linear size. Each of the 8 boxes is further subdivided into 8 yet smaller boxes, and so on. The data structure looks like a tree. The trunk divides into 8 branches, each of which divides into a further 8 branches etc. Each particle is assigned to every box that contains it. So every particle appears in the largest box, but as each branch is subdivided, a stage is reached where boxes contain individual particles. Each branch is continually subdivided until each particle has been given its own box at the uppermost level of the tree.

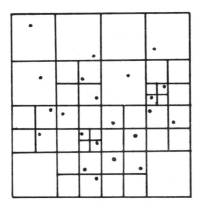

Fig. 2. Box structure built by a tree algorithm for a system of particles in 2−D. Each point is a particle. The boxes are subdivided until each particle is the sole occupant of a box.

Once generated, the tree can be used to locate all particles within a certain distance. In this sense, it is similar to a linked list, but it is more flexible than the linked list method given above. Nearby interaction can be calculated exactly by following the tree up to its highest levels where individual particles are located. For interactions which are less close, it is possible to follow the tree up to intermediate levels to calculate the electric field produced by small collections of particles. Going to the most distant particles, it is only necessary to follow the tree up to relatively large boxes and calculate the field produced by relatively large collections of particles. The number of operations is $\sim NlogN$ where N is the number of particles.

Because these methods model binary interactions, the actual mass and charge of the particles is important, whereas for PIC codes modelling collective effects it is only necessary that the charge to mass ratio should be correct. Hence, it is not possible to lump particles together into macro−particles. As a consequence, it is impossible to model the relatively large plasmas modelled with PIC codes. On the other hand, if the details of binary collisions are important then the system of interest is probably small, and this limitation is not too severe. It does mean however that it is difficult to model both large scale collective effects and small scale binary interactions at the same time.

Tree methods have yet to be widely used in plasma physics. They are unlikely to replace PIC codes for collective effects since they are less efficient, but the rising interest in dense plasmas which are strongly coupled in varying degrees suggests that Linked−List and/or Tree methods are going to increase in importance. It should be noted that they are not easily vectorised. The generation and use of Linked−Lists and especially trees involves a large amount of conditional branching within the program. Algorithms suitable for a serial machine may look very different when optimised for a vector machine.

D. FLUID CODES

D.1 The fluid model

The fluid model can be used whenever particles are localised by collisions or magnetic field. It is in fact used in many cases where its validity is doubtful, but more accurate models are computationally too slow. It is widely used in the simulation of a great variety of experiments. At its lowest level, the fluid model expresses the conservation of mass, momentum and energy. Since these conservation laws are basic features of all systems, the fluid model can do surprisingly well in circumstances where at first sight it ought not. Where the model fails, it is often still usable given some adjustment to the transport of energy, momentum etc. By definition, transport is included to model small departures from the complete localisation of particles to a fluid element. Problems arise when the departures cease to be small, but even then, given sufficient physical insight, it is often possible for the modeller to coax meaningful results from the simulation.

D.2 A Lagrangian fluid code

Consider the simplest fluid model in which there is no magnetic field, the fluid is adiabatic (no heat flow) and all quantities are a function of x and t only. In the Lagrangian method, the fluid is divided into a series of moving slabs which are accelerated by the pressure differences across them. The code calculates the velocity and position of each of the slabs.

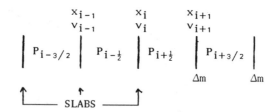

Fig. 3 Lagrangian finite difference model.

The slabs each have a mass Δm. They can be considered to be infinitely thin. The thermal energy can be thought of as sitting in the space between the slabs. The interslab thermal energy produces a pressure which accelerates the slabs. Equivalently, the system consists of a series of cells containing thermal energy, with the position and velocity of the cell boundaries (= slabs) being calculated by the code.

The equations of motion for the ith slab are:

$$\Delta m \frac{dv_i}{dt} = P_{i-\frac{1}{2}} - P_{i+\frac{1}{2}} \qquad\qquad \frac{dx_i}{dt} = v_i$$

For an adiabatic fluid, $P \propto V^{-\gamma}$ where γ is the ratio of specific heats and V is the volume occupied by unit mass. Hence the pressures between the slabs are given by

$$P_{i+\frac{1}{2}} = K \ (x_{i+1}-x_i)^{-\gamma}$$

where K is constant in time, but could vary between different cells.

The equations of motion can be differenced by the leap—frog method similar to that described in the section on particle codes. The complete set of difference equations is then

$$v_i^{n+\frac{1}{2}} = v_i^{n-\frac{1}{2}} + (P_{i-\frac{1}{2}}^n - P_{i+\frac{1}{2}}^n)\Delta t/\Delta m \qquad x_i^{n+1} = x_i^n + v_i^{n+\frac{1}{2}}\Delta t$$

$$P_{i+\frac{1}{2}}^{n+1} = K \ (x_{i+1}^{n+1} - x_i^{n+1})^{-\gamma}$$

where the superscripts n and n+1 denote the timelevels $n\Delta t$ and $(n+1)\Delta t$ respectively.

The Lagrangian difference equations centre naturally in both time and space. Hence they are accurate. The finite difference model is closely related to the physics, i.e. it can be interpreted in terms of the motion of physically real slabs. This leads to a robust code since the code behaves well if the physics is well—behaved, as indeed it must if the problem is well—formulated. As a result, Lagrangian fluid codes are very powerful tools. A good example is the MEDUSA fluid code (Christiansen et al, 1974) which is used very successfully to model laser—produced plasmas. Such codes as MEDUSA often support a lot of extra physics on top of basic hydrodynamics. After many years of development (e.g. Evans et al, 1982; Evans, 1985), MEDUSA supports radiation transport, atomic physics, equation of state, energy transport by thermal and superthermal electrons, and thermonuclear fusion reactions. Any physics which is important in an experiment is added to the code to make the simulation as real as possible. Indeed, large simulation codes become a very good way of storing the understanding of plasmas.

An important addition to basic fluid codes is viscosity. Shock fronts occur frequently in plasmas. A shock consists of a thin region in space in which the kinetic energy of large scale fluid motions is converted into randomised thermal energy. The conversion occurs through viscosity. The viscosity of plasmas is usually so small that the conversion takes place in a very thin layer, much thinner than the computational grid. It is therefore necessary to artificially increase the viscosity until the conversion layer is a few times the cell—size. This is known as an 'artificial viscosity' (e.g. Potter, 1973; Richtmyer & Morton, 1967). Without artificial viscosity in some form, it is not possible to model systems containing shocks.

Most 1—dimensional fluid simulations are Lagrangian, but in 2 or 3 dimensions they run into problems. In 2 dimensions, the building blocks are no longer slabs, but quadrilaterals or triangles (e.g. Atzeni, 1986; Verdon et al, 1982). The sides and vertices of the mesh move as the fluid moves, and an initially well—ordered mesh can distort into a disordered mesh. If this is allowed to continue, vertices eventually cross cell boundaries, the mesh becomes tangled, and the calculation becomes meaningless.

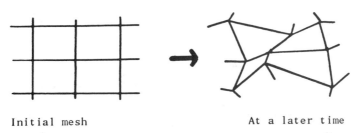

Initial mesh   At a later time

Fig. 4. Distortion of Lagrangain mesh in 2—dimensions.

Mesh distortion can be counteracted by rezoning (e.g. Horak et al, 1978), i.e. re−siting all mesh points on a rectangular grid, but the necessary interpolation introduces errors.

D.3 Eulerian fluid methods

In Lagrangian methods the mesh moves with the fluid. In contrast, in Eulerian methods the mesh or grid remains fixed while the fluid moves relative to it. The x−coordinate is divided into a series of cells of width Δx. The fluid quantities of density, pressure and velocity are ρ_i, P_i and v_i in the ith cell. ρ_i, P_i and v_i then change as mass, energy and momentum are transferred across boundaries between neighbouring cells. The fluid equations in 1−dimension can be written as:

$$\frac{\partial \rho}{\partial t} + \frac{\partial(\rho v)}{\partial x} = 0 \quad \text{(mass eq}^n\text{)}, \qquad \frac{\partial(\rho v)}{\partial t} + \frac{\partial(v(\rho v))}{\partial x} = -\frac{\partial P}{\partial x} \quad \text{(momentum eq}^n\text{)},$$

$$\frac{\partial U}{\partial t} + \frac{\partial(Uv)}{\partial x} = -P\frac{\partial v}{\partial x} \quad \text{(energy eq}^n\text{)}$$

where ρ is the mass density, v is the fluid flow velocity, P is the pressure, and U is the thermal energy density ($= 3P/2$ for a perfect gas). Each of these conservation equations takes the general form:

$$\frac{\partial f}{\partial t} + \frac{\partial(vf)}{\partial x} = -\frac{\partial F}{\partial x}$$

The left hand side of the equation represents advection, i.e. it moves the quantity f ($= \rho$, ρv or U) at velocity v in the x direction. This can easily be seen in the case of the mass equation with uniform flow velocity. The resulting equation, $\partial\rho/\partial t + v\partial\rho/\partial x = 0$, has the general solution $\rho = \rho(x-vt)$ which describes the translation of an initial density profile $\rho(x)$ into a profile at time t of $\rho = \rho(x-x_0)$ where $x_0 = vt$. The right hand sides of the equations are source terms. A pressure gradient acts as a source of momentum, and compression $P\partial v/\partial x$ acts as a source of energy through PdV work. Writing the equations in this form brings out the importance of advection. The advection equation is a basic element of fluid simulation since fluid motion advects mass, momentum and energy across the grid. This apparently simple differential equation is very difficult to solve accurately. It is the cause of many of the difficulties with Eulerian codes.

The naively obvious way to difference the advection equation $\partial f/\partial t + v\partial f/\partial x = 0$ is to centre difference in space and forward difference in time, but this method is unconditionally unstable. The next most obvious method is to forward difference in time but backward difference in space (or forward difference if $v < 0$). This is known as the Donor−cell method because the spatial difference is extended into the adjacent cell from which fluid is flowing (being donated). The Donor−cell method is stable for $\Delta t \leqslant \Delta x/v$, but very diffusive as shown in Fig. 5.

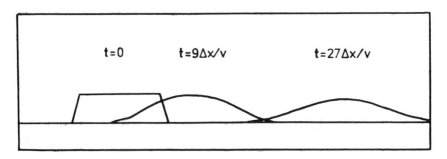

Fig. 5. Advection of a square pulse at velocity v by the Donor−Cell method. The pulse is initially 11 cells wide. The length of the grid is 50 cells.

A better advection algorithm is the Lax—Wendroff method (Potter, 1973; Richtmyer & Morton, 1967) which is 2nd order accurate in Δt and Δx, but it is strongly dispersive, i.e. different spatial Fourier components travel at different velocities as shown in Fig. 6.

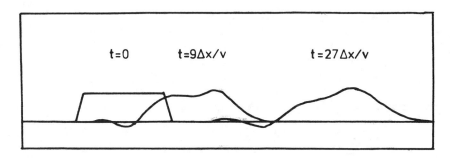

Fig. 6. Lax—Wendroff advection. Same parameters as in Fig. 5.

Accurate solution of the fluid equations is in fact very difficult. It is an active field of research and there is no one algorithm which is universally agreed as being the best. A good comparison of the different methods is given by Woodward and Colella (1984). Two of the more popular algorithms are FCT (Boris & Book, 1973) and Van Leer (1977).

FCT stands for Flux Corrected Transport. It is in fact a general method rather than one precise algorithm. The underlying principle is to pick a fairly simple advection algorithm which is dominated by diffusion, allow the diffusion to occur, but then correct for the diffusion by applying anti—diffusion. Boris and Book call the diffusive advection algorithm the 'transport stage' and they choose:

$$f_i^{n+1} = (Q_+ + Q_-)f_i^n + \tfrac{1}{2}Q_-^2(f_{i-1}^n - f_i^n) + \tfrac{1}{2}Q_+^2(f_{i+1}^n - f_i^n)$$

where $Q_\pm = (\tfrac{1}{2} \mp v_i^{\frac{1}{2}}\Delta t/\Delta x) / (1 \pm (v_{i\pm1}^{\frac{1}{2}} - v_i^{\frac{1}{2}})\Delta t/\Delta x)$

and $v_i^{\frac{1}{2}}$ are the velocities at time—level $n+\tfrac{1}{2}$. If v is a constant, as in our examples above, the algorithm becomes:

$$\bar{f}_i^{n+1} = f_i^n - \tfrac{1}{2}\epsilon(f_{i+1}^n - f_{i-1}^n) + (\tfrac{1}{8}+\tfrac{1}{2}\epsilon^2)(f_{i+1}^n - 2f_i^n + f_{i-1}^n)$$

where $\epsilon = v\Delta t/\Delta x$ and we have put a $^-$ over f_i^{n+1} because it is not the final value. ϵ is the distance moved in one timestep divided by the cell—size. On dividing by Δt and rearranging, the last equation can be shown to be a difference form of the differential equation:

$$\frac{\partial f}{\partial t} = -v\frac{\partial f}{\partial x} + D\frac{\partial^2 f}{\partial x^2} + O(\Delta x^2) + O(\Delta t^2) \quad \text{where } D = \tfrac{1}{8}\Delta x^2/\Delta t$$

The first term on the right hand side is the required advective term. The 2nd term is a diffusion term which is unwanted in the final solution. The diffusion could be counteracted by applying straight anti—diffusion $\partial f/\partial t = -D\partial^2 f/\partial x^2$, or in finite difference terms

$$f_i^{n+1} = \bar{f}_i^{n+1} - \tfrac{1}{8}(\bar{f}_{i+1}^{n+1} - 2\bar{f}_i^{n+1} + \bar{f}_{i-1}^{n+1})$$

Alternatively, this can be rewritten in terms of fluxes $J_{i\pm\frac{1}{2}}$ which move mass etc across cell boundaries.

$$f_i^{n+1} = \bar{f}_i^{n+1} + J_{i-\frac{1}{2}} - J_{i+\frac{1}{2}} \quad \text{where } J_{i\pm\frac{1}{2}} = \pm\tfrac{1}{8}(\bar{f}_{i\pm1}^{n+1} - \bar{f}_i^{n+1})$$

Straight antidiffusion counteracts the diffusion, but also introduces new errors by creating new maxima and minima in the solution, sometimes producing negative densities or energies. Boris and Book showed that there is a simple rule which keeps the advantages of antidiffusion but removes the disadvantages. The aim of their rule is that it 'should generate no new maxima or minima in the solution, nor should it accentuate already existing extrema'. Positivity is thereby also maintained.

The FCT algorithm applies the antidiffusive fluxes everywhere unless to do so would create or accentuate extrema. The rule which achieves this is to apply 'corrected' fluxes:

$$J^c_{i+\frac{1}{2}} = \sigma_{i+\frac{1}{2}} \; MAX[MIN(8\sigma_{i+\frac{1}{2}}J_{i-\frac{1}{2}}, 8\sigma_{i+\frac{1}{2}}J_{i+3/2}, |J_{i+\frac{1}{2}}|), 0]$$

where $\sigma_{i+\frac{1}{2}} = sgn(J_{i+\frac{1}{2}})$, i.e. σ is ± 1 depending on whether J is positive or negative. The new value of f is then

$$f^{n+1}_i = \bar{f}^{n+1}_i + J^c_{i-\frac{1}{2}} - J^c_{i+\frac{1}{2}}$$

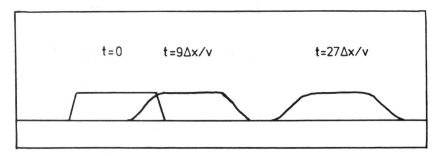

Fig. 7. Advection by FCT. Parameters same as in Fig. 5 and 6.

Figure 7 shows the application of FCT to the square wave advection problem. Boris and Book show that modifications to the method produce even better results. FCT is capable of advecting sharp edges without them spreading over more than 2 or 3 grid−points. However, the algorithm is a non−linear difference solution to a linear problem. Difficulties do arise. A significant problem is 'staircasing'. FCT treats discontinuities very well, but it can distort more gentle gradients into a series of sharp jumps looking like a staircase (e.g. Woodward and Colella, 1984). The original algorithm was known as SHASTA. It has since been improved by a number of authors (e.g. Book, Boris & Hain, 1975; Zalesak, 1979). Since FCT is a general principle rather than a specific algorithm, it can be applied to improve other advection schemes.

Another very successful advection algorithm is the Van Leer method (Van Leer, 1977). This is an improvement on the much earlier FLIC scheme (Gentry et al, 1966). It is presented clearly by Youngs (1982). It uses high order differencing to calculate the flux of mass etc across cell boundaries. As in the FCT method, non−linear cut−offs are applied to the fluxes to maintain positivity and avoid the generation of oscillations. Fig. 8 gives an example (Town, private communication) of the application of Van Leer's method.

Although the FCT and Van Leer algorithms both include conditional branching in the decision whether to apply the cut−offs on the fluxes, this is easily adapted to a vector machine by using MAX and MIN operations as given above in the equation for J^c.

If heat flow is important, then it appears in the energy equation as a diffusive term. This usually has to be solved implicitly to avoid undue limitation on the timestep. In 2−dimensions this requires solution of a quin−diagonal matrix equation. Fortunately, efficient matrix solvers such ICCG (Kershaw, 1978) are available.

We have described Lagrangian and Eulerian methods as though they were completely separate. In fact, there are intermediate schemes in which the mesh is allowed to move but is not completely fixed into the fluid. For example, an orthogonal mesh can be maintained but the grid allowed to move with the fluid in some average sense (e.g. Pert, 1983). Mesh tangling is thereby avoided whilst retaining, at least in part, the advantages of the Lagrangian method.

For many applications in plasma physics, magnetic field is important. The hydrodynamic problem then becomes a magnetohydrodynamic (MHD) problem. Magnetic forces and the generation, advection and diffusion of magnetic field have to be added to the fluid equations. This is clearly very important in Tokamaks and pinches in which the plasma is contained by magnetic pressure. If the plasma is dominated by externally imposed magnetic field, i.e. internally generated field is neglected, the MHD equations (Potter, 1973, Roberts & Potter, 1970) are:

$$\frac{\partial \rho}{\partial t} = -\nabla \cdot (\rho v) \quad \text{(mass eq}^n\text{)}, \qquad \frac{\partial (\rho v)}{\partial t} = -\nabla \cdot (\rho v v + P) + j \times B \quad \text{(momentum eq}^n\text{)},$$

$$\frac{\partial U}{\partial t} = -P\nabla \cdot v - \nabla \cdot (Uv) + \eta j^2 \quad \text{(energy eq}^n\text{)},$$

$$\frac{\partial B}{\partial t} = \nabla \times (v \times B) - \mu_0^{-1}\nabla \times (\eta \nabla \times B) \quad \text{(magnetic field)}, \qquad j = \mu_0^{-1}\nabla \times B \quad \text{(current)}$$

where j is the electric current density, and η is the resistivity. The equations are similar to the fluid equations given above except for the addition of a) the magnetic force on the RHS of the momentum equation, b) Ohmic (resistive) current dissipation on the RHS of the energy equation, and c) an extra equation for the evolution of the magnetic field.

The 1st term in the magnetic field equation represents advection and the 2nd represents resistive diffusion of field. Hence time−dependent MHD contains the familiar elements of advection and diffusion which dominate non−magnetic fluid codes. For greater generality, a number of other effects need including in the equations: a) magnetic source terms (e.g. Pert, 1981), b) the effect of magnetic field on transport (Epperlein & Haines, 1986), and c) an equation for magnetic field in a vacuum.

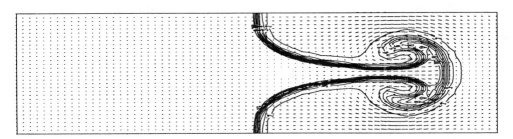

Fig. 8. Density (contours) and velocities (vectors) showing the growth of a small perturbation in a density interface which is overtaken by a shock (Richtmyer−Meshkov instability). The code uses the Van Leer method. (courtesy of RPJ Town)

E) FOKKER–PLANCK SIMULATIONS

The PIC method is appropriate if a plasma is collisionless. If particles are localised by collisions or magnetic field, a fluid model can be used. However, there is an intermediate regime in which collisions are important but they are not strong enough to make the fluid model valid. This regime is best decribed by the Fokker−Planck equation for the electron distribution function $f(x,v,t)$:

$$\frac{\partial f}{\partial t} + v \cdot \frac{\partial f}{\partial x} + (q/m)(E + v \times B) \cdot \frac{\partial f}{\partial v} = \left[\frac{\partial f}{\partial t}\right]_c$$

143

The term on the right hand side represents collisions. It consists of advection and diffusion terms in velocity space:

$$\left[\frac{\partial f}{\partial t}\right]_c = \frac{\partial}{\partial v}\cdot(\mathbf{F}f) + \frac{\partial}{\partial v}\cdot\left[\mathbf{T}\cdot\frac{\partial f}{\partial v}\right]$$

where $\mathbf{F}$ is a vector function of v, and $\mathbf{T}$ is a tensor function of v. $\mathbf{F}$ and $\mathbf{T}$ are derived from the Rosenbluth potentials which are integrals of f over velocity space (e.g. Tidman et al, 1964). We have recently found it necessary to solve this equation as an initial value problem in two spatial dimensions. After some simplification and approximation, the problem can be reduced to a 2nd order differential equation in x and z (the spatial dimensions) and v (magnitude of velocity) (Epperlein et al, 1988). Diffusion is important in both space and velocity so an unconditionally stable solution is needed. The naive method would be to make it fully implicit and invert the resulting matrix equation. However, the problem is 3−dimensional in (x,z,v), so the matrix is large with 15 non−zero diagonals if magnetic field is neglected and 19 if it is included. Instead we decided to use an Alternating Direction Implicit (ADI) method and neglect the magnetic field which was acceptable for our applications. The differential equation can be written in the form:

$$\frac{\partial f}{\partial t} = L_{xz}(f) + L_v(f) + L_{xzv}(f)$$

where L_{xz} is an operator containing $\partial/\partial x$ and $\partial/\partial z$ but not $\partial/\partial v$, L_v is an operator containing $\partial/\partial v$ but not $\partial/\partial x$ or $\partial/\partial z$, and L_{xzv} is an operator containing cross−terms $(\partial/\partial x)(\partial/\partial v)$ and $(\partial/\partial z)(\partial/\partial v)$. The ADI scheme then alternates between treating a) L_{xz} implicitly and L_v explicitly, and b) L_{xz} explicitly and L_v implicitly. L_{xzv} is always treated explicitly, but the term is relatively small and careful choice of differencing avoids instability.

L_{xz} and L_v contain diffusion and dominate the calculation. The ADI differencing of L_{xz} and L_v is unconditionally stable and 2nd order accurate. The first step (implicit in x and z) still requires solution of a large matrix equation. This is performed with the ICCG method of Kershaw (1978). The ADI method is not as accurate as matrix solution of the fully implicit equation, but it allows 2−dimensional simulation where it would otherwise be impractical. Details of the method are given in Epperlein et al (1988). An example of its application is given by Rickard et al (1989).

F) CONCLUSIONS

We have discussed some of the main classes of simulation of plasmas. We have particularly concentrated on those techniques relevant to basic plasma physics. Fluid and PIC codes have played a very important role in the understanding of plasmas. As algorithms are improved, new algorithms developed, and the speed of computers increase, we can expect many more fruitful years of plasma simulation.

ACKNOWLEDGEMENTS

Development of simulation techniques is a community activity, and I would particularly like to thank RPJ Town, Drs. GJ Rickard, P Gibbon, EM Epperlein, RG Evans, Prof GJ Pert, and other members of the Collaborative Computing Project in Plasma Physics (CCP10) for our many useful discussions.

REFERENCES

S.Atzeni, Comments Plasma Phys. Controlled Fusion, *10*, 129 (1986).
J. Barnes & P. Hutt, Nature, *324*, 446 (1986).
C.K. Birdsall & A.B. Langdon, 'Plasma Physics via Computer Simulation', McGraw Hill, Singapore (1985).

D.L. Book, J.P. Boris & K. Hain, J. Comp. Phys., *18*, 248 (1975).

J.P. Boris & D.L. Book, J. Comp. Phys., *11*, 38 (1973).

J.P. Christiansen, D.E.T.F. Ashby & K.V. Roberts, Comp. Phys. Comm, 7, 271 (1974).

J. Clerouin, J−P. Hansen, B. Piller, Phys. Rev. A, *36,* 2793 (1987).

A.E. Dangor, A.K.L. Dymoke−Bradshaw, A.E. Dyson, P. Gibbon & S.J. Kartunnen, 19th Anomalous Absorption Conf., paper I6, Durango, Colorado, June 1989.

E.M. Epperlein & M.G. Haines, Phys. Fluids, *29*, 1029 (1986).

E.M. Epperlein, G.J. Rickard & A.R. Bell, Comp. Phys. Comm., *52*, 7 (1988).

R.G. Evans, Proc. 3rd SUSSP Summer School on Laser−Plasma Interactions, ed. M.B. Hooper (1985).

R.G. Evans, A.R. Bell & B.J. MacGowan, J. Phys. d, *15*, 711 (1982).

R.A. Gentry, R.E. Martin & B.J. Daly, J. Comp. Phys., *1*, 87 (1966).

L. Hernquist, Comp. Phys. Comm. (special issue), *48(1)*, 107 (1987).

R.W. Hockney & J.W. Eastwood, *'Computer Simulation Using Particles'*, McGraw−Hill (1981).

H.G. Horak, E.M. Jones, J.W. Kodis & M.T. Stanford, J. Comp. Phys., *26*, 277 (1978).

D.S. Kershaw, J. Comp. Phys., *26*, 43 (1978).

R.J. Mason, Phys. Fluids, *23*, 2204 (1980).

G.J. Pert, J. Comp. Phys., *43*, 111 (1981).

G.J. Pert, J. Comp. Phys., *49*, 1 (1983).

D. Pesme, S.J. Kartunnen, R.R.E. Salomaa, G. Laval, N. Silvestre, Laser & Part. Beams, *6*, 199 (1988).

D. Potter, *Computational Physics*, Wiley−Interscience (1973).

R.D. Richtmyer & K.W. Morton, *Difference Methods for Initial Value Problems,* Interscience (1967).

G.J. Rickard, A.R. Bell & E.M. Epperlein, Phys. Rev. Lett., *62*, 2687 (1989).

K.V. Roberts & D.E. Potter, in *'Methods of Computational Physics'*, Vol. 9, ed. B. Alder, S. Fernbach & M. Rotenberg, Academic Press (1970).

D.A. Tidman, R.L. Guernsey & D. Montgomery, Phys. Fluids, 7, 1089 (1964).

B. Van Leer, J. Comp. Phys., *23*, 276 (1977).

C.P. Verdon, R.L. McCrory, R.L. Morse, G.R. Baker, D.I. Meiron & S.A. Orszag, Phys. Fluids, *25*, 1653 (1982).

P. Woodward & P. Colella, J. Comp. Phys., *54*, 115 (1984).

D.L. Youngs, in *Numerical Methods for Fluid Dynamics*, ed. K.W. Morton & M.J. Baines, Academic Press (1982).

S.T. Zalesak, J. Comp. Phys., *31*, 335 (1979).

COMPUTATIONAL IMPLEMENTATION OF THE R–MATRIX METHOD IN

ATOMIC AND MOLECULAR COLLISION PROBLEMS

K.A. Berrington

Department of Applied Mathematics and Theoretical Physics
Queen's University Belfast, BT7 1NN, U.K.

THE R–MATRIX METHOD

Whilst working on a contract for the Manhatten Project, Wigner and Eisenbud (1947) published a new theoretical method for interpreting resonances which had been observed in nuclear reactions. These resonances could be explained in terms of a compound nucleus interaction, in which the colliding nuclei "stick" temporarily in a compound state; the total wavefunction can therefore be expanded in a set of such states, and a many–body problem solved using nuclear structure techniques. This reaction zone was labelled the "internal region" of configuration space and delineated by a sphere of radius r = a around the scattering centre. In the "external region" however, where the colliding or separating nuclei are further apart, the system reduces to a two–body problem, the interaction being a simple function of the radial separation r. In order to connect the two regions, Wigner and Eisenbud introduced a matrix, which they called curly R, to relate the wavefunction to its derivative on the boundary r = a. Thus was R–matrix theory born.

COLLISION PROCESSES IN ATOMS AND MOLECULES

The interaction of electrons and photons with atoms and molecules is a fundamental feature of the commonest state of matter in the universe: plasma. From stellar atmospheres to planetary atmospheres to the inter–stellar medium, atomic processes such as electron excitation followed by radiative decay give rise to the emission of electromagnetic radiation which we can observe; indeed the very light sustaining us here on earth comes from such processes in the sun's atmosphere (the photosphere). Most of what we know about the composition, density, temperature, opacity etc. of the sun and other areas of the universe has to be deduced from the observed emission and absorption lines in their spectra – and these spectral lines can be interpreted only by knowing the basic atomic processes which are occurring.

Other important applications of atomic physics are in the laboratory. For example in fusion experiments, electron interactions with atoms and atomic ions can give important diagnostic information on the plasma – and can also lead to serious heat losses in the case of atomic contaminants from the vessel walls etc. The development of certain lasing schemes, for example X–ray lasers, requires a detailed knowledge of resonance behaviour in atomic collision processes. Yet further applications lie in current laboratory experiments using synchrotron radiation or electron beams, and in laser induced atomic excitation and ionization experiments.

Supercomputational Science
Edited by R.G. Evans and S. Wilson
Plenum Press, New York, 1990

In all of these applications a large variety of high quality atomic data is required, particularly on the interaction of photons and electrons with atoms and ions, to understand and predict laboratory or astrophysical processes. This gives a tremendous motivation to exploit powerful computational methods, such as the R—matrix method, and powerful supercomputers to provide such data. It is not the only motivation of course – there is clearly an aesthetic interest in being able to understand and calculate *ab initio* the basic interactions between quantum—mechanical particles.

SCME THEORY

It was Burke and collaborators (eg Burke et al, 1971; Burke and Robb, 1975) who realised that an understanding of processes involving the scattering of low energy electrons from an atomic or molecular target (A):

$$e^- + A \rightarrow A^{-*} \rightarrow e^- + A, \tag{1}$$

and related processes such as photoionization:

$$h\upsilon + A \rightarrow A^* \rightarrow e^- + A^+, \tag{2}$$

where the * indicates intermediate resonance states, could be understood in terms of an R—matrix type theory.

Configuration space describing the electron—atom, ion or molecule complex is divided into two regions by a sphere of radius $r = a$ around the atomic or molecular target. In the internal region the electron interaction with the target is strong, electron exchange and correlation effects are important and the intermediate complex can be considered as an atomic or molecular structure problem. On the other hand in the external region, if the radius of the sphere $(r = a)$ is chosen just to envelope the charge distribution of the target, the electron interaction with the target can be described by a simple potential. Sometimes analytic solutions are possible, for example in electron—ion scttering where it is often possible to include just the Coulomb interaction of the scattered electron with the ion core.

The link between these two regions is provided by the R—matrix which is defined by the equation

$$F_i(a) = \sum_j R_{ij}(E) (a\, dF_j/dr - b_j F_j)_{r=a} \tag{3}$$

where $F_i(r)$ is the radial wavefunction describing the motion of the scattered electron in the i—th channel and the b_j are arbitrary parameters. E is the total energy. Let E_i be the energy of target state i and ϵ_i the energy of the added electron. Then

$$E = E_i + \epsilon_i \tag{4}$$

At energies giving bound states for the whole system, $\epsilon_i < 0$ for all channels i, and the radial functions $u_i(r)$ go to zero exponentially in the limit of $r \rightarrow \infty$. The collision states are such that $\epsilon_i > 0$ for some (or all) values of i. Channel i is said to be open if $\epsilon_i > 0$ and closed if $\epsilon_i < 0$.

Although the R-matrix method has been formulated in a number of different ways for different situations, for simplicity here assume an atom or atomic ion target and an LS coupling scheme. The formulation is as in Burke et al (1971), Burke and Robb (1975) and Berrington et al (1987). For a relativistic treatment see Scott and Burke (1980), Scott and Taylor (1982) and Norrington and Grant (1981).

The R-matrix, for an electron scattered by an N electron target, is calculated by solving the Schrödinger equation (atomic units are used: $e = m_e = c = 1$)

$$H \Psi_E = E \Psi_E \qquad (5)$$

in the internal region. The complete wavefunction Ψ_E is expanded in terms of a discrete basis defined by

$$\Psi_k = A \sum_{i,j} \Phi_i(X,\hat{r}) \, U_j(r) \, c_{ijk} + \sum_j \varphi_j(X,r) \, d_{jk} \qquad (6)$$

where X stands for the coordinates of the N electrons of the target, r for the coordinates of the added electron, $r = (\hat{r}, r)$, and the antisymmetrization operator

$$A = (N+1)^{-1/2} \sum_{n=1}^{N+1} (-1)^n. \qquad (7)$$

The Φ_i in (6) are vector coupled products of the N-electron target state wavefunctions with the spin-angle functions of the scattering electron, and the φ_j are (N+1)-electron correlation functions which are insignificant on the boundary (the boundary radius $r = a$ is chosen to completely enclose the N-electron target, i.e. all the target radial orbitals are negligible for $r = a$).

The $U_j(r)$ in (6) are radial basis orbitals representing the scattering electron and are non-zero on the boundary at $r = a$. In the Burke et al (1971) and Burke and Robb (1975) formulation the $U_j(r)$ are chosen to be members of a complete set of orthonormal solutions of a radial wave equation with some suitably chosen potential, and which satisfy fixed boundary conditions

$$b_j = \frac{a}{U_j(a)} \left. \frac{dU_j}{dr} \right|_{r=a} \qquad (8)$$

where the b_j in equations (8) and (3) are usually taken to be zero. The truncation of this complete set of solutions represents an approximation in the method over and above the truncation in the number of target states included in (6); however a "Buttle" correction can be applied to the R-matrix to allow for this truncation (Burke and Robb, 1975).

The coefficients c_{ijk} and d_{jk} in the truncated expansion (6) are obtained by a diagonalization of the Hamiltonian in this basis:

$$e_k \delta_{kk'} = (\Psi_k | H | \Psi_{k'}) \qquad (9)$$

where the integral is taken over all the N+1 electronic coordinates in the internal region.

The non—relativistic Hamiltonian in atomic units takes the form

$$H = \sum_{n=1}^{N+1} -(\nabla_n^2 / 2 + Z / r_n) + \sum_{n>n'=1}^{N+1} 1 / r_{nn'}, \qquad (10)$$

where Z is the nuclear charge. This Hamiltonian is diagonal in the total orbital angular momentum L of the system, the total spin S and the total parity Π. The wavefunction basis defined by (6) is therefore determined for each choice of L S Π. Having diagonalized the Hamiltonian matrix (9), the R—matrix for each energy can be determined from

$$R_{ii'}(E) = \frac{1}{2 a} \sum_{k} W_{ik}(a) (e_k - E)^{-1} W_{i'k}(a) \qquad (11)$$

where the surface amplitudes

$$W_{ik}(a) = \sum_{j} U_j(a) c_{ijk}. \qquad (12)$$

An important aspect of the R matrix method is that the main part of the work required to calculate the R—matrix is in setting up and diagonalizing the Hamiltonian matrix in the internal region, to obtain the eigenvalues e_k and eigenvectors c_{ijk} used in (11) and (12). This needs to be done only once for each L S Π in order to determine the R—matrix at all energies. The evaluation of the matrix elements of H is similar to a bound state calculation, the main difference being that integrals involving the radial coordinates are over a finite rather than an infinite range. This is a relatively trivial difference and therefore bound state codes can be readily modified to carry out R—matrix calculations.

In the external region ($r > a$) electron exchange between the scattered electron and the target electrons is by definition negligible, and the potential matrix coupling channels i and i' has assumed its asymptotic form:

$$V_{ii'}(r) = \sum_{\lambda=1} v_{ii'\lambda} \; r^{-\lambda-1}, \quad r \to \infty. \qquad (13)$$

The resultant radial Schrödinger equation reduces to coupled second—order ordinary differential equations. These must be solved at each energy, and matched to the R—matrix on the boundary, in order to calculate observable quantities such as the collision cross section (Burke and Robb, 1972).

COMPUTATIONAL IMPLEMENTATION

A suite of computer programs for electron—atom and electron—ion collision processes based on the approach of Burke et al (1971) and Burke and Robb (1975) was published by Berrington et al (1978). A later version of the programs, to treat radiative bound—bound and bound—free absorption processes in atoms and ions was published by Berrington et al (1987). This latter version is being used in the Opacity Project, an international collaborative effort to calculate all atomic data required for the *ab initio* determination of stellar opacities (Seaton, 1987).

Both versions of the atomic R–matrix program are in regular use throughout the world on a variety of computers and supercomputers – Crays being the most popular. The programs are run in modular form. To obtain electron collision data four such modules are run sequentially (additional modules are required for radiative processes – see Berrington et al, 1987):

STG1 calculates the radial basis functions $U_j(r)$ and performs all radial integrals in the internal region required for the Hamiltonian matrix;

STG2 defined the configurations Φ_j and φ_j in (6) and calculates all angular and spin integrals to constuct the Hamiltonian matrix for each L S Π;

STGH diagonalizes the Hamiltonian matrices and calculates the surface amplitudes W_{ik} in (12);

STGF solves the external region problem, matching to the R–matrix on the boundary, and calculates collision cross sections for each energy.

On scalar computers these modules can take roughly equal amounts of computer time. However, the supercomputer behaviour of these modules is rather different. Although the programs are somewhat large (around 10 000 statements each), it is interesting to examine some of the main features.

The most time consuming steps in STG1 and STG2 involve the electron–electron repulsive terms in the Hamiltonian (the right hand terms of eq 10). The resulting matrix elements can be written as a sum of weighted radial integrals:

$$(\psi / V / \psi') = \sum_k a_k \, R_k(1,2,3,4) \qquad (14)$$

where the ψ are individual terms in (6) and V is the two–electron operator in (10). The evaluation of the R_k radial integrals in STG1 shows good vectorisation properties. The integral is actually a double integral over the two electron coordinates r and r':

$$R_k(1,2,3,4) = \int_0^a dr \int_0^a dr' \, U_1(r) \, U_2(r') \, (r_<^k / r_>^{k+1}) \, U_3(r) \, U_4(r') \qquad (15)$$

where $r_< = \min(r,r')$; $r_> = \max(r,r')$.

These integrals are most easily evaluated by defining

$$Y_k(2,4;r) = r^{-(k+1)} \int_0^r dr' \, (r')^k \, U_2(r') \, U_4(r')$$

$$+ r^k \int_r^a dr' \, (r')^{-k+1)} \, U_2(r') \, U_4(r') \qquad (16)$$

$$\therefore \quad R_k = \int_0^a dr \, U_1(r) \, U_3(r) \, Y_k(2,4;r) \qquad (17)$$

Now the evaluation of Y_k in (16) is not well optimised for vector operation, since the vector lengths vary as r goes from o to a. However, once calculated, Y_k can be used to evaluate a number of different R_k integrals where orbitals 2 and 4 are in common, but orbitals 1 and 3 allowed to loop over all possible orbitals (often there are about 20 orbitals per angular momentum).

The evaluation of R_k in (15) is however highly optimum for a vector computer. The integral can be represented as a quadrature summation over a set of radial mesh points m:

$$R_k = \sum_m U_1(r_m)\, U_3(r_m)\, Y_k'(r_m), \qquad (18)$$

where the prime indicates that the Y_k has been pre–multiplied by the integration weights at each mesh point k (normally Simpson's rule is used). At each mesh point then there are three floating point operations. Since the addition can be chained with one of the multiplications on Cray computers, the operation need only take two clock periods per mesh point (the number of mesh points is typically a few hundred). On a CRAY X–MP/48, with an 8.5 ns clock period, one would expect a peak execution rate of up to 160 Mflops in the evaluation of (18).

In the programs published by Berrington et al (1978 and 1987) all radial integrals R_k are first evaluated and stored on disk. However, such a procedure can lead to I/0 bottlenecks on supercomputers when there are large numbers of $U_j(r)$ orbitals, and a re–assessment of the method has lead to the conclusion that it is probably better to store the Y_k functions (a much smaller amount of data, which could be held in a few Mwords of memory) and to use (18) to calculate R_k when it is required in the evaluation of the Hamiltonian matrix. Some duplication will inevitably occur in the R_k integrals, but the vector speed is so high that any additional cost will be out–weighed by the reduction in I/0 cost. These considerations are crucial in a new development of the R–matrix method to treat intermediate energy scattering (I.E.R.M., see Burke et al, 1987) and electron impact ionization, where up to two (rather than just one) electrons are allowed in the continuum; the number of R_k integrals will then grow by at least a factor of 10^4.

The angular and spin integrals, the a_k weights of (14), are calculated in STG2. One of the most efficient methods is that due to Bar–Shalom and Klapisch (1988), who use graphical analysis to construct the formulas and evaluate them by summing products of Racah coefficients. This technique is rule based and inherently poorly vectorised, requiring instead fast conditional branch execution. Parallelization relies on the fact that large numbers of similar angular and spin integrals are required in a given calculation

In STGH the main task is the full diagonalization of the large, dense, symmetric, Hamiltonian matrices, one for each chosen $L\ S\ \Pi$. The levels of parallelism inherent in diagonalization is the subject of an accompanying lecture.

The parallelization of STGF is obvious — the external region equations have to be solved for each energy — and the code can be multi–tasked or run on separate processors. Only a small amount of memory is required once the R–matrix on the boundary is formed for a particular energy, so STGF is currently being implemented on a 20 transputer Meiko system at Belfast.

COMMENTS

In many areas of science and engineering the main computational tasks are superficially similar, for example the need to solve systems of differential equations. However there are some features peculiar to quantum mechanics which do not arise in other "classical" areas. Consider the Schrödinger wave equation, the starting point for *ab initio* quantal calculations, in its time dependent form:

$$i \hbar \frac{\partial \psi}{\partial t} = -\frac{\hbar^2}{2m} \nabla^2 \psi + V \psi \qquad (19)$$

If V = 0 we have the diffusion equation with an imaginary diffusion constant. But the potential (V) makes each quantum mechanics problem a special case. Indeed, as has been shown, the evaluation of the Hamiltonian matrix for a many–particle system, which can exist in an indefinite number of configurations, is often the dominant part of the computation. Moreover, when many identical particles are involved, such as electrons, the exchange potential makes the interactions non–local in the region of configuration space defined by the bound states of the system. Also the application of variational principles introduces integral operators into eq (19). The resulting equations are therefore integro–differential. There is a further complication for collision problems; the system must be described by a multi–channel formulation which allows for interference between the possible incoming and outgoing channels. Such interactions can give rise to coupling potentials which die off very slowly with distance from the centre of collision.

Computational techniques must therefore consider convergence, stability, accuracy, computer time and memory, as well as the need to maintain generalarity in the application of the resulting codes across a wide range of problems. Thus a typical code may have a mix of requirements ranging from fast memory and I/0, fast scalar arithmetic and conditional branches, vector processing facilities and multi–tasking — all of which are efficiently done on a supercomputer such as the CRAY X–MP/48. In these circumstances a single index such as the megaflop rate cannot on its own measure the efficient utilisation of the total computer resource for problems in quantum mechanics; the touch–stone must instead be the scientific worth of the results.

In this connection, consider the Opacity Project (Seaton, 1987), referred to earlier in the description of the R–matrix program of Berrington et al (1987). The opacity properties of a plasma are a measure of the absorption of radiation by the plasma. In stellar atmospheres and other similar plasmas the dominant photoabsorption mechanisms involve individual atoms and atomic ions:

$$h\upsilon + A_i \rightarrow A_f \qquad (\text{"bound–bound"})$$

$$h\upsilon + A_i \rightarrow A_f^+ + e^- \qquad (\text{"bound–free"})$$

$$e^- + h\upsilon + A_i \rightarrow A_f + e^- \qquad (\text{"free–free"})$$

where A_i is an atomic target in an initial state i, A_f is its final state. In the conditions of a stellar envelope, atoms can exist in a wide range of excited states, so it is necessary to have a consistent set of data for all these states, with a high photon energy resolution; a virtually impossible task for the laboratory experimentalist.

Now it has been shown that the R–matrix method is a powerful technique for solving Schrödinger's equation for a many–particle system in an *ab initio* way; the equations are solved in a local region using energy–independent basis functions such that a single diagonalization of the Hamiltonian matrix yields the wavefunction for any energy. The method is therefore highly efficient for situations where a large number of energies has to be sampled: for example when locating bound states of the total wavefunction; or when resolving the energy dependence of the bound–free process, where resonances can make a significant or even dominant contribution to the absorption cross section. Both the initial (bound) and final (free) states can be represented by a consistent wave function description, and cross sections can be routinely calculated from any initial atomic ground or excited state, over any required grid of photon frequencies.

The Opacity Project, an international collaboration involving atomic physicists and astrophysicists in London, Belfast, Paris, Nice, Munich, Caracas, Urbana, Boulder and Ohio is using the R–matrix method and programs to systematically calculate hundreds of thousands of atomic energy levels, tens of millions of bound–bound oscillator strengths and hundreds of millions of frequency–dependent bound–free cross sections from every calculated atomic level, for around 100 astrophysically abundant atomic ions required for the accurate calculation of stellar opacities. Of course once calculated the data will have many other applications in astrophysics and in the laboratory, and will form the most reliable and systematic collection of such data ever assembled.

It should be emphasised that the Opacity Project is a product both of sophisticated theoretical and programming treatment and of supercomputing power.

REFERENCES

Bar–Shalom, A. and Klapisch, M., 1988, Comp. Phys. Commun. **50**, 375.
Berrington, K. A. Burke, P. G., le Dourneuf, M., Robb, W. D., Taylor, K. T. and Vo Ky Lan, 1978, Comp. Phys. Commun., **14**, 367.
Berrington, K. A., Burke, P. G., Butler, K., Seaton, M. J., Storey, P.J., Taylor, K. T. and Yu Yan, 1987, J. Phys. B: At. Mol. Phys., **20**, 6379.
Burke. P. G., Hibbert, A. and Robb, W. D., 1971, J. Phys. B: At. Mol. Phys., **4**, 153.
Burke, P. G. and Robb, W. D., 1975, Adv. in Atom. Molec. Phys., **11**, 143.
Burke, P. G., Noble, C. J. and Scott, M. P., 1987, Proc. R. Soc. A. **410**, 289.
Norrington, P. H. and Grant, I. P., 1981, J. Phys. B: At. Mol. Phys. **14**, L261.
Scott, N. S. and Burke P. G., 1980, J. Phys. B: At. Mol. Phys. **13**, 4299.
Scott, N. S. and Taylor, K. T., 1982, Comp. Phys. Commun. **25**, 347.
Wigner, E. P. and Eisenbud, L., 1947, Phys. Rev. **72**, 29.

MULTITASKING THE HOUSEHOLDER DIAGONALIZATION

ALGORITHM ON THE CRAY X–MP/48

K.A. Berrington,

Department of Applied Mathematics and Theoretical Physics,
Queen's University Belfast, BT7 1NN, U.K.

REASONS FOR MULTITASKING

In a previous lecture (computational implementation of the R–matrix method in atomic and molecular collision problems) it was mentioned that an important part of the computation in solving collision problems by R–matrix techniques was the diagonalization of the internal–region Hamiltonian matrices. These matrices are usually real, symmetric and dense (i.e. non–sparse). All eigenvalues and eigenvectors are required to define the R–matrix. the matrices can be of various sizes, up to an order of a few thousand square.

The largest matrix which can be stored in the fast memory of a CRAY X–MP/48 (*i.e.* 8 MWords) is of order 3500 (note that the matrix is symmetric and only a triangle need be stored). Such matrices were occuring frequently in current R–matrix calculations on the CRAY X–MP/48. It was therefore decided to investigate multitasking the algorithm, since it is clearly an inefficient use of resources to use all of the memory but only one processor (the computer centre charges heavily for this!). The Householder method was chosen because it is a finite iterative process (*i.e.* it is known exactly how many steps are required), and also because it requires little working space beyond that required to hold the matrix in upper triangle form (Householder and Bauer, 1959; Wilkinson, 1960; Ralston and Wilf, 1967; Gourlay and Watson, 1973).

THE ALGORITHM

Diagonalization procedes in two stages: firstly a tri–diagonalization reduction is performed (Householder's method); secondly the eigenvalues and eigenvectors are found from the tri–diagonal form.

The Householder reduction of a matrix $\mathbf{A}$ of order n is effected by n–2 similarity transformations with orthogonal matrices $\mathbf{P_1}$, $\mathbf{P_2}$, ..., $\mathbf{P_{n-2}}$ successively:

$$\mathbf{A}^{(r+1)} = \mathbf{P_r} \mathbf{A}^{(r)} \mathbf{P_r} \qquad (1)$$

here r = 1, 2, ..., n–2, and $\mathbf{A}^{(1)}$ is the orginal matrix $\mathbf{A}$. At each step, a row and a column is set to zero (except for the diagonal and adjacent element). Clearly (1) is recursive and cannot be executed in parallel. However, within one cycle of the reduction the transformation acts on rows independently. Consider a cycle at step r.

Matrix $A^{(r)}$ consists of $r-1$ rows and columns already tri–diagonalized, with a square submatrix starting in the rth row and column remaining to be transformed.

First sum the squares of the off–diagonal elements down the rth column (or row – the matrix is symmetric) of $A^{(r)}$:

$$S^2 = \sum_{i=r+1}^{n} A^2_{i,r} \quad \text{and set } a = \frac{1}{S(S \pm A_{r+1,r})}. \tag{2}$$

(The sign in the denominator is arbitrary and is chosen to avoid subtraction errors).

Then define a column vector u with zeros in the first $r+1$ elements and the remaining elements taken from the rth column of $A^{(r)}$:

$$u^T = (0,...,0, A_{r+1,r} \pm S, A_{r+2,r},..., A_{n,r}) \tag{3}$$

which implies that $u^T u = 2/\alpha$. It can be easily shown that

$$P_r = I - \alpha\,u\,u$$

is an orthogonal matrix (i.e. $P_r^T P_r = I$). Using P_r in (1) we find

$$A^{(r+1)} = A^{(r)} - u\,q^T - q\,u^T \tag{4}$$

where $q = p - K\,u$, $K = \dfrac{\alpha}{2}\,u^T p$ and $p = \alpha\,A^{(r)}u.$ \qquad (5)

This transformation of $A^{(r)}$ ensures that the first $r-1$ rows and columns (which have already been tri–diagonalized in previous cycles) remain unaltered, the rth diagonal element remains the same and its adjacent element becomes $\mp S$, and the rest of the rth row and column is made zero.

In (5), since u and q are both column vectors, the evaluation of q and the scalar quantity K are single–loop vector operations. However, writing out as elements, we see that

$$p_i = a \sum_{j=r+1}^{n} A_{ij}\,u_j \tag{6}$$

consists of two nested loops: the inner loop (j) can be vectorised; the outer loop (i) can be multitasked. (Strictly, summing the elements of an array is a recursive operation; however, Cray computers can partially vectorise this).

Similarly, the evaluation of (4) consists of two nested loops:

$$A_{ij} = A_{ij} - u_i\,q_j - q_i\,u_j \quad (i,j=r+1,n). \tag{7}$$

PARALLELIZATION

It is clear that the tri–diagonalization process consists of three levels of nested loops (it is said to be an "n³ process" — computing time normally increasing with the cube of the order of matrix, n):

the outer loop (over r in equation (1)) is recursive;

the middle loops can be multitasked;

the inner loops can be vectorised.

The next stage in the operation is to determine the eigenvalues and eigenvectors from the tri–diagonal matrix. There are several methods to do this (see, for example, Gourlay and Watson, 1973), but the crucial point is that the commonest methods (*e.g.* bisection followed by back–substitution) evaluate eigenvalues and eigenvectors *independently* of one another. This process naturally multitasks, and again there is a vectorisation within each task. It should be emphasised that multitasking should never be employed at the expense of vectorisation on Cray computers; partly because the vector speed is so valuable, and partly because of the high overheads involved in initiating tasks. This general rule has been applied in the current discussion.

THE PROGRAM

A micro–tasked, vectorised program has been written (Sawey and Berrington, 1989) to implement the full diagonalization of a symmetric matrix using the Householder algorithm on a four processor CRAY X–MP/48, enitrely within memory. In a typical run to diagonalize a matrix of order 3500, the following timings were obtained:

```
Processor 1 :  12m 05s
Processor 2 :  12m 27s
Processor 3 :  11m 57s
Processor 4 :  14m 39s
Total         51m 08s
```

These timings show reasonable load balance between the processors, though one processor (number 4) is clearly having to execute code which cannot be parallelized: such work will dominate the overall time if an infinite number of processors are available (cf Amdahl's Law). 69 MFlops per processor was achieved, which is little more than half of peak vector speed on the CRAY X–MP. The degradation comes partly from inherently unvectorisable code, which means that vector processing cannot be continuous; and partly from the difficulty of addressing a complete row of a matrix, which is stored in upper triangle form in a linear array to save space. (Using a two–dimensional arrary to hold the matrix would improve the performance here, but at the expense of memory).

It is interesting to examine the clock–time as a function of the number of processors, again for diagonalizing a matrix of size 3500, but now on a CRAY Y–MP/832:

```
1 processor  :  1644 s.   (113 MFlops)
6 processors :   279 s.   (112 MFlops)
8 processors :   229 s.   (102 MFlops)
```

Clearly, it is possible to envisage a full diagonalization of a symmetric matrix of size up to 7500 in less than one hour on the CRAY Y–MP/832, using all eight processors and working entirely within the fast memory.

This micro–tasked and vectorised program is now in regular use in R–matrix calculations on electron–atom and electron–ion scattering, and is interfaced to the R–matrix programs of Berrington et al (1978).

SHARED vs DISTRIBUTED MEMORY

The above program relies on a large fast memory shared amongst all the processors. However, it is possible to envisage diagonalizing a large matrix held in a distributed form over a number of local–memory processors. The Householder algorithm is currently being implemented on a twenty–transputer Meiko computer at Belfast, in which each transputer has 4 Mbytes of (local) memory. The procedure is to distribute the original matrix row–by–row onto the processors, and to recognise that after each step in the iteration (1), only a single vector (the first row, see eq. 2 and 3) has to be retrieved and transmitted to each processor to start the next cycle. Thus the amount of inter–processor communication is kept to a minimun, maintaining a high processor utilisation.

REFERENCES

Berrington, K.A., Burke, P.G., Le Dourneuf M, Robb, W.D., Taylor, K.T. and
    Vo Ky Lan, 1978, Comp. Phys. Commun. **14**, 367.
Gourlay, A.R. and Watson, G.A., 1973, Computational methods for matrix
    eigenproblems. Wiley & Sons.
Householder, A.S. and Bauer, F.L., 1959, Numerische Math. 1 Band **1**. Heft, p29.
Ralston, A. and Wilf, H.S., 1967, Mathematical methods for digital computers. II
    Wiley & Sons.
Sawey, M. and Berrington, K.A., 1989, Comp. Phys. Commun.: submitted.
Wilkinson, J.H. 1960, Computer J. **3**, 23.

RELATIVISTIC ATOMIC STRUCTURE CALCULATIONS I:

BASIC THEORY AND THE FINITE BASIS SET APPROXIMATION

Harry Quiney

Department of Theoretical Chemistry, University of Oxford, Oxford OX1 3UB

INTRODUCTION

Atomic electronic structure calculations have been used to test theories of the physical laws since the advent of quantum mechanics in the 1920's. Much of the current activity in atomic structure theory involves the development of accurate and efficient computational techniques in order to model astrophysical phenomena or spectroscopic experiments of great complexity, so that atomic physics seems distant from the well–publicised areas of fundamental research into high–energy physics. It is not, however, true to suggest that the atom is no longer of service in our attempts to understand the forces in Nature. The relative simplicity of the atom has allowed the incorporation of new fundamental developments into computational models which test our understanding of the physical laws in complex systems. These models include the small effects which have been observed experimentally which arise in the theories of quantum electrodynamics (QED) and the non–conservation of parity (PNC).

Atomic spectroscopy evidently still has an important role to play in fundamental physics, but the challenges to theory are formidable in this area. The most successful experiments have been performed on elements with large values of the nuclear charge, Z, for which the small effects of QED or PNC, which vary approximately as Z^3, are most significant. For systems of this type, however, it is necessary first to overcome technical difficulties associated with the requirements of the theory of special relativity and the many–body nature of the atomic wavefunction before reliable information about these other small effects may be obtained. Such technical developments also have important applications to the interpretation of complex spectra, and to the advancement of theories of chemical bonding in systems containing heavy elements and in solid–state theories.

In this first lecture, the relativistic Hartree–Fock theory is reviewed, with particular emphasis on those aspects of the computational technique which differ substantially from the non–relativistic theory. Many–body perturbation theory will then be introduced and the features of the relativistic theory discussed. The result will be a model based on the single–particle Dirac–Hartree–Fock approximation, which can then be used to evaluate many–body corrections due to the correlation between particles, and the possibility, in a relativistic theory, of the creation and annihilation of electron–positron pairs. The model will be discussed in the context of a recently–developed method which employs finite–dimensional basis sets of analytic functions, with a detailed discussion of the computational features of this approach

Supercomputational Science
Edited by R.G. Evans and S. Wilson
Plenum Press, New York, 1990

when implemented on vector–processing machines. In the second lecture, we will examine how the structure of computational algorithms may be adapted to suit the architecture of a vector–processing computer, in particular, the CRAY X–MP/48.

AN INTRODUCTION TO RELATIVISTIC QUANTUM MECHANICS

The relativistic equation describing the motion of an electron in an external field was presented by Dirac (1928). He arrived at the wave equation which now bears his name by arguing that a relativistic quantum theory must treat the four components of space–time equally. This is a fundamental objection to the familiar Schrödinger equation, which contains the first derivative of the time coordinate, but the second derivative of the spatial variables. The flaw lies in the assumptions which led to the non–relativistic theory, particularly the reliance on the classical wave equation to justify the form of the Hamiltonian operator. Dirac indicated that the requirement of relativistic invariance under a Lorentz transformation leads naturally to a complicated form for the wavefunction containing four components, and the relativistic Hamiltonian operator must exhibit transformation properties which are absent in the Schrodinger operator. If we consider a classical electromagnetic four–potential, $A^\mu(x)$, such that

$$A^\mu(x) = \left[\frac{\phi(x)}{c}, A(x) \right] \qquad [2.1]$$

comprising the scalar and vector potentials $\phi(x)$ and $A(x)$, respectively, the Dirac equation for an electron of charge $-e$ can be written in the covariant form

$$[\gamma_\mu(p^\mu + eA^\mu) - mc]\psi(x) = 0 \qquad [2.2]$$

The wavefunction, $\psi(x)$, is a four–component vector, known as a spinor. The 4×4 matrices, γ_μ, are chosen to satisfy the commutation relations

$$\{\gamma_\mu, \gamma_\nu\} = \gamma_\mu\gamma_\nu + \gamma_\nu\gamma_\mu = 2g_{\mu\nu} \qquad [2.3]$$

where $g_{\mu\nu}$ is the the metric tensor, which has non–zero elements only for $\mu = \nu$ such that $g_{00} = 1 = -g_{11} = g_{22} = g_{33}$, and $p_\mu = i\partial/\partial x^\mu$.

The first derivation of the Dirac–Hartree–Fock (DHF) equations was given by Bertha Swirles (Lady Jeffreys) in 1935. She followed the established practices of that time and formed a relativistic many–electron Hamiltonian operator from the sum of the single–particle operators for each electron coordinate and from operators which represent the interaction of pairs of electrons through an instantaneous Coulomb mechanism. This operator, which is now usually called the many–electron Dirac–Coulomb operator, H_{DC}, is similar in general form to the Hamiltonian of non–relativistic many–electron quantum mechanics. It is, in Hartree atomic units,

$$H_{DC} = \sum_{i=1}^{N} H_{D,i} + \frac{1}{2} \sum_{i,j=1}^{N} \frac{1}{r_{ij}} \qquad [2.4]$$

where the Dirac single–particle operator for the electron with coordinate r_i is

$$H_{D,i} = c\boldsymbol{\alpha}_i \cdot \mathbf{p}_i + (\beta_i - 1)c^2 - \frac{Z}{r_i} \qquad [2.5]$$

Here, c is the speed of light, Z is the nuclear charge, $\boldsymbol{\alpha}_i$ and β_i are 4×4 matrices

$$\alpha = \begin{bmatrix} 0 & \sigma \\ \sigma & 0 \end{bmatrix} \qquad \beta = \begin{bmatrix} I & 0 \\ 0 & -I \end{bmatrix} \qquad [2.6]$$

and $\mathbf{p}_i$ is the 3–component momentum of the ith electron. The 2 × 2 matrices, σ, are Pauli spin matrices, and I is the unit matrix of order 2. The harmonic time–dependence of the Dirac equation has been separated from the spatial coordinates using the assumption that the classical potential is independent of time. The original equation is then premultiplied by $c\gamma_0$, and the non–relativistic time variable isolated, so that we are working in a fixed single–time reference frame. The solutions of this Dirac wave equation take the general form,

$$\psi(\mathbf{r}) = \psi_k(\mathbf{r}) \exp(-iE_k t) \qquad [2.7]$$

A configuration of single–particle solutions of the eigenvalue equation

$$H_{D,i} \, \psi_k(\mathbf{r}) = E_k \psi_k(\mathbf{r}) \qquad [2.8]$$

is then formed into a determinantal product, Ψ_k, in order to satisfy the Pauli Exclusion Principle,

$$\Psi_k(\mathbf{r}_1, \mathbf{r}_2, ..., \mathbf{r}_n) = \frac{1}{\sqrt{N!}} \begin{vmatrix} \psi_1(\mathbf{r}_1) & \psi_2(\mathbf{r}_1) & .... & \psi_n(\mathbf{r}_1) \\ \psi_1(\mathbf{r}_2) & \psi_2(\mathbf{r}_2) & .... & \psi_n(\mathbf{r}_2) \\ . & . & .... & . \\ . & . & .... & . \\ \psi_1(\mathbf{r}_n) & \psi_2(\mathbf{r}_n) & .... & \psi_n(\mathbf{r}_n) \end{vmatrix}$$

$$[2.9]$$

This antisymmetrized wavefunction is taken as a trial solution of the many–electron equation

$$H_{DC} \, \Psi_m = E_m \, \Psi_m \qquad [2.10]$$

It is assumed, for simplicity, that the bare–nucleus single–particle functions will provide adequate initial approximation to the average distribution of electrons in a many–electron atom. In practice, it is often better to choose some effective value of Z, or some more representative potential, to start the procedure. Since the antisymmetrized functions, Ψ_m, are just linear combinations of single–particle functions $\psi_k(\mathbf{r}_i)$, we may separate the many–electron equation into N single–particle equations for each electron moving in the average potential due to the remaining N–1 electrons. The equations are solved to self–consistency, so that a small change in any of the single–particle functions, δ, causes a change in the total energy E_m of the Dirac–Hartree–Fock state, Ψ_m, of order δ^2. The value of δ is usually chosen so that each of the single–particle states is determined to machine accuracy. The Dirac–Hartree–Fock method, like the more familiar non–relativistic approximation, involves the iterative determination of mean–field potentials.

We also consider a generalization of H_{DC} which allows for the magnetic interactions between relativistic electron currents in atoms, and which recognises that the delay in one electron interacting with another, due to the finite speed of light, will modify the Coulomb interaction between electrons. The quantum mechanical operator for such an interaction between a pair of electrons was derived by Breit in 1929 based on earlier classical arguments presented by Darwin (1920). It is

$$H_B(1,2) = -\frac{1}{2R} \left[\alpha_1 . \alpha_2 + \frac{(\alpha_1 . R)(\alpha_2 . R)}{R^2} \right] \qquad [2.11]$$

where R is the interparticle vector and α_i is a 4×4 matrix characteristic of the Dirac theory. It is implicit in the derivation of this approximate operator that the electrons interact through the exchange of low—frequency photons, so that we may use the Breit operator only for pairs of electrons whose single—particle energies are small compared with c. The non—relativistic reduction of this operator yields a number of operators which correct for the existence of the electron spin and for magnetic interactions which arise through the coupling of orbital and spin angular momenta. These operators, which are familiar from elementary texts, are those of the orbit—orbit, spin—spin, spin—orbit and spin—other—orbit interactions. Further fine—structure effects result from the non—relativistic reduction of the single—particle Dirac equations. In a sense, we gain a real advantage in using a relativistic theory, because many of these small interactions are included to all orders in perturbation theory, and the theory becomes both simpler and more elegant.

It should be mentioned that the above argument has attracted a good—deal of criticism over the past sixty years, and particularly in the last twenty years, since people have attempted to perform relativistic electronic structure calculations based on the Dirac—Coulomb and Breit operators. A complete explanation of the problem is not appropriate here, and requires some knowledge of quantum field theory. The essence of the problem lies in the fact that the single—particle Dirac equation has solutions which are usually classified as being of either *positive* or *negative* energy.

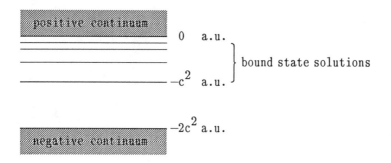

This picture is modified slightly if the nucleus is modelled as an object with a finite size, rather than as a point, but the general features remain unchanged. There is a correspondence between the positive—energy solutions of the Dirac equation and the bound and continuum solutions of the non—relativistic single—particle Schrödinger equation, with some small energy corrections and with the two—fold degeneracy of each state corresponding to two states of spin built in. The Dirac equation predicts correctly the the fine—structure of one electron systems, as well as the lowest order approximation to the value of the electron spin magnetic moment, without the arbitrary assumptions required in the Schrodinger theory.

The Dirac equation also has a continuum of negative—energy solutions, which have energies of less than $-2c^2$ atomic units, with respect to a zero of energy corresponding to an electron at rest. These states are interpreted using the Dirac hole—theory of the positron. In order that ordinary matter be stable, these negative—energy states must be considered to be filled with electrons, otherwise ordinary matter would spontaneously fill these states with the consequent emission of a photon. Everything which we observe is considered to be measured with respect to a vacuum state in which all the negative—energy states, which form a continuum, are occupied according to the Pauli Exclusion Principle. If a vacancy is created in this unobservable negative—energy sea, we interpret this event as the creation of an electron—positron pair, the original electron occupying a positive—energy state and the hole in the negative—energy density behaving like a particle with the mass of an electron but with a positive charge, which we call a positron. This description is analogous to the chemical theory of valency. On the other hand, this infinite density of electrons must distort in the presence of an external field, for example, in the neighborhood of a nucleus. This will give rise to a shielding of the nuclear charge and a modification of the Coulomb interaction. This phenomenon is called vacuum polarization, and gives rise to observable line—shifts in atomic spectra. Quantum field theory describes these processes more elegantly, without the assymetry between electrons and positrons, but the physical content is the same. In a computational model, it is necessary that the negative—energy single particle states should appear on an equal footing with the positive energy states, since it is the union of these two branches which forms the complete set of states on which the physical model is based.

The Dirac—Coulomb operator contains no information about the occupancy of the negative—energy states and so the problem regarding the stability of matter with respect to radiative decay must be faced. The Dirac—Hartree—Fock approximation is, however, a method in which single—particle states are varied one at a time, so that as long as we can define a set of states at the end of the procedure which can be classified as being of positive— or negative—energy, there is no problem in implementing the Dirac hole theory other than the purely technical one of bookkeeping. The restrictions regarding the derivation of the Breit operator mean that it may not be used in interactions involving a pair of electrons involving both positive— and negative—energy states. A more complete model of photon exchange is required in this case, but these effects are very small and may be neglected to a good approximation.

A number of points emerge from this discussion, which will serve as a description of what we require of a computational relativistic electronic structure theory. Several features which are not found in non—relativistic quantum mechanical methods place additional demands on the processing power required and on storage. The single—particle solutions are four—component vectors, called spinors. These components may be grouped together into two sets of pairs, called the large— and small—components. Within each pair, there is a degeneracy corresponding in the non—relativistic theory to the existence of two possible projections of the electron spin. Since fine—structure effects result from the non—relativistic reduction of the Dirac equation, we expect that the relativistic structure of the equations must lead to a larger number of single—particle states at zero—order in a relativistic model. If the negative—energy states are considered, the roles of the large— and small—components must be reversed so that orthogonality within the complete set of states, including both positive— and negative— energy branches, is maintained. In any method which attempts to approximate the complete set of single particle states by some discretization procedure, the negative—energy states must appear explicitly. The requirement that all of the negative—energy states are filled according to the Pauli Exclusion Principle in the vacuum state means that the complete theory of the hydrogen atom involves, by necessity, many—body interactions. In order that the bookkeeping is done correctly and that the Dirac—Hartree—Fock approximation represents a legitimate zero—order approximation to real systems, second—quantization of the model is required, particularly if interactions with the negative—energy states are considered.

The relativistic atomic Hartree—Fock method is now presented, and the reconciliation of these many fundamental requirements discussed.

THE RADIAL DIRAC–HARTREE–FOCK EQUATIONS

Due to the presence of a well–defined centre of force at the nucleus, the single–particle equations for atoms are separated into radial and spin–angular coordinates. The four–component spinors are classified according to a quantum number set $\{n_i, \kappa_i, m_i\}$ or equivalently $\{n_i, \ell_i, j_i, m_i\}$

$$\psi_{n\kappa m}(r) = \frac{1}{r} \begin{bmatrix} P_{n\kappa}(r)\, \chi_{\kappa m}(\theta, \varphi) \\ iQ_{n\kappa}(r)\, \chi_{-\kappa m}(\theta, \varphi) \end{bmatrix} \qquad [3.1]$$

where $P_{n\kappa}(r)$ and $Q_{n\kappa}(r)$ are the large and small–component radial amplitudes and the functions $\chi_{\kappa m}(\theta, \varphi)$ denote two–component angular spinors

$$\chi_{\kappa m} = \sum_{\sigma = \pm 1/2} Y_\ell^{m-\sigma}(\theta, \varphi)\, u^\sigma \langle \ell\, 1/2\, m - \sigma\, \sigma \mid \ell\, 1/2\, j\, m \rangle$$

$$[3.2]$$

$Y_\ell^{m-\sigma}(\theta, \varphi)$ is a spherical harmonic function, u^σ is a spin eigenvector and $\langle \ell\, 1/2\, m - \sigma\, \sigma \mid \ell\, 1/2\, j\, m \rangle$ is a Clebsch–Gordan coefficient. The orbital quantum number, ℓ, refers to the large component, so that it is the total angular momentum, j, which represents a true eigenstate of the system. For a given value of ℓ, the angular quantum number, κ, may take values ℓ or $-(\ell+1)$. The total angular momentum takes the value $(2|\kappa|-1)/2$. The spin–angular parts of the spinors are handled algebraically, while the radial functions depend on the precise specification of the potential. The significant computational component in relativistic atomic structure theory involves the determination of these radial functions, and the evaluation of the radial integrals which arise from the decomposition of the one– and two–electron matrix elements. The structure of the radial equations is consistent with our expectation that the number of single–particle states in a relativistic calculation will be approximately twice that in a non–relativistic calculation, since for any $\ell > 0$, the radial amplitudes for $j=\ell+1/2$ and $j=\ell-1/2$ are different and are characterized by different angular quantum numbers, κ. Moreover, instead of a single Schrödinger radial function, each fine–structure state has two radial components to be determined. The resulting closed–shell radial differential equation for each single particle state takes the form of a coupled pair of first–order ordinary differential equations of the form

$$\begin{bmatrix} -Z/r & c\left(-\dfrac{d}{dr} + \dfrac{\kappa_i}{r}\right) \\ c\left(\dfrac{d}{dr} + \dfrac{\kappa_i}{r}\right) & -2c^2 - Z/r \end{bmatrix} \begin{bmatrix} P_i(r) \\ Q_i(r) \end{bmatrix} + \sum_j \frac{U(i,j;r)}{r} \begin{bmatrix} P_j(r) \\ Q_j(r) \end{bmatrix}$$

$$= \epsilon_{ii} \begin{bmatrix} P_i(r) \\ Q_i(r) \end{bmatrix} \qquad [3.3]$$

together with the requirement that the component functions should satisfy boundary conditions at the nucleus and at infinity which ensure that observable quantities have a finite expectation value. The function $U(i,j;r)$ is constructed at each iteration from estimates of the spinor components. The Hartree–Fock potential, U_{HF}, which defines the mean–field antisymmetrized Coulomb interaction between electrons in the subshells of the atom is

$$\langle i | U_{HF} | j \rangle = \sum_k (\langle ik|g|jk \rangle - \langle ki|g|jk \rangle)$$

$$= \int_0^\infty \frac{U(i,j;r)}{r} \rho_{ij}(r) \, dr$$

[3.4]

The summation over k includes all (positive–energy) occupied spinors, and the Coulomb interaction is represented by the operator, g. The radial density, $\rho_{ij}(r)$, is given by

$$\rho_{ij}(r) = P_i(r)P_j(r) + Q_i(r)Q_j(r)$$

Here is the reconciliation of one of the most serious difficulties associated with the Dirac–Hartree–Fock approximation. The restriction of the summation over k to positive–energy single particle states contains the concealed restriction that we are assuming that the negative–energy states are both filled and inert, so that we just ignore them. The *ad hoc* derivation of the equations may be justified rigorously within quantum electrodynamical theory, so I wish to emphasise only that the relativistic atomic structure theory presented here is not flawed, but a precisely–defined model with the Dirac–Hartree–Fock method as its legitimate zero–order approximation.

This has been a brief outline of the steps involved in a closed–shell Dirac–Hartree–Fock calculation. Most of the detail has been avoided, because the usual methods of calculation, while highly accurate, are by nature very difficult to implement efficiently on vector processing machines. The search for a method which can exploit the architecture of a supercomputer and which is able to reflect all of the features of the physical model, including retarded magnetic interactions, many–body effects and the negative–energy states had led to the the development of basis set methods, which are discussed below.

The usual method which is used to compute all the required quantities, such as the radial densities and the two–electron matrix elements, is the finite difference approximation. Each pair of functions $P_i(r)$ and $Q_i(r)$ are represented as a discrete set of points in some range of r from the nucleus to a fixed outer boundary, the initial few points are approximated by a power–series expansion, and the last few points by the asymptotic behaviour of the solutions. The derivatives are approximated by weighted sums of the function values, the matrix elements are estimated by numerical quadrature, and the differential equations are solved, subject to the other approximations, by a "marching" process, in which the eigenvalue is varied until the solution functions satisfy the finite difference equations to some specified tolerance.

The finite difference approximation has been used to construct an efficient algorithm which has been implemented by hand and on a succession of mechanical and electronic computers ever since the self–consistent field was introduced by Hartree in 1928, but this traditional approach to electronic structure calculations is not ideally suited to a vector processing computer. The solution of each pair of radial functions using a "marching" algorithm is recursive (the function value depends on preceding values), as is the method of evaluating the radial two–electron integrals. Each radial function depends on the the radial functions of all the other occupied spinors, which means that there is little enhancement possible from a vector processing machine. The solution procedes from one spinor to the next, so that if a large basis of functions is required, for example, in a multi–configurational calculation, such an approach fails to exploit efficiently the architecture of a supercomputer. The fact that the method varies only one orbital at a time means that the strategies discussed in the second of these lectures in the context of the finite basis set method are of limited use in accelerating the rate of execution of a Dirac–Hartree–Fock program based on the finite–difference approximation.

MATRIX ELEMENTS OF SCALAR TWO–BODY INTERACTIONS

The most significant technical difficulty in atomic structure calculations in either the finite difference or finite basis set approximation is the evaluation of the two–body matrix elements of the Coulomb and Breit operators. These are required both in the construction of the Hartree–Fock potential and in the many–body corrections to observable quantities through the use of perturbation theory. Since the computational aim of this work is to evaluate relativistic many–body effects, the structure of relativistic two–body matrix elements must be understood before algorithms can be discussed.

The matrix element of any scalar two–body interaction, g_{12}, is given by

$$<\psi_a(1)\psi_b(2)| \; g_{12} \; |\psi_c(1)\psi_d(2)> =$$

$$\sum_{L,M}(-1)^{L-M}(-1)^{j_a-m_a}(-1)^{j_b-m_b}\begin{bmatrix} j_a & L & j_c \\ -m_a & M & m_c \end{bmatrix}\begin{bmatrix} j_b & L & j_d \\ -m_b & -M & m_d \end{bmatrix} X^L(abcd)$$

$$[4.1]$$

in the most general form, where $X^k(abcd)$, the effective interaction strength, is a radial integral which is independent of the magnetic quantum numbers m_i and M.

The quantity

$$\begin{bmatrix} j_1 & j_2 & j_3 \\ m_1 & m_2 & m_3 \end{bmatrix} \qquad\qquad [4.2]$$

is a Wigner 3–j symbol it takes the value zero unless the angular momenta satisfy the triangle condition

$$|j_1 - j_2| \le j_3 \le (j_1 + j_2) \qquad\qquad [4.3]$$

and observe the completeness condition

$$m_1 + m_2 + m_3 = 0 \qquad\qquad [4.4]$$

The 3–j symbol represents, to within a phase factor, the coefficient which couples the angular momentum vectors (j_1m_1) and (j_2m_2) to give the resultant vector (j_3m_3). It is usual to work with 3–j symbols, rather than vector–coupling coefficients (or Clebsch–Gordan coefficients), because the Wigner representation has a higher degree of symmetry with respect to interchange of the columns. The 3–j symbol is a complicated algebraic quantity, but one may circumvent these difficulties by recognizing that eigenvectors of the angular momentum operator form a complete orthonormal set, and that the algebraic properties of this set may be described by a number of compact graphical rules.

An appreciation of these rules is important, because the efficient evaluation of the angular contributions to the two–body matrix elements proves to be a bottleneck in the calculation of very complex systems, and the graphical rules are particularly valuable in resolving the phase factors involved in any arbitrary coupling.

The graphical representation of a 3–j symbol is

$$\begin{bmatrix} j_1 & j_2 & j_3 \\ m_1 & m_2 & m_3 \end{bmatrix} = \begin{array}{c} j_3 m_3 \\ \rule{2cm}{0.4pt} \end{array} \Bigg| \begin{array}{l} j_2 m_2 \\ + \\ j_1 m_1 \end{array} \qquad [4.5]$$

The + sign indicates that the angular momenta are read anticlockwise around the vertex; it doesn't matter which line you start with, because the 3–j symbol is variant with respect to an even permutation of columns. If the angular momenta are read clockwise, then the sign at the vertex is labelled −, and an additional factor is introduced. This is equivalent to the odd permutation of the columns.

$$\begin{bmatrix} j_1 & j_3 & j_2 \\ m_1 & m_3 & m_2 \end{bmatrix} = (-1)^{j_1+j_2+j_3} \begin{array}{c} j_3 m_3 \\ \rule{2cm}{0.4pt} \end{array} \Bigg| \begin{array}{l} j_2 m_2 \\ - \\ j_1 m_1 \end{array} \qquad [4.6]$$

Phase factors are accomodated by the addition of arrows to the angular momentum lines

$$(-1)^{j_3-m_3} \begin{bmatrix} j_1 & j_2 & j_3 \\ m_1 & m_2 & -m_3 \end{bmatrix} = \begin{array}{c} j_3 m_3 \\ \rule{2cm}{0.4pt}\!\!\leftarrow \end{array} \Bigg| \begin{array}{l} j_2 m_2 \\ + \\ j_1 m_1 \end{array} \qquad [4.7]$$

$$(-1)^{j_3+m_3} \begin{bmatrix} j_1 & j_2 & j_3 \\ m_1 & m_2 & m_3 \end{bmatrix} = \begin{array}{c} j_3 m_3 \\ \rule{2cm}{0.4pt}\!\!\rightarrow \end{array} \Bigg| \begin{array}{l} j_2 m_2 \\ + \\ j_1 m_1 \end{array} \qquad [4.8]$$

Note that any m value changes sign when passing through an arrow; in the above cases, m_3 takes the value $-m_3$ at the vertex. A single line is represented by

$$\begin{array}{cc} j\,m & j'm' \\ \rule{5cm}{0.4pt} \end{array} = \delta(j,j')\delta(m,m') \qquad [4.9]$$

which reflects the orthonormality of angular momentum eigenstates. The vector–coupling coefficient, $<j_1 m_1, j_2 m_2 | j_3 m_3>$ is related to the 3–j symbol through

$$<j_1 m_1, j_2 m_2 | j_3 m_3> = (-1)^{j_1-j_2+m_3}(2j+1)^{1/2} \begin{bmatrix} j_1 & j_2 & j_3 \\ m_1 & m_2 & -m_3 \end{bmatrix}$$

$$[4.10]$$

and has the graphical representation

$$\langle j_1 m_1, j_2 m_2 | j_3 m_3 \rangle = \quad \begin{array}{c} \xrightarrow{j_1 m_1} \quad + \quad \xleftarrow{j_2 m_2} \\ \Big| \\ j_3 m_3 \end{array} \qquad [4.11]$$

where the heavy lines represents the factor $(2j_3+1)^{1/2}$.

Internal lines with common magnetic quantum numbers involve an implicit summation over all magnetic substates. The product of two 3—j symbols becomes

$$\begin{array}{c} \xrightarrow{j_1 m_1} + \overline{} \xleftarrow{j_3 m_3} \\ \Big| \\ j_4 m_4 \end{array} \times \begin{array}{c} \xrightarrow{j_3 m_3} + \xleftarrow{j_2 m_2} \\ \Big| \\ j_5 m_5 \end{array} = \begin{array}{c} \xrightarrow{j_1 m_1} + \xleftarrow{j_3} + \xleftarrow{j_2 m_2} \\ \Big| \quad \Big| \\ j_4 m_4 \quad j_5 m_5 \end{array} \qquad [4.12]$$

the magnetic label on the angular momentum line j_3 is suppressed because the summation over all substates is implied by its internal position in the graph. The signs at the vertices are unchanged, as are any arrows on the original 3—j symbols and it is noted that in this context, an "internal" line is one with no free ends.

Using these graphical conventions, the two—body matrix element of any scalar two—body interaction may be written

$$\langle \psi_a(1)\psi_b(2) | g_{12} | \psi_c(1)\psi_d(2) \rangle = \quad \begin{array}{cc} j_a m_a \Big| & \Big| j_b m_b \\ - \Big|\!\xrightarrow{L}\!\Big| + \\ j_c m_c \Big| & \Big| j_d m_d \end{array} \quad X^L(abcd)$$

$$[4.13]$$

The summation over all allowed tensor orders, L, is implied. This is a remarkably useful result, particularly in the analysis of many—body effects, since we may exploit angular momentum rules to simplify the calculation. Although the algebra of angular momentum operators has been studied since the early 1930's, it is only in the last two decades that graphical techniques have found widespread use in atomic structure theory, and only in the last few years that computer programs have become available which simplify the complex couplings found in many—electron open—shell systems. The rules of Yutsis, Levinson and Vanagas, [YLVn], which reduce complicated angular momentum graphs to simple products of elementary quantities, are discussed in the section on many—body perturbation theory.

The above expression for the two—body matrix element is valid equally for either the Coulomb or Breit interaction. The only difference, from a computational viewpoint, is in the form of the effective interaction strength, $X^L(abcd)$.

The effective interaction strength of the Coulomb interaction is

$$X^L(abcd) = (-1)^L \langle j_a \| C^{(L)} \| j_c \rangle \langle j_a \| C^{(L)} \| j_c \rangle \, \Pi^e(\kappa_a, \kappa_c, L) \Pi^e(\kappa_b, \kappa_d, L) \, R^L(abcd)$$

$$[4.14]$$

The effective interaction strength of the Breit interaction is

$$X^L(abcd) = (-1)^L \langle j_a \| C^{(L)} \| j_c \rangle \langle j_a \| C^{(L)} \| j_c \rangle \sum_{\nu=L-1}^{L+1} \Pi^0(\kappa_a, \kappa_c, \nu) \Pi^0(\kappa_b, \kappa_d, \nu)$$

$$\times \sum_{\mu=1}^{8} s_\mu^{\nu L}(abcd) \, S_\mu^\nu(abcd) \qquad [4.15]$$

The associated quantities are

$$\langle j \| C^{(L)} \| j' \rangle = (-1)^{j+1/2} [j,j']^{1/2} \begin{bmatrix} j & L & j' \\ 1/2 & 0 & -1/2 \end{bmatrix} \qquad [4.16a]$$

$$\Pi^0(\kappa,\kappa',k) = \frac{1}{2}[1 - (-1)^{\ell+\ell'+k}] \qquad [4.16b]$$

$$\Pi^e(k,k',k) = 1 - \Pi^0(\kappa,\kappa',k) \qquad [4.16c]$$

$$[j] = 2j + 1 \qquad\qquad [j,j'] = [j][j'] \qquad [4.16d,e]$$

Introducing the potential functions

$$U_\nu(1,2) = \begin{cases} r_1^\nu / r_2^{\nu+1} & \text{if } r_1 < r_2 \\ 0 & \text{if } r_1 > r_2 \end{cases}$$

$$U_\nu(1,2) = \bar{U}_\nu(1,2) + \bar{U}_\nu(2,1) \qquad [4.17]$$

the radial Coulomb integral, $R^L(abcd)$, is given by

$$R^L(abcd) = \int_0^\infty\!\!\int_0^\infty [P_a(r_1)P_c(r_1) + Q_a(r_1)Q_c(r_1)]U_L(1,2)$$

$$\times \quad [P_b(r_2)P_d(r_2) + Q_b(r_2)Q_d(r_2)] \qquad [4.18]$$

The primary radial integral of the Breit interaction is $S^\nu(abcd)$, where

$$S^\nu[ac|cd] = \int_0^\infty\!\!\int_0^\infty P_a(r_1)Q_c(r_1)\,\bar{U}_\nu(1,2)\,P_b(r_2)Q_d(r_2)$$

$$[4.19]$$

The correspondence between the primary integral and the eight integrals $S_\mu^\nu(abcd)$ is established through the table

μ	$S^\nu[..\,|..]$
1	$\begin{bmatrix} ac & bd \end{bmatrix}$
2	$\begin{bmatrix} bd & ac \end{bmatrix}$
3	$\begin{bmatrix} ca & db \end{bmatrix}$
4	$\begin{bmatrix} db & ca \end{bmatrix}$
5	$\begin{bmatrix} ac & db \end{bmatrix}$
6	$\begin{bmatrix} db & ac \end{bmatrix}$
7	$\begin{bmatrix} ca & bd \end{bmatrix}$
8	$\begin{bmatrix} bd & ca \end{bmatrix}$

The coefficients which appear in the expression for the effective interaction strength of the Breit matrix elements are

The Breit coefficients, $s_\mu^\nu(abcd)$

Case I: $L = \nu$

$$s_\mu^{LL}(abcd) = -\frac{(\kappa_a + \kappa_c)(\kappa_b + \kappa_d)}{L(L+1)} \qquad \mu = 1,2,\ldots,8$$

Parity: $\ell_a + \ell_c + \nu$ and $\ell_b + \ell_d + \nu$ both odd

---

Case II: $L = \nu \pm 1$

μ	$L = \nu + 1$	$L = \nu - 1$
1	$(L+K)(b' + c'K')$	$(b+cK)(K'-L-1)$
2	$(L+K')(b' + c'K)$	$(b+cK')(K-L-1)$
3	$(L-K)(b' - c'K')$	$(b-cK)(-K'-L-1)$
4	$(L-K')(b' - c'K)$	$(b-cK')(-K-L-1)$
5	$-(L+K)(b' - c'K')$	$-(b+cK)(-K'-L-1)$
6	$-(L-K')(b' + c'K)$	$-(b-cK')(K-L-1)$
7	$-(L-K)(b' + c'K')$	$-(b-cK)(K'-L-1)$
8	$-(L+K')(b' - c'K)$	$-(b+cK')(-K-L-1)$

Parity: $\ell_a + \ell_c + \nu$ and $\ell_b + \ell_d + \nu$ both odd

$K = \kappa_a - \kappa_c \qquad\qquad K' = \kappa_b - \kappa_d$

$$b' = \frac{\nu+2}{2(2\nu+1)} \qquad c' = -\frac{\nu-1}{(2\nu+1)(2\nu+2)} \qquad \nu \ge 0$$

$$b = \frac{\nu-1}{2(2\nu+1)} \qquad c = -\frac{\nu+2}{2\nu(2\nu+1)} \qquad \nu \ge 1$$

The general features of this structure must be reflected in the computational algorithm. The component structure of relativistic spinors gives rise to blocks of two—electron integrals coupling certain combinations of radial components. The selection rules relating to the Coulomb and Breit interactions are different, as are the integral—types required to calculate their interaction strengths. We will find that the finite basis set method is readily adapted to this structure, because the large and small component ampitudes for any symmetry—type always share common functional elements. The distinction between Coulomb and Breit matrix elements is made through the straightforward application of linear algebra, which is ideally suited to implementation on a supercomputer.

THE MATRIX DIRAC—HARTREE—FOCK METHOD FOR ATOMS

The basis set approach to the solution of the non—relativistic radial equations was proposed by Roothaan. Rather than represent a wavefunction as a discrete set of points, Roothaan presented the algebraic equations which result if we assume that the wavefunctions may be represented by linear combinations of analytic functions. The basis set of functions that is used is necessarily finite and incomplete, but in the case of bound—state problems, this represents no practical problem because most atomic phenomena of interest are represented by localized wave—packets, which do not sample space which is far removed from the nucleus and which are not highly oscillatory. This should not be thought of as an unacceptable restriction, since the same problem is present in finite—difference approximations, where a physical boundary must be set for the atom, and some finite number of mesh—points chosen to represent each radial function. For each angular symmetry—type, κ, it is assumed that the radial functions may be expanded in a finite basis of functions of dimension N_κ, such that

$$P_{\kappa i}(r) = \sum_{j=1}^{N_\kappa} X_{\kappa i}^{Lj} f_{\kappa j}^{L}(r) \qquad [5.1]$$

$$Q_{\kappa i}(r) = \sum_{j=1}^{N_\kappa} X_{\kappa i}^{Sj} f_{\kappa j}^{S}(r) \qquad [5.2]$$

A great deal of research over the past ten years has been based on the above form of the expansions for the radial large and small components. Note that the dimension of the large and small component basis sets are equal. Careful analysis has shown that this is necessary to maintain the symmetry of the positive— and negative—energy branches of the spectrum. More importantly, it should be noted that the radial large and small component basis sets $\{f_{\kappa j}^{L}(r)\}$ and $\{f_{\kappa j}^{S}(r)\}$ need not have the same elements. In fact, it is found that stable approximations to the Dirac spectrum are obtained only if the basis functions are chosen in a special way, which matches basis functions in a pairwise sense, and which imposes physical boundary conditions on the space of trial functions. These constraints avoid the "variational collapse" of the spectrum, where the notions of positive— and negative—energy become meaningless, but prove to be the greatest obstacle to the development of efficient relativistic many—body methods, since we need to be able to extend systematically any approximation toward completeness, yet maintain variational stability at each step in the calculation.

After a lengthy analysis, it can be shown that acceptable basis sets for relativistic electronic structure calculations within the point nuclear approximation may be derived from the pairwise relationship between components

$$f_{\kappa n}^T(r) = r^\gamma \exp(-\lambda r)\left\{ -(1-\delta_{n0})L_{n-1}^{2\gamma}(2\lambda r) \pm \frac{(N_n - \kappa)}{(n + 2\gamma)} L_n^{2\gamma}(2\lambda r)\right\}$$

$$
\begin{aligned}
n &= 0,1,2,\ldots \quad \text{for } \kappa < 0\\
n &= 1,2,3,\ldots \quad \text{for } \kappa > 0
\end{aligned}
\qquad [5.3]
$$

The completeness requirement is achieved in this case by increasing the maximum value of n, the relativistic principal quantum number, but keeping the value of λ constant, which fixes an effective scale of length for the basis. This set is called the L–spinor basis because of the presence of the generalized Laguerre polynomial elements $L_k^{2\gamma}(z)$. The upper sign refers to the large component radial basis function, and the lower to the small component function. The quantities γ and N_n are

$$\gamma = \sqrt{\kappa^2 - (Z/c)^2} \qquad [5.4]$$

$$N_n = \sqrt{n^2 - 2(n - |\kappa|)(|\kappa| - (Z/c)^2)} \qquad [5.5]$$

and the generalized Laguerre polynomial has the explicit form

$$L_k^{2\gamma}(z) = \sum_{m=0}^{k}(-1)^m \begin{bmatrix} k + 2\gamma \\ k - m \end{bmatrix} \frac{z^m}{m!} \qquad [5.6]$$

Alternatively, we may fix the value of n at the ground–state value (either n=0 or n=1) for a given value of κ, and then extend the basis by considering a set of functions characterized by a set of parameters, $\{\lambda_i\}$. A set of functions formed in this way is called an S–spinor basis (S for "Slater") because of its similarity to the basis of exponential–type functions introduced by Slater in early studies of electronic structure. The parameters $\{\lambda_i\}$ must be chosen according to a systematic prescription so that the basis tends towards completeness, and avoids, and much as possible, computational linear dependence. A compact definition of the S–spinor basis is

$$f_{\kappa i}^T(r) = r^\gamma \exp(-\lambda_i r)\left\{ -(1-\delta_{p0})L_{p-1}^{2\gamma}(2\lambda_i r) \pm \frac{(N_p - \kappa)}{(p + 2\gamma)} L_p^{2\gamma}(2\lambda_i r)\right\}$$

$$i = 1,2,3,\ldots N_\kappa \qquad [5.7]$$

where $p = 0$ for $\kappa < 0$ and $p = 1$ for $\kappa > 0$, and N_κ is the dimension of the radial basis for this symmetry–type. Note that the basis set parameter sets $\{\lambda_i\}$ may be different for each of the symmetry types. If we consider the explicit form of the Laguerre polynomials, these basis functions may be written in the equivalent form

$$f^T = \begin{cases} r^\gamma \exp(-\lambda_i r) & \text{for } \kappa < 0 \\ (A^T + \xi_i r)\, r^\gamma \exp(-\lambda_i r) & \text{for } \kappa > 0 \quad i = 1,2,\ldots N_\kappa \end{cases}$$

$$[5.8]$$

This reasonably simple basis possesses all the properties which are required to avoid variational collapse problems, and provides a set which may, in principle, be extended towards completeness in the limit $N_{max} \rightarrow \infty$. For $\kappa = +1$, for example, the required coefficients are

$$A^L = (2 - N)(2\gamma + 1)/(2N - 2)$$

$$A^S = -N(2\gamma + 1)/(2N - 2) \qquad \qquad [5.9]$$

where

$$\gamma = (1 - Z^2/c^2)^{1/2} \text{ and } N^2 = 2 + 2\gamma$$

Similar coefficients may been derived for higher angular momenta directly from the general expression for the S–spinor.

For closed–shell systems, the matrix Dirac–Hartree–Fock equations may be written as a set of block–diagonal generalized matrix eigenvalue equations of the form

$$F_\kappa X_\kappa = E_\kappa S_\kappa X_\kappa \qquad \qquad [5.10]$$

in which F_κ is the matrix representation of the Fock operator, X_κ is the matrix of expansion coefficients, E_κ is a diagonal matrix of eigenvalues and S_κ is a block–diagonal basis set overlap matrix for relativistic symmetry–type κ. The matching of large and small component basis functions in pairs means that each of the matrices in the generalized eigenvalue problem have dimension $2N_\kappa \times 2N_\kappa$.

When we diagonalize the Fock matrix for each symmetry type, the discrete spectrum which is obtained has the general form

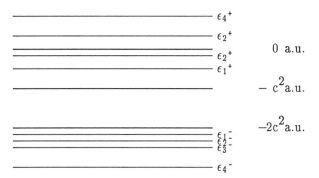

Here, the spectrum corresponds to a basis of 4 large–component and 4 small–component functions. Two of the single particle eigenstates have energies in the region $0 > \epsilon > -c^2$; these are interpreted as representations of bound states. The remainder of the states form a discrete representation of the upper and lower continua. In practice, many more than four S–spinor functions are used. The representation of the spectrum becomes more detailed as the dimension of the basis set is enlarged. It is usual to use around twenty S–spinor functions per symmetry, and for very high precision, it is possible to use up 500 L–spinors, yielding a rich representation of all regions of the spectrum.

The structure of the two–electron interaction matrices reflects the decomposition of the relativistic two–body matrix elements into radial and spin–angular components described above. The block–diagonal Fock matrix ,F_κ, may be written

173

$$F_\kappa = h_\kappa + g_\kappa + b_\kappa \qquad [5.11]$$

The matrices which must be constructed for each angular symmetry–type, κ, of the matrix Dirac–Fock problem are:

The overlap matrix, S_κ

$$S_\kappa = \begin{bmatrix} S_\kappa^{LL} & 0 \\ 0 & S_\kappa^{SS} \end{bmatrix} \qquad [5.12]$$

The bare–nucleus Dirac matrix, h_κ

$$h_\kappa = \begin{bmatrix} V_\kappa^{LL} & c\,\Pi_\kappa^{LS} \\ c\,\Pi_\kappa^{SL} & V_\kappa^{SS} - 2c^2 S_\kappa^{SS} \end{bmatrix} \qquad [5.13]$$

The matrix of the instantaneous Coulomb interaction, g_κ

$$g_\kappa = \begin{bmatrix} J_\kappa^{LL} - K_\kappa^{LL} & -K_\kappa^{LS} \\ -K_\kappa^{SL} & J_\kappa^{SS} - K_\kappa^{SS} \end{bmatrix} \qquad [5.14]$$

The matrix of the low–frequency Breit interaction, b_κ

$$b_\kappa = \begin{bmatrix} B_\kappa^{LL} & B_\kappa^{LS} \\ B_\kappa^{SL} & B_\kappa^{SS} \end{bmatrix} \qquad [5.15]$$

The submatrices are evaluated with respect to a given basis of square–integrable functions, in this case, the large– and small–components of the radial S–spinor set. We may write the general form of a single element of a radial S–spinor set $\{\psi_{\kappa,i}(r)\}$ as

$$\psi_{\kappa,i}(r) = \begin{bmatrix} f_{\kappa,i}^{L}(r) \\ f_{\kappa,i}^{S}(r) \end{bmatrix} \qquad [5.16]$$

The submatrices then have the elements

$$S_{\kappa,ij}^{TT} = \int_0^\infty dr\; f_{\kappa,i}^{T}(r)\, f_{\kappa,j}^{T}(r) \qquad [5.17]$$

$$V^{TT}_{\kappa,ij} = \int_0^\infty dr\, f^{T}_{\kappa,i}(r)\,(-Z/r)\, f^{T}_{\kappa,j}(r) \qquad [5.18]$$

$$\Pi^{SL}_{\kappa,ij} = \int_0^\infty dr\, f^{S}_{\kappa,i}(r)\left[\frac{d}{dr} + \frac{\kappa}{r}\right] f^{L}_{\kappa,j}(r) \qquad [5.19]$$

$$J^{TT}_{\kappa,ij} = \sum_{\kappa'kl}(2j'+1)[D^{TT}_{\kappa'kl}\,\mathcal{J}^{0,TT,TT}_{\kappa ij,\kappa'kl} + D^{\overline{TT}}_{\kappa'kl}\,\mathcal{J}^{0,TT,\overline{TT}}_{\kappa ij,\kappa'kl}]$$

$$[5.20]$$

$$K^{TT'}_{\kappa,ij} = \sum_{\nu}\sum_{\kappa'kl}(2j'+1)\,b_\nu(\kappa\kappa')D^{TT'}_{\kappa'kl}\,\mathcal{K}^{\nu,TT',TT'}_{\kappa ij,k'kl}\ .$$

$$[5.21]$$

The superscripts TT represent a pair LS or SL, TT′ may be LL, LS, SL or SS, and TT may be either LL or SS. The two–electron integrals $\mathcal{J}$ and $\mathcal{K}$ are Coulomb and exchange integrals over the radial basis

$$\mathcal{J}^{\nu,TT,T'T'}_{\kappa ij,\kappa'kl} = \int_0^\infty\int_0^\infty f^{T}_{\kappa,i}(r)f^{T}_{\kappa,j}(r)\,U_\nu(r,s)\,f^{T'}_{\kappa',k}(s)f^{T'}_{\kappa',l}(s)\,ds\,dr$$

$$[5.22]$$

$$\mathcal{K}^{\nu,TT,T'T'}_{\kappa ij,\kappa'kl} = \int_0^\infty\int_0^\infty f^{T}_{\kappa,i}(r)f^{T}_{\kappa,j}(s)\,U_\nu(r,s)\,f^{T'}_{\kappa',k}(r)f^{T'}_{\kappa',l}(s)\,ds\,dr$$

$$[5.23]$$

$$U_\nu(r,s) = \begin{cases} r^\nu/s^{\nu+1} & r<s \\ s^\nu/r^{\nu+1} & s<r \end{cases} \qquad [5.24]$$

$D^{TT'}_{\kappa ij}$ is the density matrix

$$D^{TT'}_{\kappa ij} = X^{T}_{\kappa,i}X^{T'}_{\kappa,j} \qquad [5.25]$$

The general form of the Breit interaction matrices is

$$B^{TT}_{\kappa,ij} = \sum_\nu\sum_{\kappa'kl}(2j'+1)e_\nu(\kappa,\kappa')\,D^{\overline{TT}}_{\kappa'kl}\,\mathcal{K}^{\nu,TT,\overline{TT}}_{\kappa ij,\kappa'kl}$$

$$[5.26]$$

$$B_{\kappa,ij}^{T\overline{T}} = \sum_{\nu}\sum_{\kappa' kl} (2j'+1)\left[d_{\nu}(\kappa,\kappa')\, D_{\kappa'\,kl}^{\overline{T}T}\, \kappa_{\kappa i\,j\,,\,\kappa'\,kl}^{\nu,T\overline{T},\overline{T}T} + \right.$$

$$\left. g_{\kappa}(\kappa,\kappa')\, D_{\kappa'\,kl}^{\overline{T}T}\, \mu_{\kappa i\,j\,,\,\kappa'\,kl}^{\nu,T\overline{T},\overline{T}T}\right]$$

[5.27]

where

$$\mu_{\kappa i\,j\,,\,\kappa'\,kl}^{\nu,T\overline{T},\overline{T}T} = \int_0^\infty \int_r^\infty f_{\kappa,i}^{T}(r)f_{\kappa,j}^{\overline{T}}(s)\, U_{\nu}(r,s)\, f_{\kappa',k}^{\overline{T}}(r)f_{\kappa',l}^{T}(s)\ ds\ dr$$

[5.28]

The angular coefficients $b_{\nu}(\kappa\kappa')$, $e_{\nu}(\kappa\kappa')$, $g_{\nu}(\kappa\kappa')$ and $d_{\nu}(\kappa\kappa')$ are derived the graphical techniques described above.

The advantages of employing the finite basis set method in a supercomputing environment are at last apparent. The radial basis functions may always be written as linear combinations of primitive exponential functions, so that the only computational difference between the large and small components lies in the values of the contraction coefficients. The various blocks of two–electron integrals which are required for a Dirac–Hartree–Fock calculation all share a common set of intermediates, the integrals involving exponential functions and the operator $U_k(1,2)$, so that the individual blocks may be constructed using a series of matrix multiplications. The matrix elements vary throughout a self–consistent field calculation, but the basis function integrals are determined once and for all, at the start of the calculation. By the use of linear algebra, the construction of self–consistent fields becomes particularly efficient, and the fact that Coulomb and Breit integrals are constructed from common parts means that there is virtually no computational overhead in treating these effects together. This is a major feature of the method, since the Breit interaction has usually been excluded from the definition of the self–consistent field in finite–diffence calculations because of the cost of evaluating large numbers of additional two–electron integrals at each stage in the iterative procedure.

RADIAL INTEGRAL EVALUATION IN THE MATRIX APPROXIMATION

The use of an analytic basis greatly facilitates the evaluation of the two–electron interaction matrix elements encountered in both Dirac–Hartree–Fock and perturbation theory calculations. Any radial integral involving the Coulomb or low–frequency Breit interactions may be obtained from primitive integrals of the form

$$I_{pqrs}^{\nu,ijkl} = \int_0^\infty \int_0^\infty dr\ ds\ g_p^i(r)\, g_q^j(r)\, U_{\nu}(r,s)\, g_r^k(s)\, g_s^l(s)$$

[6.1]

where

$$g_p^i(r) = r^{\gamma_p + i} \exp(-\xi_p r) \qquad [6.2]$$

$$\gamma_p = (\kappa_p^2 - (Z/c)^2)^{1/2} \qquad [6.3]$$

An expression for this integral is known in terms of elementary functions

$$I_{pqrs}^{\nu,ijkl} = \Gamma(a+b) \left\{ (\xi_{pq})^{-a}(\xi_{rs})^{-b} B(a,b;z) + (\xi_{pq})^{-a'}(\xi_{rs})^{-b'} B(b',a';z') \right\}$$

$$[6.4]$$

where

$$\xi_{pq} = \xi_p + \xi_q \qquad\qquad \xi_{rs} = \xi_r + \xi_s$$

$$a = \gamma_p + \gamma_q + i + j + \nu + 1 \qquad b = \gamma_r + \gamma_s + k + 1 - \nu$$

$$a' = \gamma_p + \gamma_q + i + j - \nu \qquad b' = \gamma_r + \gamma_s + k + 1 + \nu + 1$$

$$z = x/(1 + x) \qquad\qquad z' = x'/(1 + x')$$

$$x = \xi_{pq}/\xi_{rs} \qquad\qquad x' = \xi_{rs}/\xi_{pq} \qquad [6.5]$$

$\Gamma(x)$ is the gamma function and $B(a,b;z)$ is the unnormalized, incomplete beta function

$$\Gamma(x) \qquad = \int_0^\infty t^{x-1}\exp(-t)\, dt \qquad\qquad \mathscr{R}e(x) > 0,$$

$$B(a,b;z) \qquad = \int_0^z t^{a-1}(1-t)^{b-1}\, dt \qquad\qquad 0 \le z \le 1,\ a > 0$$

$$[6.6]$$

The $\mathcal{M}$–type integrals which occur in the Breit matrix elements are readily obtained from the primitive integral by retaining only half of the expression for an $\mathcal{I}$–type integral. The number of evaluations of $\Gamma(x)$ which are required is very small, and standard methods may be employed. The efficient and accurate evaluation of $B(a,b;z)$, however, is central to the success of the relativistic finite basis set method for atoms. The continued fraction representation

$$B(a,b;z) = a^{-1} z^a (1 - z)^b \left[\frac{1}{1\ +} \ \frac{k_1}{1\ +} \ \frac{k_2}{1\ +} \cdots \right] \qquad [6.7]$$

where

$$k_{2m+1} = -\frac{(a + m)(a + b + m)z}{(a + m)(a + 2m + 1)} \qquad [6.8]$$

$$k_{2m} = -\frac{m(b-m)z}{(a+2m-1)(a+2m)} \qquad [6.9]$$

has proved to be efficient in the numerical evaluation of the incomplete beta function. The program SWIRLES also makes use of the linear transformation

$$B(a,b;z) = B(a,b) - B(b,a;1-z) \qquad [6.10]$$

where $B(a,b)$ is the complete beta function. This transformation accelerates the convergence of the calculation of the incomplete beta function for $z > (a-1)/(a+b+2)$, and greatly reduces the effects of accumulated numerical errors.

The radial matrix elements of the Coulomb and low—frequency Breit interactions for a particular index set $\{p,q,r,s\}$ depend on primitive integrals which differ in tensor order, ν, and on each of the indices in the set $\{i,j,k,l\}$ which typically take all four—index combinations of 0 and 1. The sixteen allowed combinations of the indices $\{i,j,k,l\}$, which arise as a consequence of the contraction of exponential functions may be reduced to nine unique cases by exploiting integral symmetry. At both the Dirac—Hartree—Fock and many—body perturbation theory levels of approximation, the two—electron supermatrices for all the allowed combinations of radial components may be generated simultaneously, because the primitive integrals are stored as tables of intermediates which are later formed into integral lists. The set of integral lists which is required to perform a relativistic matrix calculation has the labels [LL|LL], [LL|SS], [SS|LL], [SS|SS], [SL|SL] and [SL|LS], but each of the lists differ only in the combination of contraction coefficients for the large— and small—components, and may be constructed from a common set of intermediates.

As a further feature of this approach, we may allow the numerical value of the speed of light, c, to become very much larger than its real value ($c \simeq 137$). It may be shown that the matrix representation of the Dirac—Hartree—Fock equations is equivalent to the representation of the non—relativistic Hartree—Fock approximation in a corresponding basis of exponential—type radial functions. A large numerical value for c corresponds to the classical limit of signals being transmitted instantaneously between two separated points.

A series of stable recurrence relations have been implemented in SWIRLES which connect all the incomplete beta functions implied by the indices $\{i,j,k,l,\nu\}$ for a given argument z or z', so that calculations involving f—orbitals which typically require ninety values of the incomplete beta function for a given set of indices $\{p,q,r,s\}$ actually requires the explicit evaluation of only four elements in the list. In terms of the normalized incomplete beta function,

$$I(a,b;z) = B(a,b;z)/B(a,b) \qquad [6.11]$$

a table of values may be generated by repeated use of the rules

$$I(a,b;z) = zI(a-1,b;z) + (1-z) I(a,b-1;z)$$

$$(a + b - ab)I(a,b;z) = a(1-z)I(a+1,b-1;z) + bI(a,b+1;z)$$

$$(a + b)I(a,b;z) = a\, I(a+1,b;z) + b\, I(a,b+1;z) \qquad [6.12]$$

starting from $I(a_0,b_0;z)$ and $I(a_0+1,b_0;z)$ and then stepping through all the functions $I(a_0+m,b_0+n;z)$ for $0 \leq m \leq M$ and $0 \leq n \leq N$ and predetermined values of a_0, b_0, M and N.

A unique feature of the use of analytic finite basis set methods and a recursive strategy for integral evaluation is that the inclusion of the both the Coulomb and

Breit interactions at all stages of a self–consistent field calculation is actually *preferred* to the usual approach, which is based on the Dirac–Coulomb operator and the perturbative evaluation of magnetic and retarded interaction, on the grounds of computational economy. The diagonal submatrices of the Coulomb and Breit matrices share the same integral lists and so there is no need to store the Coulomb and Breit integrals separately. Only the Breit submatrix B_κ^{SL} requires an additional integral list which is distinct from those required in calculations based on the Dirac–Coulomb hamiltonian. This additional list is not prohibitively long and may often be shortened by the use of integral symmetry.

The computational feature of both schemes which are proposed above for the evaluation of two–electron radial integrals is that they are recursive. Each step in the continued fraction evaluation of the incomplete beta function depends on the value from the previous step, so that the algorithm is not a promising candidate for efficient processing on a supercomputer. The subsequent use of linear recurrence relations greatly reduces the number of arithmetic operations involved in generating the the two–electron integrals list, but their recursive structure may take no advantage of vector architecture in the form that they are presented above. In the second of these lectures, we will see how a rearrangement of the data may be used to free these methods of their recursive dependencies, leading to a scheme which makes efficient use of a vector–processing machine.

MANY–BODY PERTURBATION THEORY

The evaluation of many–body corrections to observable quantities through the use of perturbation theory requires all the features discussed above, together with new methods which generate long lists of matrix elements with the fewest possible number of floating point operations. The new feature is the need to perform a four–index transformation, from integrals over basis functions, $<ij|kl>$, to matrix elements over spinors, $<ab|cd>$. A naive representation of this is

$$<ab|cd> = \sum_{ijkl} C_a^i \cdot C_b^j \cdot C_c^k \cdot C_d^l <ij|kl> \qquad [7.1]$$

where C_a^i is the expansion coefficient of the state $|a>$ in terms of the ith basis function. It is assumed that the coefficients are real, which is true in the present case because of the convention which has been adopted in the definition of the radial Dirac equation. Each of the labels a,b,c,d,i,j,k,l may takes any value 1,2,3,...,N, so that a complete transformation of this type depends varies as N^8. The situation is actually worse than it appears, because, the component labels have been suppressed. The complete matrix element $<AB|CD>$ is a sum of eight allowed combinations of radial functions involved in the effective interaction strengths of the Coulomb and Breit interactions and there is a further summation over the allowed values of the tensor order, L, with an associated angular factor at each order. The problem may be streamlined by the use of a series of matrix multiplications

$$<ij|kd> = \sum_l C_d^l <ij|kl> \qquad [7.2a]$$

$$<ij|cd> = \sum_k C_c^k <ij|kd> \qquad [7.2b]$$

$$<ib|cd> = \sum_j C_b^j <ij|cd> \qquad\qquad [7.2c]$$

$$<ab|cd> = \sum_i C_a^i <ib|cd> \qquad\qquad [7.2d]$$

The component labels (large or small) have again been suppressed in the indices a,b,c,d,i,j,k,l. In general, this transformation, which scales as $4N^5$, must be performed blockwise for each of the allowed combinations $<LL|LL>$, $<LL|SS>$, $<SS|LL>$, $<SS|SS>$, $<SL|SL>$, $<SL|LS>$, $<LS|LS>$ and $<LS|SL>$. Significant savings in both storage requirement and computational volume may be made by generating the basis function integrals and performing simultaneously the first two partial transformations. The lists $\{<LL|LL> + <LL|SS>\}$, $\{<SS|LL> + <SS|SS>\}$, $\{<SL|SL> + <SL|LS>\}$ and $\{<LS|LS> + <LS|SL>\}$ may then be stored in a combined format, because the subsequent partial transformations of the $<LL|$, $<LS|$, $<SL|$ and $<SS|$ pair–densities are independent of the preceding transformations.

Once a list of matrix elements has been assembled, energy corrections may be evaluated using many–body perturbation theory. At second–order in perturbation theory, the correction to the Dirac–Hartree–Fock energy, E_2, is given by

$$E_2 = \frac{1}{2} \sum_{abrs} \frac{<ab|rs><rs|ab>}{\epsilon_a + \epsilon_b - \epsilon_r - \epsilon_s} - \frac{1}{2} \sum_{abrs} \frac{<ab|rs><rs|ba>}{\epsilon_a + \epsilon_b - \epsilon_r - \epsilon_s}$$

$$[7.3]$$

The first summation is the so–called direct term, and the second is the exchange term. We may now exploit the graphical methods which were developed earlier, and introduce the theorems of Yutsis, Levinson and Vanagas to simplify the calculation of angular factors.

The direct term has the graphical representation

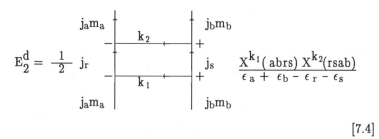

$$[7.4]$$

The exchange term has the graphical representation

$$E_2^e = -\frac{1}{2} \ j_r \qquad \frac{X^{k_1}(abrs)\, X^{k_2}(rsba)}{\epsilon_a + \epsilon_b - \epsilon_r - \epsilon_s}$$

$$[7.5]$$

where we have used the rule that there is an implicit summation over internal magnetic substates. Both of these diagrams are then closed by joining the free ends of the diagrams with common angular momentum labels, so that the dependence on the magnetic quantum numbers vanishes. Note that the summation over the tensor indices k_1 and k_2 is implicit.

The evaluation of these diagrams, and the more complicated examples which arise in higher orders of perturbation theory, is simplified by graphical rules, which are easy to implement in special cases such as the above, and which have been coded in published computer programs which are able to deal with difficult cases involving the coupling of up to sixty angular momenta. A selection of these rules, which are relevent to second–order perturbation theory calculations are

$$\{j_1, j_2, j_3\} = \quad j_3 \left(\!\! \begin{array}{c} + \\ j_2 \\ - \end{array} \!\! \right) j_1 \qquad \qquad [7.6]$$

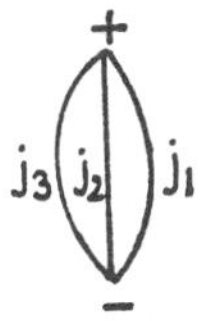

which takes the value zero, unless the triangular delta condition, $|j_1 - j_2| \leq j_3 \leq (j_1 + j_2)$ is satisfied, when it takes the value one. A Wigner 6–j symbol is written

$$\begin{Bmatrix} j_1 & j_2 & j_3 \\ j_4 & j_5 & j_6 \end{Bmatrix} = + \quad \text{} \quad + \qquad [7.7]$$

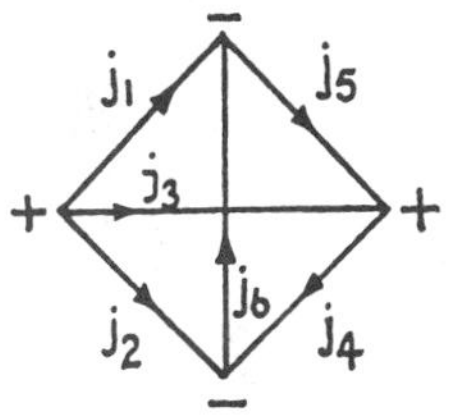

These are the primary structures to which any angular momentum diagram is reduced. The rules of reduction are based on a theorem which states that the angular momentum of the connecting line labelled j in the diagram

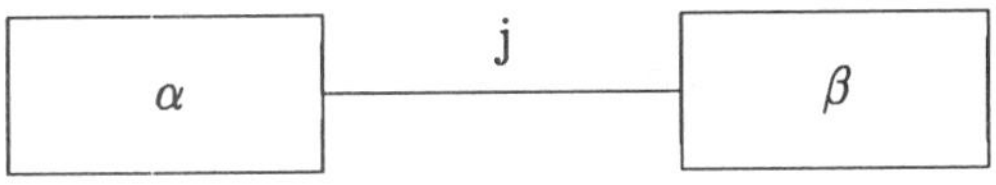

$$[7.8]$$

must be equal to zero. The boxes represent parts of a complete angular diagram, and it is required that one of them, α, contains no free lines, and that each of its internal lines has precisely one arrow. A number of results based on this theorem are known. We require, at second–order in perturbation theory, the theorem for diagrams separable on one line (called YLV1)

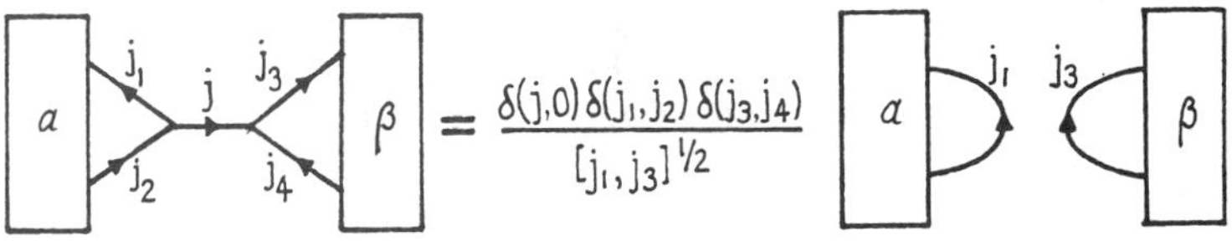

$$\text{} = \frac{\delta(j,0)\,\delta(j_1,j_2)\,\delta(j_3,j_4)}{[j_1,j_3]^{1/2}} \quad \text{} \qquad [7.9]$$

and the theorem for diagrams separable on two lines (YLV2)

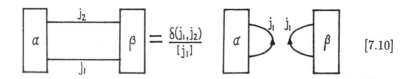

$$\frac{\delta(j_1,j_2)}{[j_1]}$$

[7.10]

The direct and exchange diagrams then take the explicit algebraic forms

$$E_2^d = -\frac{1}{2} \sum_{\substack{abrs \\ k}} (-1)^{j_a + j_b + j_r + j_s} \{j_a, j_r, k\}\{j_b, j_s, k\} \frac{1}{[k]} \frac{X^k(abrs)X^k(rsab)}{\epsilon_a + \epsilon_b - \epsilon_r - \epsilon_s}$$

[7.11]

$$E_2^e = -\frac{1}{2} \sum_{\substack{abrs \\ k_1 k_2}} (-1)^{j_a + j_b + j_r + j_s} \begin{bmatrix} j_r & j_b & k_2 \\ j_s & j_a & k_1 \end{bmatrix} \frac{X^{k_1}(abrs)X^{k_2}(rsba)}{\epsilon_a + \epsilon_b - \epsilon_r - \epsilon_s}$$

[7.12]

In general, the evaluation of the terms in relativistic many–body theory are reduced to formulae involving the calculation of effective interaction strengths, $X^k(abcd)$, phase factors, and Wigner n–j symbols. These features have been assembled into a FORTRAN module, XKABCD, which evaluates lists of effective interaction strengths using continued fraction representations and recurrence relations in the calculation of basis set integrals, together with the linear transformation of the basis integrals using a series of partial transformations. The use of CRAY Assembler Language (CAL) subroutines for the matrix multiplications involved in the four–index transformation and for the sums–over–states in each of the many–body diagrams relieves the bottleneck in this most expensive part of a relativistic many–body calculation, at the expense of abandoning standard FORTRAN and the consequent loss of program portability. The very high rate of computation which may be achieved by matching numerical algorithms to the architecture of a supercomputing machine has made possible the routine evaluation of relativistic many–body effects.

SUMMARY

The contents of this lecture provide a fairly complete account of the relativistic finite basis set method for atoms, so I will summarize briefly the aims and difficulties of the method with a minimum of technical detail.

The relativistic theory of atomic structure is based on the expansion of the many–electron wavefunction in a complete set of single–particle states. In the finite basis set method, this complete set is represented by a discrete, square–integrable set, which is constructed from linear combinations of radial exponential–type functions and an implicit representation of the angular functions. The major computational components in any model of atomic structure are the determination of the radial amplitudes, and the evaluation of radial two–body effective interaction strengths. Radial integrals over basis functions are expressed in terms of higher transcendental functions and linear recurrence relations, so that all quadrature is performed to machine accuracy. All errors are confined to the truncation of the finite basis and the limitations of computers with a finite wordlength. The angular dependencies are handled algebraically, and may be expressed in terms of graphs with well–defined values.

Recursive dependencies in the evaluation of the two–body reduced matrix elements limit the performance which could be expected from the direct implementation of the methods which have described in this lecture. Most of the operations are on scalar quantities, rather than on the vector–valued entities which reflect the architecture of a supercomputer. I wish to emphasize that it is the matching of the algorithm to the capabilities of the machine which yields the greatest benefit; a reliance on the current generation of compilers to "work it out" is doomed to failure if the source code which is presented to them contains essentially scalar structures.

As an illustration, very early versions of the methods described above were so slow, even on the CRAY X–MP/48, that modest self–consistent field calculations were prohibitively expensive. In the current implementaton of these algorithms, self–consistent field and all–electron many–body perturbation theory calculations are possible for elements as heavy as radon, with further refinements opening up the possibility of modelling observable effects due to the subtle interplay of relativity and quantum electrodynamics. The implementation of these numerical techniques in the atomic structure program, SWIRLES, is the subject of the second lecture.

RELATIVISTIC ATOMIC STRUCTURE CALCULATIONS II:

COMPUTATIONAL ASPECTS OF THE FINITE BASIS SET METHOD

Harry Quiney

Department of Theoretical Chemistry, Unversity of Oxford, Oxford OX1 3UB

INTRODUCTION

In the first of these lectures, we examined the basic theory of relativistic electronic structure calculations. The principal computational requirement in the determination of Dirac spinors within the Dirac–Hartree–Fock (DHF) approximation involves the solution of coupled first–order integro–differential equations. The traditional approach employs the finite–difference techniques introduced by Hartree in the calculation of non–relativistic self–consistent fields. The scheme is highly accurate and has been implemented by hand, on mechanical calculators and on electronic computers, for which many FORTRAN programs have been published. The first successful relativistic mean–field calculation using the finite–difference approximation, but which approximated the exchange potential, was performed by Williams in 1940. Today, a number of sophisticated programs are freely available as black–box atomic structure models which perform self–consistent field and multi–configurational calculations, but which are are not suited ideally to the calculation of relativistic many–body effects and which do not exhibit a computational structure which is compatible with the architecture of supercomputing machines.

The radial modules of the computer program SWIRLES represent a departure from the traditional finite–difference methods of atomic physics. The radial DHF equations are solved using a variant of the Rayleigh–Ritz method which has been developed to overcome a number of problems associated with relativistic finite basis set expansions. The finite basis set form of the DHF equations was presented by Synek (1964) and Kim (1967) and an extensive review of the special problems associated with the method was given by Kutzelnigg (1984). SWIRLES utilizes a basis set which suffers from none of the shortcomings of earlier attempts to implement the finite basis set method for relativistic problems, and which gives energies and expectation values which are comparable in accuracy with finite–difference techniques. The algorithm is structured to exploit the architecture of modern parallel computers, and the representation of the complete Dirac spectrum allows the rapid evaluation of many–body effects using perturbative expansions. The scheme fits naturally within modern formulations of quantum electrodynamics, since the square–integrable representation of the spectrum allows the evaluation of Feynman–like diagrams by a finite summation over intermediate states of both positive– and negative–energy. Quadrature is carried out to machine accuracy because all integrals over basis functions which are required for DHF or MBPT

Supercomputational Science
Edited by R.G. Evans and S. Wilson
Plenum Press, New York, 1990

calculations may be reduced to simple linear combinations of higher transcendental functions.

PROGRAM ORGANIZATION

The calculation of atomic properties using the finite basis set approximation may be divided into three major sections. The calculation of relativistic atomic structures may be described by the following set of procedures

STAGE 1: Determination of relativistic self—consistent fields

1. Input specification of the atom or ion to be modelled. The specification includes the nuclear charge, the choice of Hamiltonian, the basis set parameters for the reference orbitals and the reference configuration

2. Calculate all one— and two—electron integrals required for the determination of the specified self—consistent field, and store in external files in supervector format

3. Initialize expansion coefficients of the reference orbitals based on a guess for the atomic potential. A bare nucleus potential is used, but a screened potential is preferable, and would yield more rapidly convergent results

4. The expansion coefficients of the reference orbitals of each symmetry— type are updated, by constructing the Fock matrix from the current estimates of the expansion coefficients.

5. There is an iterative cycle through the symmetry—types until the change in the expansion coefficients is less than some specified tolerance. If the convergence criterion is not satisfied, return to step 4, otherwise proceed to step 6

6. Calculate expectation values of operators, such as the Hamiltonian, r^k and the Breit operator. A complete specification of the Dirac—Hartree— Fock atom, including the expansion coefficients of the reference orbitals and the orbital eigenvalues, is written to an external master file.

A rather special feature of the DHF method is that the total energy need not approach the converged energy from above, as it does in non—relativistic theory. This is because some intermediate approximations to the DHF states contain admixtures of the negative energy spectrum corresponding to the converged self—consistent field potential. This presents no fundamental difficulty, since the DHF approximation represents a stationary point in energy with repect to the variation of the expansion coefficients, rather than an absolute minimum, as is found in the non—relativistic Schrodinger theory.

The second major section of the scheme evaluates the virtual spectrum of the Dirac operator with the specified external self—consistent field potential. The procedure is

STAGE II: Calculation of the virtual spectrum

1. Input the specification of each of the virtual symmetry—types, and the corresponding description of the basis set parameters. This information is appended to the master file, containing the definition of the system and the coefficients and energies which constitute the reference orbitals.

2. Generate the two–electron integral list required for each virtual symmetry–type, construct the corresponding Fock matrix, and determine the expansion coefficients and orbital energies for each of the states in the spectrum.

3. Write the expansion coefficients and orbital energies for each state in each symmetry–type to the master file

The master file now contains a specification of the atom, in terms of the number of bound–state electrons, the nuclear charge, the physical effects contained in the Hamiltonian, the reference orbitals and orbital energies, and a discrete representation of the virtual–state spectrum of the Dirac equation corresponding to a specified static external field. This list, containing a few thousand numbers, may be thought of as a very compact and detailed definition of the underlying physical model which is central to the relativistic theory of atomic structure. Usually known as the Furry bound–state interaction picture, the many–electron wavefunction of a complex atom is expanded in a complete set of single–particle Dirac spinors, where it is emphasized that such a set contains states of both "positive" and "negative" energy in a relativistic theory.

The contents of the master file may be regarded as a discrete representation of the fundamental theory, which we may refine by increasing the dimension of the radial basis set used for each symmetry–type, and by increasing the number of symmetry–types included in the spectral list. In either case, it is the completeness of the set of single–particle states which is sought, so that the asymptotic behaviour of a sequence of finite representations may be used to estimate the value of observable quantities calculated using a complete set.

All other operations which are encountered are of a purely computational nature. The usual presentation of relativistic quantum field theory emphasizes the calculation of the terms in a perturbation series represented by an infinite set of Feynman diagrams. Once a potential has been chosen, and the spectrum determined (in Stages I and II), a sequence of approximations to the many–body wavefunction is generated by constructing linear combinations of the single–particle states (Stage III).

The choice of potential determines the rate of convergence of the perturbation expansion, and we have chosen a self–consistent field potential because it seems reasonable that this should provide a good approximation to the true atomic potential. Now that the file of single–particle state exists, we could emphasize the integrated nature of the formalism, by calculating the zero– and first–order energies in many–body perturbation theory. We would find that the zero–order energy was numerically equal to the classical Dirac–Hartree–Fock energy, the first–order energy correction would vanish, since this is actually a restatement of the self–consistency requirement, and many–body corrections would begin at second–order in perturbation theory. In practice there is little point in recalculating quantities whose values are already known from Stage I of the procedure.

We are left with Stage III, which, from a formal viewpoint, summarizes the entire computational content of relativistic atomic structure theory

STAGE III: Relativistic Many–Body Perturbation Theory

1. Specify a set of many–body diagrams. It is usual to use the DHF results as the zero–order approximation, and to ignore the first–order term if a self–consistent field potential is employed. If we choose the set of bare nuclear states, by suppressing the iterative determination of the self–consistent field potential, then the lower–order diagrams must be specified.

2. Generate all the basis set integrals which are required to evaluate a given diagram and perform a series of linear transformations to construct blocks of matrix elements

3. Evaluate the diagrams by summing over complete sets of single–particle states

At high–order in perturbation theory, this simple prescription becomes prohibitively expensive, because of the increasingly deep nesting of the summation variables. Experience has shown that highly accurate electronic structure approximations are obtained at fourth–order in perturbation theory, which is within the technical limitations of current supercomputers. The particular advantage of this method, compared with a "configuration interaction" approach, which approximates the complete Dirac matrix and then performs a diagonalization to yield a many–body spectrum, is that each of the diagrams may be thought of as a sequence of matrix multiplications, which are particularly efficient operations on a supercomputer. An additional advantage is gained by the partitioning of the many–body problem into diagrams, and symmetry classifications, because the storage requirements are modest and the calculation may be performed entirely in fast–core memory.

If we analyse each of the Stages in a relativistic atomic structure calculation, two operations dominate the total computational requirement; the generation of two–electron integrals over the primary basis functions, and the subsequent transformation of these integrals into relativistic matrix elements. The second of these topics is identical to the problem encountered in non–relativistic quantum chemistry, and will be discussed by other lecturers at this Summer School. The rate of calculation of the two–electron integrals is determined largely by the efficiency with which the incomplete beta functions are generated. The discussion of this problem follows closely the sequence of refinements which I have made to an essentially scalar algorithm in order to extract an acceptable performance on the CRAY XMP/48. I make no claim that these changes are optimal; the overall improvement in performance, however, has made possible calculations which were prohibitively expensive using a scalar algorithm and the general principles involved are of value for a large number of similar problems unconnected with atomic structure theory. The modifications have been restricted to standard FORTRAN 77, in order to preserve portability of the program. The discussion of the evaluation of incomplete beta functions using the continued fraction and linear recurrence relations is set in the context of the FORTRAN subroutines BETAVEC and BETTAB, which are implemented in the atomic structure program, SWIRLES.

SUBROUTINE BETAVEC(ZT,BTEMP,ID,IZZ,NZZ,ITRAN)

BETAVEC evaluates blocks of normalized incomplete beta functions using a continued fraction algorithm. In order to minimise the number of steps involved in the continued fraction representation of the function, use has been made of the transformation

$$I(a,b;Z) = 1 - I(b,a;1-Z) \qquad [3.1]$$

where $I(A,B;Z)$ is the normalized incomplete beta function, which has the integral representation

$$I(a,b;Z) = \frac{1}{B(a,b)} \int_0^x t^{a-1}(1-t)^{b-1} dt \qquad [3.2]$$

where B(a,b) is the (complete) beta function

$$B(a,b) = \frac{\Gamma(a)\ \Gamma(b)}{\Gamma(a+b)}$$ [3.3]

Some intermediate quantities used in BETAVEC are initialized in a prior call to the module BETASET.

ZT(128) is a list of up to 128 values of the argument Z for fixed values of A and B for which the incomplete beta function is required. They must all be in the range 0–1 and sorted so that the function is to be evaluated using either the transformed or untransformed representation. The values of Z, which are unordered, will all be either greater or less than some critical value, which is stored as ZTEST in the initialization call to BETASET.

BTEMP(128) contains the output list of incomplete beta functions in correspondence to the input argument values in ZT(M)

ID is a label indicating the appropriate set of coefficients for the incomplete beta function representation. The label takes the values 1–8 (inclusive), corresponding to up to 4 classes of incomplete beta function per symmetry block with an additional factor of two arising from the transformed variants

IZZ is a label indicating which of the parameter sets (pairs {A,B}) is being used. This defines the "class" of incomplete beta function required for a block of integrals.

NZZ is the number of non–zero values of the argument stored in the vector ZT(M). May take values in the range 0–128 (inclusive).

ITRAN is a label indicating whether the transformed (ITRAN=1) or untransformed (ITRAN=0) representation is being used

The argument values are calculated from the exponential parameters and lie in the range 0–1. A call to BETAVEC is made when the list ZT is full (containing 128 elements) or at the end of a block to complete the list (containing less than 128 elements). The value of 128 was chosen as a reasonable compromise between the desire to vectorize this section of the code and the need to minimise the additional storage requirements of efficient vector code.

The value of ZMATCH (the change–over point between the untransformed and transformed representations of I(A,B;Z)) is chosen to be the value of Z for which the number of arithmetic operations for the two forms is approximately equal. The "textbook" value of ZMATCH is (A+1)/(A+B−2) but in practice it was found that this was only a rough guide if either parameter takes a value greater than 5. It is found that the number of continued fraction steps is a very slowly varying function of Z up to the matching point. Only very small values of the argument require substantially fewer terms, but the number of such integrals is small and their numerical values contribute negligibly to electronic matrix elements. Values of Z close to either zero or one occur when two–electron integrals are required between two exponential charge distributions, one of which has a small characteristic length while the other is very diffuse. The interaction is small, because the overlap is small. The decision was made to choose a single value of ITMAX (the number of continued fraction convergents evaluated) for all functions of a given "class". This introduces no numerically significant error, and eliminates the need to place the arguments into rank order and the sorting processes that would accompany such a procedure. This is a compromise which was made to simplify the code and to enhance the vectorizability of the algorithm.

The implementation of the continued fraction algorithm used in this module provides an interesting example of how a recursive algorithm, which is not a promising candidate for efficient vector processing, may be adapted to exploit the architecture of a supercomputer if it is recognised that the procedure is to be executed for a large number of independent values of the argument. The recursive part of the algorithm, which requires values computed in previous passes through the iterative procedure is moved to an outer loop. The computation of intermediate quantities for a vector of independent values of the argument is moved to the inner loop, and processed as a vector. It is not the continued fraction algorithm which is being adapted to the requirements of vector processing, because the recursive structure remains as an outer non–vectorizable loop. The intermediate quantities in the algorithm, which contribute to the convergents of the continued fraction, are generated as vectors of length NZZ, and it is here that improvements to execution rate of the program may be made, at the expense of increased storage requirements.

The continued fraction representation of the normalized incomplete beta function is

$$I(a,b;z) = \frac{z^a(1-z)^b}{a\,B(a,b)} \left\{ \frac{1}{1+} \frac{d_1}{1+} \frac{d_2}{1+} \cdots \right\} \qquad [3.3]$$

where

$$d_{2m+1} = -\frac{(a+m)(a+b+m)}{(a+2m)(a+2m+1)} \qquad [3.4a]$$

$$d_{2m} = \frac{m(b-m)}{(a+2m-1)(a+2m)} \qquad [3.4b]$$

The continued fraction representation is then expressed as a rational function approximation, such that

$$f_n = \frac{A_n}{B_n} \qquad [3.5]$$

where A_n and B_n are given by the recurrence relations

$$A_{-1} = 0 \qquad B_{-1} = 0$$

$$A_0 = 1 \qquad B_0 = 1$$

$$A_j = A_{j-1} + d_j A_{j-2}$$

$$B_j = B_{j-1} + d_j B_{j-2} \qquad j=1,2,\ldots, n \qquad [3.6]$$

The quantity f_n is called the nth convergent of the function f, which is currently the incomplete beta function. A FORTRAN subroutine of this representation has been published recently, as part of the set of "Numerical Recipes".

With some scalar optimization, this sub—program could be placed in a loop and a table of incomplete beta functions evaluated with few additional changes. The values of A and B are preset, and are not whole numbers.

```
C
C*** ASSIGN SCALAR VARIABLES (REPRESENTATIVE VALUES ARE SHOWN)
C
      ITMAX=15
      ONE=1.0
      EPS=1.0E-14
      QAB=A+B
      QAP=A+ONE
      QAM=A-ONE
      QABP=QAB/QAP
C
C*** STORE ODD AND EVEN CONTINUED FRACTION COEFFICIENTS
C*** DODD(M) AND DEVEN(M), RESPECTIVELY
C
      DO 10 I=1,ITMAX
      EM=FLOAT(M)
      EM2=EM+EM
      DODD(I)=-(A+EM)*(A+B+EM2)/((A+EM)*(A*EM2+ONE))
      DEVEN(I)=EM*(B-EM)/((A+EM2-ONE)*(A+EM2))
10    CONTINUE
C
C*** LOOP OVER ALL VALUES OF Z=ZT(IZ), STORE THE FINAL CONTINUED FRACTION
C*** IN BTEMP(IZ)
C
      DO 40 IZ=1,NZZ
      Z=ZT(IZ)
C
C*** ASSIGN INITIAL VALUES OF THE CONVERGENTS
C
      AM=ONE
      BM=ONE
      AZ=ONE
      BZ=ONE-QABP*Z
      DO 20 M=1,ITMAX
      D=DEVEN(M)*Z
      AP=AZ+D*AM
      BP=BZ+D*BM
      D=DODD(M)*Z
      APP=AP+D*AZ
      BPP=BP+D*BZ
      AOLD=AZ
      AM=AP/BPP
      BM=BP/BPP
      AZ=APP/BPP
      BZ=ONE
C*** TEST FOR CONVERGENCE (EPS = CONVERGENCE PARAMETER)
      IF(ABS(AZ-AOLD).LT.EPS*ABS(AZ)) GO TO 30
20    CONTINUE
30    CONTINUE
      BTEMP(IZ)=AZ
40    CONTINUE
```

We could make some scalar improvement to this by assuming that ITMAX=ITMAX(Z), although this will have little effect unless Z is very close to zero, and it is further assumed that none of the elements of ZT(M) has a value greater than $(A-1)/(A+B-2)$. Whatever we do, the rate of execution of the above code will be far less than maximum on any vector–processing machine, because the assignment to the numerator and denominator of each convergent, APP and BPP, respectively, depends on quantities which were calculated in the previous iteration. To make matters worse, the minimum value of ITMAX which is required to evaluate a continued fraction to machine accuracy is typically far less than 10, so that even if the contents of the loop with label 20 contained only vector instructions, the overheads in starting the loop would probably minimize any improvements which might occur due to vector processing. The length of the vector is at the "break–even" point for a CRAY–XMP, and for older machines, the cost of initializing the loop would far outweigh any gains.

Atomic structure calculations require the evaluation of lists of incomplete beta functions with around 1 million elements; the actual number scales as N^4 where N is the number of radial basis functions. Early experiments using a naive implementation of the continued fraction algorithm similar in structure to the code shown above indicated that the execution rate on the CRAY/XMP at RAL is about 1–2 MFLOP, the overall rate of execution of the atomic structure program was less than 10 MFlop, the difference being attributable to some sections which performed linear algebra operations. If it is recalled that the maximum rate of execution quoted by CRAY Research ("the rate you are guaranteed never to exceed") is 235 MFlop on a single processor, then it is clear that such a program wastes an extremely valuable and expensive resource.

An effective general strategy for the efficient vector processing of an algorithm which seems to have recursive dependencies is to identify long, non–recursive loops containing only operations on the elements of vectors and to move these to the inner–most locations in nests. In the current case, the only option is to move the loop labelled 40 to the innermost position. The parameter NZZ typically takes the value 128, so we have fulfilled the requirement that the loop should be longer than the "break–even" value, and satisfied a subsidiary condition that it should be a multiple of 64, which reflects the particular architecture of a CRAY/XMP. It is certain that the inner loop of this structure need contain no recursive assignments, because we know that the values of ZT(M) are independent, but some of the intermediate quantities need to stored, if the convergents for each of the values of the argument are to be vector–processed. The test for convergence will also inhibit vectorization, so ITMAX is set to the number of terms required for the largest value in the vector ZT(M).

Examination of the code above reveals that the variables AM, BM and AZ are set to unity for the first iteration, and that BZ is set to unity for all subsequent iterations. Since the only operation performed by these variables is multiplication, we can avoid redundant multiplications by unity by splitting the loop which evaluates the convergents into two sections; the first initializes the convergents given that AM, BM and AZ all equal unity on entry, and the second updates the values of these variables, and recognises that BZ (which represents the denominator of each level of the rational function approximation) is unity for each subsequent iteration. Since AM, BM and AZ are the only variables whose values are required from the previous iteration, we store these values for each value of Z in a vector. The variable BZ must be initialized at the first iteration for each Z, so the additional storage which is required to enable efficient vectorization of the algorithm consists of four vectors, so we require the additional DIMENSION statement

```
      DIMENSION AM(128),BM(128),AZ(128),BZ(128)
C
C*** INITIALIZE THE VECTOR BZ(M)
C
      DO 1 M=1,NZZ
1     BZ(M)=ONE-QABP*ZT(M)
```

```
C
C*** INITIALIZE THE VECTORS AM,BM,AZ, CORRESPONDING TO THE FIRST
C    ITERATION OF THE ORIGINAL CODE: THEIR ORIGINAL VALUE OF UNITY
C    IS IMPLICIT
C
      DE=DEVEN(1)
      DO=DODD(1)
      DO 4 M=1,NZZ
       DDE=DE*ZT(M)
       DDO=DO*ZT(M)
       AP=ONE+DDE
       BP=BZ(M)+DDE
       APP=AP+DDO
       BPP=BP+DDO*BZ(M)
       AM(M)=AP/BPP
       BM(M)=BP/BPP
       AZ(M)=APP/BPP
4     CONTINUE
C
C*** THE VALUE BZ(M) IS NOW UNITY: THIS VALUE IS IMPLIED BUT NOT
C*** OPERATED ON.
C
      DO 5 IM=2,NZSUM
      DE=DEVEN(IM)
      DO=DODD(IM)
      DO 3 M=1,NZZ
       DDE=DE*ZT(M)
       DDO=DO*ZT(M)
       AP=AZ(M)+DDE*AM(M)
       BP=ONE+DDE*BM(M)
       APP=AP+DDE*BM(M)
       BPPOO=ONE/(BPZ+DDO)
       AM(M)=AP*BPPOO
       BM(M)=BP*BPPOO
       AZ(M)=APP*BPPOO
3     CONTINUE
5     CONTINUE
```

Not much can be done with the factor $(Z{**}A)*((ONE{-}Z){**}(ONE{-}B))$ which multiplies the continued fraction, since the values of A and B are unrelated, and are not whole numbers. Some exponentiation is unavoidable and this becomes an important component in the total computing time.

The overall gain in computation rate of the second section of code compared to the first is remarkable. The rate of execution of BETAVEC is approximately 130 MFlops, which represents an increase in speed by a factor of 100 compared to the scalar code. In early versions of the atomic program SWIRLES, the evaluation of the incomplete beta functions represented the rate–limiting step in the calculation of electronic wavefunctions. The most expensive parts of the calculation of self–consistent field problems are now the construction of the two–electron interaction matrix (Module GMAT) and the construction of the two–electron supervector elements (Module SUPVEC), which both contain substantial scalar code and I/O. The overall rate of computation of SWIRLES is close to 70 MFlops for large SCF problems, and typical execution times lie in the range 10–30 seconds, so that the careful development of code which exploits the machine architecture has transformed the method from an unwieldly and expensive curiosity into the "state–of–the–art".

SUBROUTINE BETTAB(NZTERM)

BETTAB exploits the linear recursions which connect incomplete beta functions with a common argument and with parameter values which differ by integers. The incomplete beta function is a special case of the hypergeometric function, and the linear recurrence relations are special cases of Gauss's "contiguous" relations connecting hypergeometric functions. In common with the relations which connect other higher transcendental functions, the recurrences are usually stable in a single direction, and over limited ranges of the parameters. The stable directions of recurrence are best determined by experiment; the propagation of error in the recurrence is attributable to the alternative forms of the solutions to the differential equations of which the higher transcendental functions are themselves solutions. The recurrences represent identities in exact arithmetic, but in a finite word—length representation it is impossible to exclude unwanted admixtures of spurious solutions.

The directions of recursion in BETTAB were determined by experiment, and have been tested for the range of parameter values which are encountered in atomic physics. Stability to machine accuracy is achieved in almost all cases. Only if the argument is very close to zero does the value obtained by recurrence differ substantially from the function value obtained by direct evaluation of the continued fraction representation. In this case, however, the value of the normalized incomplete beta function is very close to zero, and the effect of recursion is to cause the entry in the table to vanish prematurely. This causes no significant error in the execution of the atomic physics program as a whole, because a very small value of Z corresponds to the interaction of two exponential charge distributions with negligible overlap, which could be excluded by a physical argument and which gives no numerically significant contribution to the electronic energy or the functional form of any single—particle function.

NZTERM is the number of values of Z for which tables of incomplete beta functions are to be constructed.

The coefficients which are required for the recursive evaluation of the blocks are generated and stored by module BETASET; a call to this routine must precede a call to either BETAVEC or BETTAB for each set of angular quantum numbers.

The linear recurrence relations which are used in this module are

$$I(a,b;z) = zI(a-1,b;z) + (1-z)I(a,b-1;z) \qquad [4.1]$$

$$I(a,b;z) = \frac{1}{a+b} \left\{ a(I(a+1,b;z) + bI(a,b+1;z) \right\} \qquad [4.2]$$

The parameters a and b depend on the symmetry—types involved in the matrix element and on the value of ν in the multipole expansion of the electron—electron interaction. In SWIRLES, this interaction may contain both the instantaneous Coulomb and low—frequency Breit interactions, whose matrix elements may be constructed from a common table of incomplete beta—functions. If ν_{max} is the largest value of ν encountered in the evaluation of a given block of matrix elements, then the number of incomplete beta functions for a given value of z is approximately $2(\nu_{max} + 3)^2$. This is a slight over—estimate of the minimimal permissible list, but a more robust and straightforward algorithm results if two square tables are generated, each with $(\nu_{max} + 3)^2$ elements, the factor of two arising because each two—electron integral involves two values of the argument, z. Each table is generated from two starting points, which have been evaluated previously and stored in the module BETAVEC. The starting values for each table are $I(A_0,B_0;z)$ and $I(A_0+1,B;z)$, where

$$A_0 = (\gamma + \gamma') + 1 \qquad\qquad B_0 = (\gamma'' + \gamma''') - \nu_{max} \qquad\qquad [4.3]$$

The parameters set $\{\gamma\}$ depends on the angular quantum number of the symmetry–types under investigation, $\{\kappa\}$, the nuclear charge, Z, and the speed of light, c. Specifically

$$\gamma = \overline{\sqrt{(\kappa^2 - (Z/c)^2)}} \qquad\qquad [4.4]$$

It is easiest to describe the algorithm which generates the tables using a symbolic representation for 3 rules which are applied successively, starting with two initial points. The rules are:

Rule A $\{I(a,b;z),\ I(a,b+1;z)\} \rightarrow I(a+1,b;z)$

Rule B $\{I(a,b;z),\ I(a+1,b;z)\} \rightarrow I(a,b+1;z)$

Rule C $\{I(a,b+1;z), I(a+1,b;z)\} \rightarrow I(a+1,b+1;z)$

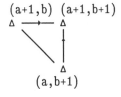

to find $I(A_0, B_0+1;z)$, and then the square of values is completed by the determination of $I(A_0+1, B_0+1;z)$ using Rule C. The index count of the first parameter is increased by 1 by the use of Rule A, and we have recreated the initial conditions of the recurrence for a new square of values. The procedure is repeated, and the rows $I(A_0+M, B_0;Z)$ and $I(A_0+M, B_0+1;Z)$ are completed by the final use of Rule C.

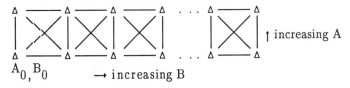

A new row is built starting from $I(A_0, B_0+1;Z)$ and $I(A_0+1, B_0+1;Z)$ as the new initial values with the repeated use of Rule B and the final use of Rule C to complete the row. The building of new rows may be represented diagrammatically by

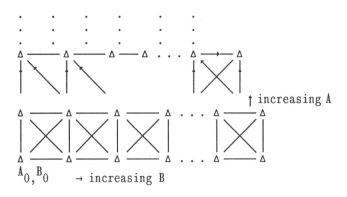

↑ increasing A

A_0, B_0 → increasing B

This procedure is repeated until the table is completed. Each new row of I(a,b;z) is found using only a small number of floating point operations, and its stability is independent of the value of Z, so we avoid the complication of having to have special versions of the algorithm for different ranges of the argument. The recursive approach is very efficient of we consider scalar speed, but the dependence on values of the incomplete beta function evaluated in previous stages of the algorithm inhibits vectorization.

The implementation of this method on a vector–processing machine follows the approach adopted in BETAVEC. Each of the tables is independent, and each is generated using common intermediates, except those which depend on the argument, z. The strategy which has been adopted generates NZTERM tables of incomplete beta functions simultaneously. The diagrammatic representation of the recursion now has depth, with each layer corresponding to a different value of z. The major computational operations are performed on the vectors which lie in the out of plane direction and pass through the nodes of the above schematic representation; an outer loop moves from one vector to the next, in a pattern dictated by the recursive formulae.

The decision to generate 2*324 tables of incomplete beta functions (each comprising up to to 100 elements) reflects the structure of the supervector module SUPVEC. The maximum permissible dimension of the basis is 18 functions per component, so that the maximum number of index pairs (ij) and (kl) is 324*324. Unlike nonrelativistic electronic structure programs, it is not always possible to use symmetrized (and hence, shorter) integral lists because the off–diagonal density matrix (connecting large and small–component densities) is not symmetric. Only the diagonal blocks of two–electron integrals may be stored in triangular storage mode (j>i), (l>k) (kl>ij). The implication of this strategy in the evaluation of the incomplete beta function is the introduction of about 60K Words of additional core storage. This seems to be a tolerable compromise, consistent with the need to exploit the vector processing capabilities of the CRAY and a desire to construct a straightforward and reliable algorithm. This additional storage is substantially less than that required to store the end–product of this procedure, the relativistic supervector for a given set of angular quantum numbers.

Below is a condensed version of the code which generates tables of incomplete beta functions using the linear recursions which connect adjacent members with common values of the argument. The tables are stored in BABZ(I,J) where I labels the value of Z and J labels the index pair (A,B) for that entry. The values of the arguments are stored in ZIJKL(M). ZIJKL1(M) has as its entries 1.0−ZIJKL(M). The contents of COMMON/BETINT are the coefficients which define the recursion for a given set of initial parameter values. The values of IND0, IND1 and IND2 at each stage in the calculation define the index pairs (A,B) in the table, which is a square matrix of dimension NSTEPS2.

```
      DIMENSION BABZ(324,100),ZIJKL(324),ZIJKL1(324)
      COMMON/BETINT/AB1(10),AB2(10),OAN1(10),OAN2(10),A1I(10),A2I(10),
     & OB1I(10),OB2I(10),ABIJ1(20),ABIJ2(20),NRECUR,A1P1,A2P1,AB10,
     & AB20,OB1,OB2

C
      NSTEPS2=NRECUR
      NSTEPS1=NRECUR-1
      NSTEPS=NRECUR-2
C
      IND1=1
      IND2=NSTEPS2+1
C
C*** START RECURSION USING 'RULE B'
C
      DO 101 M=1,NZTERM
      BABZ(M,2)=(AB10*BABZ(M,IND1)-A1*BABZ(M,IND2))*OB1
101   CONTINUE
C
C*** GENERATE TWO ROWS OF VALUES INCREASING THE VALUE OF THE FIRST
C*** PARAMETER
C
      DO 104 II=1,NSTEPS
      I1=II+1
      I2=I1+1
      IND0=((II-1)*NSTEPS2)+2
      IND1=(II*NSTEPS2)+1
      IND2=IND1+1
C
C*** APPLY 'RULE C'
C
      DO 102 M=1,NZTERM
      BABZ(M,IND2)=ZIJKL(M)*BABZ(M,IND0)+ZIJKL1(M)*BABZ(M,IND1)
102   CONTINUE
C
C*** APPLY 'RULE A'
C
      AB1II=AB1(II)
      AB2II=AB2(II)
      OAN1II=OAN1(II)
      OAN2II=OAN2(II)
      IND3=(I1*NSTEPS2)+1
C
      DO 103 M=1,NZTERM
      BABZ(M,IND3)=(AB1II*BABZ(M,IND1)-B1*BABZ(M,IND2))*OAN1II
103   CONTINUE
C
104   CONTINUE
C
C*** APPLY 'RULE C' TO COMPLETE THE ROW
C
      IND0=(NSTEPS*NSTEPS2)+2
      IND1=(NSTEPS1*NSTEPS2)+1
      IND2=(NSTEPS1*NSTEPS2)+2
C
      DO 105 M=1,NZTERM
```

```
      BABZ(M,IND2)=ZIJKL(M)*BABZ(M,IND0)+ZIJKL1(M)*BABZ(M,IND1)
105   CONTINUE
C
C*** FILL OUT ROWS BY REPEATED USE OF 'RULE B'
C*** THERE ARE NSTEPS+2 ROWS, 2 OF WHICH ARE NOW KNOWN
C
      IJ=0
      DO 109 II=1,NSTEPS
      I1=II+1
      I2=I1+1
      BB1=0B1I(II)
      BB2=0B2I(II)
      DO 107 JJ=1,NSTEPS1
      IJ=II+JJ-1
      J1=JJ+1
      IND0=((JJ-1)*NSTEPS2)+I1
      IND1=((J1-1)*NSTEPS2)+I1
      IND2=((JJ-1)*NSTEPS2)+I2
C
      AB1IJ=ABIJ1(IJ)
      AB2IJ=ABIJ2(IJ)
      A1JJ=A1I(JJ)
      A2JJ=A2I(JJ)
C
      DO 106 M=1,NZTERM
      BABZ(M,IND2)=(AB1IJ*BABZ(M,IND0)-A1JJ*BABZ(M,IND1))*BB1
106   CONTINUE
107   CONTINUE
C
C     APPLY 'RULE C' TO COMPLETE THE ROW
C
      IND0=(NSTEPS*NSTEPS2)+I2
      IND1=(NSTEPS1*NSTEPS2)+I1
      IND2=(NSTEPS1*NSTEPS2)+I2
C
      DO 108 M=1,NZTERM
      BABZ(M,IND2)=ZIJKL(M)*BABZ(M,IND0)+ZIJKL1(M)*BABZ(M,IND1)
108   CONTINUE
109   CONTINUE
C
```

The loops which contain vectorizable instructions have the labels 101–103 and 105–108 and use the index M. Notice that only consecutive entries in the vectors ZIJKL(M) and ZIJKL1(M) and the array BABZ(M,J) are accessed. It is easy to recognise the scalar code from which this module was developed, since it is necessary only to enclose the active sections in a loop of length NZTERM and index M, and to delete the loops 101–103 and 105–108 (some scalar optimization and removal of redundant storage is then possible). The difference between the scalar approach to this problem and the vector approach is similar to that found in the module BETAVEC, with an enhancement factor of slightly less than 100 being achieved due to efficient vectorization.

SUMMARY

        The computational details contained in this report resulted from the need to improve the efficiency of an existing code in order to extend the range of applicability of a promising theoretical development; the relativistic finite basis set method. This aim has been fulfilled and a working FORTRAN program has resulted which is able to model atomic systems containing many electrons to very high accuracy. It could be argued that the program is not in an optimal state and that there are still many areas where improvements could be made. This is certainly true, but in terms of overall efficiency SWIRLES far exceeds the performance of most published atomic physics programs, and has the potential to model a wider range of physical phenomena than has been possible previously. The use of the CRAY diagnostic tools SPY and PERFMON indicated particularly poor areas of coding, which were isolated and refined to a point where correlated relativistic atomic structure calculations are now routine. Increases in efficiency may not be made indefinitely since even the CRAY X–MP has a maximum rate of computation of 235 Mflops for a single processor. Realistic goals should be set in program development, which aim for a respectable fraction of the maximum rate. Any further improvements to the code would be guided by a need to treat larger and more complicated systems to a higher level of accuracy, but may necessitate the use of library routines written in CRAY Assembler Language. There is a loss of program portability if this course is taken, but it is possible to minimize this problem by confining all such code to short subroutines which may be replaced by versions written in standard FORTRAN.

ACKNOWLEDGEMENTS

I wish to acknowledge the help and guidance provided by Ian Grant over the past few years in these studies of relativistic electronic structure theory. Some of his insights are embodied in the material contained in the first of these lectures. The material in the second lecture was prepared in collaboration with Stephen Wilson, and I wish to thank him for his assistance in the solution of many of the practical difficulties encountered in this work.

This work is supported financially by the Science and Engineering Research Council.

REFERENCES

M.Abramowitz, I Stegun, Handbook of Mathematical Functions, Dover Publications
    (seventh edition, 1970)
G.Breit, Phys.Rev., **34**, 553 (1929)
C.G.Darwin, Phil Mag, **39**, 537 (1920)
P.A.M.Dirac, Proc.Roy.Soc (London), **A117**, 610 (1928)
P.A.M.Dirac, Proc.Roy.Soc (London), **A118**, 351 (1928)
I.P.Grant and H.M.Quiney, Adv.At.Mol.Phys, **23**, 37 (1987)
Y–K.Kim, Phys.Rev., **154**, 17 (1967)
W.Kutzelnigg, Int.Journ.Quant.Chem., **25**, 107 (1984)
I.Lindgren and J.Morrison, Atomic Many–Body Theory, Springer–Verlag (1982)
W.Press, B.Flannery, S.Teukolsky and W.Vetterling, Numerical Recipes,
    Cambridge University Press (1986)
H.M.Quiney, I.P.Grant and S.Wilson, J.Phys.B, **20**, 1413 (1987)
H.M.Quiney, I.P.Grant and S.Wilson, Lecture Notes in Chemistry **52**, 307,
    edited by U.Kaldor, Springer–Verlag (1989)
H.M.Quiney, Meth.Comp.Chem., **2**, 227 (1988)
B.Swirles, Proc.Roy.Soc (London), **A152**, 625 (1935)
M.Synek, Phys.Rev., **136**, 1556 (1964)
A.D.Williams, Phys.Rev., **58**, 723 (1940)

VECTOR PROCESSING AND PARALLEL PROCESSING IN MANY–BODY PERTURBATION THEORY CALCULATIONS OF ELECTRON CORRELATION EFFECTS IN ATOMS AND MOLECULES

D.J. Baker

Rutherford Appleton Laboratory, Chilton, Oxfordshire OX11 0QX, England

D. Moncrieff

ANU Supercomputer Facility, Australian National University, GPO Box 4, Canberra ACT 2601, Australia

S.C.R.I., Florida State University, Tallahassee, Florida 32306–4052, U.S.A.[§]

S. Wilson

Rutherford Appleton Laboratory, Chilton, Oxfordshire OX11 0QX, England

INTRODUCTION

The accurate treatment of electron correlation effects is central to atomic and molecular physics and to modern quantum chemistry. Over recent years, the trend in the development of techniques for handling the effects of electron correlation in atoms and molecules has been towards an increasing significance of perturbation theory both in practical applications and in the analysis and comparision of methods used in contemporary studies of many–electron systems. The rising popularity of many–body perturbation theory for quantum chemical calculations which go beyond the Hartree–Fock model is attributable to both the theoretical and the computational properties of the method. It is the close connection between these two properties that we wish to emphasize here.

Theoretically, the linked diagram theorem of many–body perturbation theory ensures that calculated electron correlation energies scale linearly with the number of electrons in the system (Brueckner 1955, Goldstone 1957, March, Young and Sampanthar 1967), a property which is widely recognized to be important in atomic and molecular electronic structure calculations, especially in comparisons of systems of differing sizes and in studies of extended systems (Čársky and Urban 1980, Jankowski 1987, Lindgren and Morrison 1982, Urban et al. 1987, Wilson 1984, 1985, 1990, Wilson and Silver 1976).

Computationally, the many–body perturbation theory not only affords a non–iterative algorithm for the calculation of accurate electron correlation energies (Silver 1978ab, Wilson 1978b, Wilson and Silver 1979) but also leads to algorithms which are particularly well suited to vector processing and parallel processing

---

[§] Permanent address

Supercomputational Science
Edited by R.G. Evans and S. Wilson
Plenum Press, New York, 1990

computing machines (Guest and Wilson 1981, Wilson 1981, 1983, 1985, Wilson and Saunders 1980). The linked diagram theorem ensures that the many–electron problem is effectively decoupled into a series of smaller problems each of which can be treated on a separate processor.

The equivalence of many–body perturbation theory formulated within the algebraic approximation (Wilson and Silver 1976) and the Møller–Plesset perturbation theory (Møller and Plesset 1932, Pople *et al.* 1978) is sometimes noted. Whilst this equivalence holds up to a point — the actual energy expressions in each order of perturbation theory are equivalent — in one very important respect the methods are radically different. The Møller–Plesset theory is a *first* quantized form of Rayleigh–Schrödinger perturbation theory with respect to a Hartree–Fock reference. Many–body perturbation theory, which was devised by Brueckner and Goldstone in the 1950's is *second* quantized, so that the cancellation of unwanted non–linear terms is a feature of the formalism, unlike the Møller–Plesset theory, where the "unlinked" diagrams must be cancelled "by hand". In molecular electronic structure studies the use of the second quantized many–body perturbation theory is clearly preferable in studies of extended systems (Wilson 1990) and mandatory in relativistic studies Quiney, Grant and Wilson, 1987, 1989, 1990, Wilson 1990) where one is dealing with and "infinitely many–bodied" problem.

In this paper, we outline some experiments in vector processing and parallel processing for

the second–order many–body perturbation theory energy which represents the dominant contribution to the correlation energy. Low order many–body perturbation theory calculations are often quite accurate; for example, the second–order energy of the argon atom in its ground state accounts for in excess of 99% of the empirically estimated total electron correlation energy if a sufficiently extended basis set is employed (Wells and Wilson 1986). On the other hand, for systems such as the beryllium atom in which there are substantial non–dynamical correlation effects, the second–order energy may account for only 80% of the correlation energy (Silver, Wilson and Bunge 1979). Second–order energy calculations can often yield molecular spectroscopic constants to an accuracy beyond that afforded by most other contemporary approaches (Wilson 1977, 1978c). Second–order calculations of the correlation energy for a closed shell system is no more demanding than a self–consistent field calculations; indeed both scale as the fourth power of the number of basis functions.

the fourth–order many–body perturbation theory energy terms involving triply excited intermediate states. Early calculations (Guest and Wilson 1980, Wilson 1979, Wilson and Guest 1980, 1981, Wilson and Saunders 1979) established that

these terms can be quite large particularly for multiple bonded systems such as N_2;

they can have quite a pronounced geometry dependence;

they are more sensitive to the quality of the basis set employed than some other fourth–order terms.

These terms are the computationally most demanding of the fourth order terms leading to an algorithm which scales as the seventh power of the number of basis functions. The development of highly efficient algorithms for the determination of these terms is crucial since the use of large basis sets, particularly in molecular calculations, is almost obligatory if basis set truncation errors are to be reduced to a point at which they become negligible.

We note that although fifth and higher order many–body perturbation theory calculations are technically feasible with basis sets of very modest size (see for example Handy *et al.* 1985 or Laidig *et al.* 1985), such studies are often futile since basis sets truncation errors are often far more significant than the error arising from truncation of the perturbation series and, moreover, can radically affect, for example, the convergence properties of the perturbation series (Wilson 1987a). Some recent publications (see, for example, Bartlett *et al.* 1989) discuss the inclusion of triple excitations in the coupled cluster expansion, which higher order terms in the many–body perturbation series are selectively summed, but this either required the use of a less than adequate basis set or the introduction of further approximations

SECOND–ORDER ENERGY COMPONENT.

The second–order energy for a closed shell system may be represented by the diagram shown in Figure 1. The corresponding algebraic expression may be written

$$E_2 = \tfrac{1}{4} \sum <ij|\hat{O}|ab> <ab|\hat{O}|ij>/(\epsilon_i+\epsilon_j-\epsilon_a-\epsilon_b)$$

where the two–electron integrals in the numerator are defined by

$$<pq|\hat{O}|rs> = \iint dr_1\, dr_2\, \phi_p(r_1)\, \phi_q(r_2)\, r_{12}^{-1} \{\phi_r(r_1)\, \phi_s(r_2)$$
$$- \phi_s(r_1)\, \phi_r(r_2)\}$$

in which ϕ_p is a spin–orbital and r_p denotes the coordinates, space and spin, of the p th. electron, and the ϵ_p are orbital energies. In this work we use lower case indices p, q, r, ... to denote arbitrary spin–orbitals, the indices i, j, k,... are employed for occupied spin–orbitals and a, b, c, ... are used for unoccupied spin–orbitals. The corresponding upper case indices are used to label the spatial orbitals.

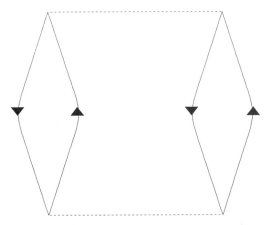

Figure 1 Diagrammatic representation of the second order energy component for a closed–shell system described in zero order by the self–consistent field wave function constructed from canonical orbitals.

Computationally efficient schemes for evaluating the energy coefficients in any non-relativistic many-body perturbation theory calculation depend on explicitly carrying out the spin integrations. For the two-electron integral defined above, we have

$$\langle pq|\hat{O}|rs\rangle = \langle PQ|r_{12}^{-1}|RS\rangle \, \delta(\sigma_p, \sigma_r) \, \delta(\sigma_q, \sigma_s)$$

$$- \langle PQ|r_{12}^{-1}|SR\rangle \, \delta(\sigma_p, \sigma_s) \, \delta(\sigma_q, \sigma_r)$$

where δ is the Kronecker delta.

We will employ the usual charge-cloud notation; that is, $[PR|QS] = \langle PQ|r_{12}^{-1}|RS\rangle$. It should be noted that only integrals of the type

$$[IA|JB]$$

arise in a second-order energy calculation and, therefore, only a partial transformation of two-electron integrals is required prior to the second-order energy calculation (Pendergast and Fink 1974, Saunders and van Lenthe 1983, Wilson 1987b). For real orbitals the two-electron integrals have certain permutational symmetry properties which can be effectively used to simplify calculations. In the case of the integrals which arise in the second-order energy expression when real orbitals are used, we have

$$[IA|JB] = [JB|IA] = [AI|BJ] = [BJ|IA]$$

Exploiting this permutational symmetry, the second order energy expression becomes

$$E_2 = \sum_{IJ} \sum_{AB} \{ [IA|JB]^2 + [IB|JA]^2 - [IA|JB] \, [IB|JA] \}$$

$$/(\epsilon_I + \epsilon_J - \epsilon_A - \epsilon_B)$$

which can be rewritten as

$$E_2 = \sum_{I \geq J} (1 + (1 - \delta(I,J))) \sum_{AB} \{ 2[IA|JB]^2 - [IA|JB] \, [IB|JA] \}$$

$$/(\epsilon_I + \epsilon_J - \epsilon_A - \epsilon_B)$$

The second-order energy may, therefore, be written as a sum of pair energies

$$E_2 = \sum_{I \geq J} E_{IJ}$$

with

$$E_{IJ} = (1 + (1 - \delta(I,J))) \sum_{A > B} \Big[[IA|JB] \, (2[IA|JB] - [IB|JA]) + $$

$$[IB|JA] \, (2[IB|JA] - [IA|JB]) \Big] / (\epsilon_I + \epsilon_J - \epsilon_A - \epsilon_B) + $$

$$\sum_A [IB|JA]^2 / (\epsilon_I + \epsilon_J - 2\epsilon_A)$$

These two expressions define the correlation energy component whose evaluation on a parallel processing machine we now consider.

The second order energy expression involves summation over the indices I, J, A and B with I≥J and A≥B. The total number of pairs energies is

$$M_0 = N_0 (N_0 + 1)/2$$

where N_0 is the number of occupied orbitals, and the number of terms arising in the summation over the A and B is

$$M_v = N_v (N_v + 1)/2$$

where N_v is the number of virtual orbitals.

Let us consider in detail the algebraic complexity of the second order expression. Performing the sum over I and J requires $\frac{1}{2}N_0(N_0+1) - 1$ floating point additions. The computation of a pair energy requires 2 additions, 1 subtractions, 1 multiplication and 1 division (a total of 5 floating point operations when A=B and 3 additions, 4 subtractions, 2 multiplications and 1 division (a total of 10 floating point operations) when A≠B. An extra addition is required when I≠J. Thus the total number of floating point operations required in the evaluation of a pair energy is

$$N_{pair}(I,J) = 5N_v + \frac{1}{2}N_v(N_v-1).10 + (1-\delta(I,J))$$

The evaluation of the second order energy component on a serial computer will take a time T_{serial} given by

$$T_{serial} = \left[\frac{1}{2}N_0(N_0+1)-1 + (5N_v+\frac{1}{2}N_v(N_v-1).10+1).\frac{1}{2}N_0(N_0+1) - N_0\right].\tau$$

$$= \left[\frac{1}{2}N_0(N_0+1).(5N_v{}^2 + 2) - (N_0+1)\right].\tau$$

where τ is the time required for a single floating point operation.

On a parallel computer with P processors a straightforward parallel algorithm is to evaluate the pair energies on separate processors. The time required can be shown to be shown to be a sum of three terms

$$T_{parallel} = \left[\left[5N_v + \frac{1}{2}N_v(N_v-1).10\right].\left[int[M_0,P]+1\right] + \left[\frac{1}{2}N_0(N_0-1)\right] + \left[\frac{1}{2}N_0(N_0+1)-1\right]\right] \tau$$

where the first term is associated with the evaluation of the pair energies, the second with the factor of 2 required when I≠J, and the third with the summation of the pair energies. $int[M_0,P]$ is the largest integer in M_0/P. In a typical application $N_v \gg N_0$ and the first term is dominant. If the number of available processors is much less than the number of distinct pair energies, $M_0 \gg P$ then the computation is performed approximately P times faster on a P processor machine than it would be on a single processor.

The calculation of an individual pair energy is well suitable to vector processing since it essentially involves matrix multiplication. On a parallel processor such as the

CRAY X–MP or CRAY Y–MP, which have four and eight processors, respectively, not only can the calculation of different pair energies proceed in parallel but the calculation of an individual pair energy can exploit the vector processing capabilities of these machines. For further details the reader is referred to our original publiction (Moncrieff, Baker and Wilson 1989).

FOURTH ORDER ENERGY COMPONENTS INVOLVING TRIPLE EXCITATIONS.

The fourth order diagrams in the many–body perturbation expansion for the correlation energy of closed–shell systems were given, for the first time by Wilson (1978a) (see also Wilson and Silver (1979)). Of the 39 diagrams which arise 16 involve intermediate states which are triply excited with respect to the single determinant reference function. An efficient scheme for evaluating these terms on the CRAY 1S computer has been reported by Wilson and Saunders (1980) Here we re–examined the efficient implementation on vector processor and consider the use of parallel processing techniques.

Let us consider as an example of a fourth order diagram involving triply excited intermediate states the energy expression corresponding to diagram F_t shown in Figure 2. The algebraic expressions corresponding to this diagram may be written as

$$
E_4(F_t) = \frac{1}{4} \sum_{\substack{ijk \\ abcde}} \frac{\langle ij|\hat{O}|ab\rangle \ \langle ak|\hat{O}|cd\rangle \ \langle cd|\hat{O}|ek\rangle \ \langle eb|\hat{O}|ij\rangle}{D_{ijab} \ D_{ijkbcd} \ D_{ijbe}}
$$

where the numerators are products of two–electron integrals and the denominators are products of sums of orbital energies

$$
D_{ij\ldots ab\ldots} = \epsilon_i + \epsilon_j + \ldots - \epsilon_a - \epsilon_b - \ldots
$$

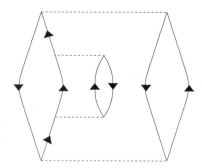

Figure 2 The fourth order triple excitation diagrams labelled F_t in previous work (Wilson 1978a)

An algorithm which scales as the seventh power of the number of basis functions may be devised to evaluate the energy component corresponding to diagram F_t by first defining the intermediate

$$f_{ijk;abc} = \sum_d \langle ij|\hat{\theta}|db\rangle \langle dk|\hat{\theta}|ac\rangle / D_{ijbd}$$

and then writing the energy component as

$$E_4(F_t) = \frac{1}{4} \sum_{ijkabc} f_{ijk;abc}\, f_{ijk;abc} / D_{ijkabc}$$

Spin–free intermediates corresponding to $f_{ijk;abc}$ may be defined as follows

$$F_{IJK;ABC}^{\alpha\alpha\alpha;\alpha\alpha\alpha} = T_1^f + T_2^f + T_3^f + T_4^f$$

$$F_{IJK;ABC}^{\alpha\alpha\beta;\alpha\alpha\beta} = T_1^f + T_3^f$$

$$F_{IJK;ABC}^{\alpha\alpha\beta;\beta\alpha\alpha} = T_2^f + T_4^f$$

$$F_{IJK;ABC}^{\alpha\beta\alpha;\alpha\beta\alpha} = T_1^f + T_2^f$$

$$F_{IJK;ABC}^{\alpha\beta\beta;\alpha\beta\beta} = T_1^f$$

$$F_{IJK;ABC}^{\alpha\beta\beta;\beta\beta\alpha} = T_2^f$$

$$F_{IJK;ABC}^{\beta\alpha\alpha;\alpha\beta\alpha} = T_3^f + T_4^f$$

$$F_{IJK;ABC}^{\beta\alpha\beta;\alpha\beta\beta} = T_3^f$$

$$F_{IJK;ABC}^{\beta\alpha\beta;\beta\beta\alpha} = T_4^f$$

where the following secondary intermediate quantities have been used

$$T_1^f = + \sum_D \langle IJ|r_{ij}^{-1}|DB\rangle \langle DK|r_{12}^{-1}|AC\rangle / D_{IJBD}$$

$$T_2^f = - \sum_D \langle IJ|r_{ij}^{-1}|DB\rangle \langle DK|r_{12}^{-1}|CA\rangle / D_{IJBD}$$

$$T_3^f = - \sum_D \langle IJ|r_{ij}^{-1}|BD\rangle \langle DK|r_{12}^{-1}|AC\rangle / D_{IJBD}$$

$$T_4^f = + \sum_D \langle IJ | r_{ij}^{-1} | BD \rangle \langle DK | r_{12}^{-1} | CA \rangle / D_{IJBD}$$

The energy components corresponding to the diagram F_t may then be written as

$$E_4(F_t) = \frac{1}{2} \sum_{IJKABC} \{ F^{\alpha\alpha\alpha;\,\alpha\alpha\alpha}_{IJK;ABC} \cdot F^{\alpha\alpha\alpha;\,\alpha\alpha\alpha}_{IJK;ABC} + F^{\alpha\alpha\beta;\,\alpha\alpha\beta}_{IJK;ABC} \cdot F^{\alpha\alpha\beta;\,\alpha\alpha\beta}_{IJK;ABC} +$$

$$F^{\alpha\alpha\beta;\,\beta\alpha\alpha}_{IJK;ABC} \cdot F^{\alpha\alpha\beta;\,\beta\alpha\alpha}_{IJK;ABC} + F^{\alpha\beta\alpha;\,\alpha\beta\alpha}_{IJK;ABC} \cdot F^{\alpha\beta\alpha;\,\alpha\beta\alpha}_{IJK;ABC} +$$

$$F^{\alpha\beta\beta;\,\alpha\beta\beta}_{IJK;ABC} \cdot F^{\alpha\beta\beta;\,\alpha\beta\beta}_{IJK;ABC} + F^{\alpha\beta\beta;\,\beta\beta\alpha}_{IJK;ABC} \cdot F^{\alpha\beta\beta;\,\beta\beta\alpha}_{IJK;ABC} +$$

$$F^{\beta\alpha\alpha;\,\alpha\beta\alpha}_{IJK;ABC} \cdot F^{\beta\alpha\alpha;\,\alpha\beta\alpha}_{IJK;ABC} + F^{\beta\alpha\beta;\,\alpha\beta\beta}_{IJK;ABC} \cdot F^{\beta\alpha\beta;\,\alpha\beta\beta}_{IJK;ABC} +$$

$$F^{\beta\alpha\beta;\,\beta\beta\alpha}_{IJK;ABC} \cdot F^{\beta\alpha\beta;\,\beta\beta\alpha}_{IJK;ABC} \}$$

The intermediates $F_{IJK;ABC}$ have the following permutational symmetry

$$F_{IJK;ABC} = -F_{JIK;ABC} = -F_{IJK;CBA} = F_{JIK;CBA}$$

By exploiting these symmetries, we can restrict the summations to $I \geq J \geq K$ and $A \geq B \geq C$. 36 contributions arise for each IJK;ABC which can be arranged as a 6x6 matrix as follows

	IJK	IKJ	JIK	JKI	KIJ	KJI
ABC	+1	+4	−1	+7	−4	−7
ACB	+2	+5	−2	+8	−5	−8
BAC	+3	+6	−3	+9	−6	−9
BCA	−2	−5	+2	−8	+5	+8
CAB	−3	−6	+3	−9	+6	+9
CBA	−1	−4	+1	−7	+4	+7

However, because of the permutational symmetry properties of the F intermediates there are only 9 unique cases. The numbers in italics above indicate these unique cases together with the sign. The uniques case may be taken to be the following :

1. IJK;ABC
2. IJK;ACB
3. IJK;BAC
4. IKJ;ABC
5. IKJ;ACB
6. IKJ;BAC
7. JKI;ABC
8. JKI;ACB
9. JKI;BAC

Thus, although considerably more complicated than the second order energy expression, the fourth–order triple excitation energy component can be written as a sum of terms each of which can be evaluated simultaneously on separate processors. The particular subdivision of the expression between the available processors will depend on the computational resources available. On the CRAY X–MP/48 at the Rutherford Appleton Laboratory, for example, we have found it useful to define a subproblem for each value of I and A. Each subproblem is well suited to vector processing. Full details of these experiments are reported elsewhere (Baker et al. 1990).

FINAL REMARKS

The linked diagram theorem ensures that calculations of electron correlation effects based on the many–body pertubration theory are well suited to vector processing and, more importantly, parallel processing. Efficient algorithms which exploit the capabilities of modern supercomputers is crucial to the development of computational schemes for extend molecules (Wilson 1990) and molecules containing heavy atoms (Quiney, Grant and Wilson 1987, 1989, 1990).

References

Baker D.J., Moncrieff, D., Saunders, V.R., and Wilson, S., 1989, Comput. Phys. Commun. *(to be submitted)*
Bartlett, R.J., Kucharski, S.A., Noga, J., Watts, J.D., and Trucks, G.W., 1989, Many–Body Methods in Quantum Chemistry, Lecture Notes in Chemistry 52 125, ed. U. Kaldor, (Springer, Berlin)
Brueckner, K.A., 1955, Phys. Rev. **100** 36.
Čàrsky, P., and Urban, M., 1980, Ab initio Calculations. Methods and Applications in Chemistry (Springer, Berlin)
Goldstone, J., 1957, Proc. Roy. Soc. (London) **A 239** 267.
Guest, M.F., and Wilson, S., 1980, Chem. Phys. Lett. 72 49.
Guest, M.F., and Wilson, S., 1981, in: Supercomputers in Chemistry, ed. P. Lykos and I. Shavitt (American Chemical Society, Washington D.C.) p.1.
Handy, N.C., Knowles, P.J., and Somasundram, K., 1985, Theoret. chim. Acta **68**, 87; see also Knowles, P.J., Somasundram, K., Handy, N.C., and Hirao, K., 1985, Chem. Phys. Lett. **113**, 8.
Jankowski, K., 1987, Meth. Comput. Chem. 1 1
Laidig, W., Fitzgerald, G., and Bartlett, R.J., 1985, Chem. Phys. Lett. **113**, 151
Lindgren, I., and Morrison, J., 1982, Atomic Many–Body Theory (Springer, Berlin)
March, N.H., Young, W.H., and Sampanthar, S., 1967, The many body problem in quantum mechanics, Cambridge University Press.
Møller, Chr., and Plesset, M.S., 1934, Phys. Rev. 46 618
Moncrieff, D., Baker D.J., and Wilson, S., 1989, Comput. Phys. Commun. **55**, 31
Pendergast, P., and Fink, W.H., 1974, J. Comput. Phys. **14**, 286.
Pople, J.A., Krishnan, R., Schlegel, H.B., and Binkley, J.S., 1978, Intern. J. Quantum Chem. 14 545.
Quiney, H.M., Grant, I.P., and Wilson, S., 1987, Physcia Scripta **36**, 460.
Quiney, H.M., Grant, I.P., and Wilson, S. 1989, in: Many–Body Methods in Quantum Chemistry, Lecture Notes in Chemistry 52 307, ed. U. Kaldor, (Springer, Berlin)

Quiney, H.M., Grant, I.P., and Wilson, S., J. Phys. B: At. Mol. Opt. Phys. *(submitted for publication)*

Silver, D.M., 1978a, Comput. Phys. Commun. **14** 71.

Silver, D.M., 1978b, Comput. Phys. Commun. **14** 81

Silver, D.M., Wilosn, S., and Bunge, C.F., 1979, Phys. Rev. **A19**, 1375.

Urban, M., Černušák, I., Kellö, V., and Noga, J., 1987, Meth. Comput. Chem **1** 117.

Wells, B.H., and Wilson, S., 1986, J. Phys. B: At. Mol. Phys. **19** 2411

Wilson, S., 1977, Intern. J. Quantum Chem. **12**, 609.

Wilson, S., 1978a, Correlated Wavefunctions, Proceeding of a Study Weekend, December 1977, edited by V.R. Saunders, Daresbury Laboratory.

Wilson, S., 1978b, Comput. Phys. Commun. **14** 91.

Wilson, S., 1978c, Molec. Phys. **35**, 1

Wilson, S., 1979, J. Phys. B: At. Mol. Phys. **12** L657; 1979 **13** 1505.

Wilson, S., 1981, in: Proceedings of Fifth Seminar on Computational Problems in Quantum Chemistry, Groningen, eds. P.Th. van Duijknen and W.C. Nieuwpoort.

Wilson, S., 1983, in: Methods in Computational Molecular Physics, eds. G.H.F. Diercksen and S. Wilson, (Reidel, Dordrecht)

Wilson, S., 1984, Electron correlation in molecules (Clarendon, Oxford).

Wilson, S., 1985, Comput. Phys. Reports **2** 389.

Wilson, S., 1987a, Adv. Chem. Phys. **67**, 439.

Wilson, S., 1987b, Meth. Comput. Chem **1** 117.

Wilson, S., 1990, The many–body perturbation theory of atoms and molecules, (Hilger, Bristol)

Wilson, S., and Guest, M.F., 1980, Chem. Phys. Lett. **73** 607.

Wilson, S., and Guest, M.F., 1981, Molec. Phys. **43**, 1331

Wilson, S, and Saunders, V.R., 1979, J. Phys. B: At. Mol. Phys. **12** 403; 1980, **15** 683.

Wilson, S., and Saunders, V.R., 1980, Comput. Phys. Commun. **19** 293.

Wilson, S., and Silver, D.M., 1976, Phys. Rev. **A14** 1949.

Wilson, S., and Silver, D.M., 1979, Comput. Phys. Commun. **17** 47.

Wilson, S., and Silver, D.M., 1979, Intern. J. Quantum Chem. **15** 683.

ELECTRON CORRELATION IN SMALL MOLECULES AND

THE CONFIGURATION INTERACTION METHOD

Peter J. Knowles

School of Chemistry and Molecular Sciences
University of Sussex
Brighton, BN1 9QJ
UK

INTRODUCTION

These lectures are concerned with the quantum chemistry of small molecules, and the techniques which are applicable for the calculation of molecular properties. Throughout, the emphasis will be on attaining the highest possible accuracy for rather small systems, typically with up to about six atoms or around 10 to 20 valence electrons.

Ignoring relativistic effects (which are known to be small for light elements), we are in the fortunate position of knowing the equations of motion for the electrons and nuclei (the Schrödinger equation). A further approximation which is usually made is to separate the motions of nuclei and electrons; in this Born–Oppenheimer approximation, the wavefunction is assumed to be a product of a nuclear function and an electronic function; the first step of a calculation, which will be the main concern of these lectures, is the solution of an electronic Schrödinger equation, in which it is assumed that the nuclei are stationary. The electronic energy obtained is a function of the (fixed) nuclear positions, and so forms a potential energy surface, on which the nuclei move, and so in the second step of the calculation, this potential energy function appears in a Schrödinger equation for the nuclei. The final eigensolutions correspond to the complete rotational–vibrational–electronic states of the molecule.

The electronic Schrödinger equation takes the form

$$\hat{H}\Psi = E\Psi \tag{1}$$

where the electronic Hamiltonian operator $\hat{H}$ depends on the nuclear repulsion energy Z, the separations r_{ij} of all N electrons, and the single particle Hamiltonian $\hat{h}(i)$ for each electron

$$\hat{H} = Z + \sum_i^N \hat{h}(i) + \sum_{i>j}^N r_{ij}^{-1} \tag{2}$$

The one electron operator $\hat{h}$ contains the kinetic energy and the attraction between the electron and the nuclei.

Supercomputational Science
Edited by R.G. Evans and S. Wilson
Plenum Press, New York, 1990

The usual starting point for the approximate solution of the electronic Schrödinger equation is the *self consistent field* (SCF) method. In the SCF method, the wavefunction Ψ is a simple product of N one electron functions ϕ_i, or *orbitals*, with fermion symmetry enforced with an antisymmetrising operator $\mathcal{A}$, which gives the wavefunction the form of a *Slater determinant*.

$$\Psi = \mathcal{A}(\phi_1(1)\phi_2(2)\ldots\phi_N(N)) = \frac{1}{\sqrt{N!}} \begin{vmatrix} \phi_1(1) & \phi_2(1) & \ldots & \phi_N(1) \\ \phi_1(2) & \phi_2(2) & \ldots & \phi_N(2) \\ \vdots & \vdots & \ddots & \vdots \\ \phi_1(N) & \phi_2(N) & \ldots & \phi_N(N) \end{vmatrix} \qquad (3)$$

Since electrons are spin-$\frac{1}{2}$ particles, the orbitals have the form of a spatial function multiplied by either an α or a β spin function. The orbitals can be taken to be orthogonal, and the Pauli principle allows double occupancy of one orbital provided each occurrence is associated with different spin. For a large class of molecules, the ground state is well described by a wavefunction containing only pairs of doubly occupied orbitals; for others, there may be one or more singly occupied orbitals.

Optimisation of the energy with respect to variations in the orbitals is equivalent to the condition that each orbital obeys the Hartree–Fock pseudo–eigenvalue equation

$$\hat{f}\phi_p = \epsilon_p \phi_p \qquad (4)$$

where the Fock operator $\hat{f}$ depends on all the orbitals, and is an effective Hamiltonian describing motion of each electron in the average Coulomb and exchange field of all others. For atoms (and perhaps diatomic molecules) the solution of the SCF equations for the orbitals is best achieved numerically, obtaining values of the orbitals on a grid of points in space. For molecules, which have much lower symmetry, the usual approach is to formulate each orbital ϕ_p as a linear combination of fixed chosen basis functions χ_α; solution of the SCF equations within this one particle basis set becomes a matrix algebra problem (Roothaan, 1951,McWeeny and Sutcliffe, 1969), determining the best orbital coefficients $q_{\alpha p}$ in the linear combination

$$\phi_p = \sum_\alpha^m q_{\alpha p}\chi_\alpha \qquad (5)$$

For molecules, the basis functions χ_α are almost universally chosen to be gaussian type functions centered on the atoms.

ELECTRON CORRELATION

In practice it is found that the SCF approximation is often rather accurate in the sense that it yields electronic energies which are usually approximately 1% in error; this is of the same order of magnitude as chemical energy differences, but often a large part of the error cancels when energy differences are taken. Under some circumstances, however, it is not sufficiently accurate for the purposes of predictive chemistry. The main assumption involved in SCF, that each electron moves in the average field of all the others, cannot be a feature of the exact electronic wavefunction. In practice, the motions of electrons are correlated; for example, in a two electron system such as the helium atom, the electrons will correlate their motions such that one electron will tend to move to the right of the nucleus when the other is to the left. This effect is not at all described in the SCF approach, and SCF wavefunctions for helium will be particularly suspect close to $r_{12} = 0$. At $r_{12} = 0$, the Hamiltonian operator is formally singular, but it can be shown (Pack and Byers Brown, 1966) that if the wavefunction behaves as $(1 + \frac{1}{2}r_{12})$, then the singularity is removed. The cusp is not of this form in the singlet spin SCF wavefunction, and the *electron correlation energy*, defined as the difference between the SCF energy and the exact energy, is approximately 1 electron volt. For the triplet state of He, however, a different situation holds. Here, because both electrons have the same spin, they are prevented from being at the same place by the Pauli principle, and electron correlation effects have a much smaller effect. This consideration carries over to systems with more electrons, where it is found that there is approximately 1 eV of correlation energy associated with each doubly occupied orbital.

The importance of electron correlation effects in molecules can be understood on consideration of the simplest many electron molecule, H_2. Solution of the SCF equations for the ground state near equilibrium bond length gives a Slater determinant $\mathcal{A}(\phi^\alpha\phi^\beta)$ with the same orbital for α and β spins. For symmetry reasons, ϕ must be an equal combination of functions χ_A, χ_B based on each atom; the ground state solution of the SCF equations has the bonding combination $\phi = A(\chi_A + \chi_B)$ (A is a normalisation constant). As the molecule is stretched towards dissociation, χ tends to a spherical atomic orbital, and the wavefunction can be partitioned as

$$\Psi = A^2\mathcal{A}((\chi_A^\alpha + \chi_B^\alpha)(\chi_A^\beta + \chi_B^\beta) \ ) \tag{6}$$

$$= A^2 (\ \mathcal{A}(\chi_A^\alpha\chi_B^\beta) + \mathcal{A}(\chi_B^\alpha\chi_A^\beta)$$

$$+\mathcal{A}(\chi_A^\alpha\chi_A^\beta) + \mathcal{A}(\chi_B^\alpha\chi_B^\beta) \ ) \tag{7}$$

The first two terms are recognisable as wavefunctions describing one electron on each H atom; the second two, however, are 'ionic', representing $H^+ \ldots H^-$ structures. At infinite separation, χ_A and χ_B do not interact, and one can obtain the energy as $\frac{1}{2}E(H) + \frac{1}{4}E(H^+) + \frac{1}{4}E(H^-)$, which is considerably greater than the correct value $E(H)$. This failure to dissociate correctly is the typical behaviour of the rather restrictive form of the SCF wavefunction in most diatomic and triatomic molecules. The connexion with the physical idea of electron correlation discussed above is elucidated by considering a wavefunction which explicitly contains the correct cusp conditions, $(1 + \frac{1}{2}r_{12})\Psi_{SCF}$; for large internuclear distance R, $r_{12} \sim R$ for the $\chi_A^\alpha\chi_B^\beta$, $\chi_B^\alpha\chi_A^\beta$ terms, whereas r_{12} remains small for the ionic terms; thus the ionic terms vanish as $R \rightarrow \infty$ as required.

Explicit introduction into the wavefunction of the interparticle coordinates as a method of describing electron correlation has been applied with some success to atomic systems; however it has not so far found a place in mainstream molecular quantum chemistry, principally because of the computational difficulty surrounding the evaluation of large numbers of integrals over the coordinates of 3 or 4 particles. Much greater success has been achieved by taking a wavefunction which is a variable linear combination of Slater determinants, including the SCF function, as well as others, built out of the same set of molecular orbitals (including 'virtual' unoccupied orbitals), which in some sense represent excited states. This is the method of *configuration interaction* (CI). The CI wavefunction is of the form

$$\Psi = \sum_{I}^{M} c_I\Phi_I \tag{8}$$

where the Φ_I are Slater determinants (or possibly linear combinations of Slater determinants) and the c_I are coefficients to be determined. Then application of the Rayleigh–Ritz method (Jeffreys and Jeffreys, 1956), where the wavefunction is that which makes the energy expectation value

$$E = \frac{\langle \Psi | \hat{H} | \Psi \rangle}{\langle \Psi | \Psi \rangle} \tag{9}$$

stationary, determines the c_I as components of the eigenvector of the linear eigenvalue equation

$$\sum_J^M H_{IJ} c_J = E c_I \tag{10}$$

where $\mathbf{H}$ is the Hamiltonian matrix, $H_{IJ} = \langle \Phi_I | \hat{H} | \Phi_J \rangle$. For the ground state, the lowest eigenvalue of (10) is an upper bound to the exact ground state energy, with equality when the set of functions Φ_I is complete. For excited states, MacDonald's Theorem (MacDonald, 1933) gives the 'betweenness' condition that the i'th and $i-1$'th eigenvalues $E_i^{(M)}$, $E_{i-1}^{(M)}$ obtained from a variational calculation with M expansion functions bracket $E_i^{(M+1)}$ obtained by augmenting the expansion set with one function. This means that the approximate excited state energies are also upper bounds.

The way that the CI method introduces a description of electron correlation can be understood by considering again the H_2 dissociation problem. The SCF wavefunction is $\mathcal{A}(\sigma_g^\alpha \sigma_g^\beta) = \mathcal{A}(\sigma_g^2)$, where $\sigma_g = A_u(\chi_A + \chi_B)$ is the symmetric bonding orbital. In the solution of the SCF equations in the basis of two atomic orbitals χ_A, χ_B, there will be a further, antibonding, orbital $\sigma_u = A_u(\chi_A - \chi_B)$, which is not occupied in the SCF wavefunction, but which appears as an eigenfunction of the Fock operator. The CI wavefunction is built as a linear combination of the two configurations σ_g^2, σ_u^2 ($\sigma_g \sigma_u$ is not present because of symmetry)

$$\Psi_{CI} = c_g \mathcal{A}(\sigma_g^2) + c_u \mathcal{A}(\sigma_u^2) \qquad . \tag{11}$$

Near equilibrium bond length R, $c_g \simeq 1$ and $c_u \simeq 0$, but as $r \to \infty$, $c_g \to 1/\sqrt{2}$, $c_u \to -1/\sqrt{2}$, $A_g \to 1/\sqrt{2}$, $A_u \to 1/\sqrt{2}$ and thus $\Psi_{CI} \to 1/\sqrt{2} \left(\mathcal{A}(\chi_A^\alpha \chi_B^\beta) + \mathcal{A}(\chi_B^\alpha \chi_A^\beta) \right)$, containing none of the spurious ionic terms. Hence the CI wavefunction has indeed allowed for the correlation effects, and produced correct dissociation. In fact one can show that such linear combinations of Slater Determinants introduces terms in r_{12}^2 into the wavefunction; although the necessary linear r_{12} terms are not present explicitly, they are simulated if sufficient terms are included in the CI expansion. For high accuracy, very long CI expansions may be necessary, but such expansions are much more easily handled that wavefunctions explicitly containing r_{12}.

FULL CONFIGURATION SPACE AND SECOND QUANTISATION

Consider a complete (infinite) one particle basis set $\{\chi_\alpha(\mathbf{r}), \alpha = 1, 2, \ldots\}$; any function of the position $\mathbf{r}$ can be represented as a linear combination

$$\psi(\mathbf{r}) = \sum_\alpha q_\alpha \chi_\alpha(\mathbf{r}) \qquad . \tag{12}$$

For a system of N particles, a complete basis can then be generated by taking all possible products $\chi_{\alpha_1}(\mathbf{r}_1) \chi_{\alpha_2}(\mathbf{r}_2) \ldots \chi_{\alpha_N}(\mathbf{r}_N)$, i.e., any N particle function may be expanded as

$$\Psi(\mathbf{r}_1, \mathbf{r}_2, \ldots \mathbf{r}_N) = \sum_{\alpha_1 \alpha_2 \ldots \alpha_N} Q_{\alpha_1 \alpha_2 \ldots \alpha_N} \chi_{\alpha_1}(\mathbf{r}_1) \chi_{\alpha_2}(\mathbf{r}_2) \ldots \chi_{\alpha_N}(\mathbf{r}_N) \tag{13}$$

214

This fact is not much use for practical calculations, since we cannot use an infinite set of functions, but if we consider now the case of a finite one particle basis χ_α, then we see the concept of the corresponding complete N particle space, composed of all possible products of orbitals. A variational calculation in such a basis will yield the lowest possible energy eigenvalue for the given one particle basis set, and such a calculation is termed Full or Complete configuration interaction (FCI). It is, however, easily appreciated that the number of possible orbital products $(2m)^N$ (m one particle α and β spin orbitals, N particles) can become exceedingly large.

We introduce the useful concept of *second quantisation* by defining the *orbital excitation operator* as (assuming orthogonal orbitals)

$$\hat{E}_{tu} = \sum_{i=1}^{N} |\phi_t(i)\rangle\langle\phi_u(i)| \qquad . \tag{14}$$

The Dirac bracket notation means that whenever the brackets become closed, $\langle f(i)|g(i)\rangle$, integration over the coordinates of electron i is performed on the functions within the bracket, $\int d\tau_i f^*(i)g(i)$. In (14) the set $\{\phi_p\}$ is supposed to be an orthonormal linear combination of the $\{\chi_\alpha\}$, typically the set of all SCF molecular orbitals. If $\hat{E}_{tu}$ is made to act on any N electron function which is a product of orbitals, or a linear combination of such products, the effect is for each occurrence of ϕ_u to generate a function which is identical, but with ϕ_u replaced by ϕ_t. Thus if ϕ_u does not appear, $\hat{E}_{tu}$ annihilates the function.

$\hat{E}_{tu}$ is a spatial orbital excitation operator; it acts on space coordinates and does not affect spin. In fact, it can be decomposed into a sum of operators which excite α and β spin orbitals separately, $\hat{E}_{tu} = \hat{E}_{t\alpha,u\alpha} + \hat{E}_{t\beta,u\beta} = t_\alpha^\dagger u_\alpha + t_\beta^\dagger u_\beta$, where u_α destroys α spin orbital ϕ_u and $t_\alpha^\dagger$ creates α spin orbital ϕ_t. The idea of second quantisation is that the orbitals themselves now become quantum mechanical operators in this way. Further details of the properties of the second quantisation can be found in the literature (Jørgensen and Simons, 1981).

As well as the single orbital excitation operators $\hat{E}_{tu}$, it is possible to define multiple excitation operators:

$$\hat{E}_{tu,vw} = \sum_{i \neq j}^{N} |\phi_t(i)\rangle\langle\phi_u(i)|\,|\phi_v(j)\rangle\langle\phi_w(j)| \equiv \hat{E}_{vw,tu} \tag{15}$$

$$\hat{E}_{tu,vw,xy} = \sum_{i \neq j \neq k}^{N} |\phi_t(i)\rangle\langle\phi_u(i)|\,|\phi_v(j)\rangle\langle\phi_w(j)|\,|\phi_x(k)\rangle\langle\phi_y(k)| \tag{16}$$

etc.

These can all be formulated as combinations of the single excitations:

$$\hat{E}_{tu,vw} = \sum_{i,j}^{N} |\phi_t(i)\rangle\langle\phi_u(i)|\,|\phi_v(j)\rangle\langle\phi_w(j)| - \sum_{i}^{N} |\phi_t(i)\rangle\langle\phi_u(i)|\phi_v(i)\rangle\langle\phi_w(i)| \tag{17}$$

$$= \hat{E}_{tu}\hat{E}_{vw} - \delta_{uv}\hat{E}_{tw} \tag{18}$$

Similar consideration of the identical operator $\hat{E}_{vw,tu}$ yields the commutation relation for the single excitations:

$$[\hat{E}_{tu}, \hat{E}_{vw}] = \hat{E}_{tu}\hat{E}_{vw} - \hat{E}_{vw}\hat{E}_{tu} = \delta_{vu}\hat{E}_{tw} - \delta_{tw}\hat{E}_{vu} \qquad . \tag{19}$$

Given that any wavefunction Ψ we construct is ultimately composed as a linear combination in the space of orbital products, then the following completeness identity is true for all $i = 1, 2, \ldots, N$

$$\left(\sum_p^m |\phi_p(i)\rangle\langle\phi_p(i)| \right) |\Psi\rangle = |\Psi\rangle \quad . \tag{20}$$

Now we insert this identity into the electronic Hamiltonian (2), replacing $\hat{H}$ by a *model Hamiltonian* $\hat{H}_M$, on the understanding that the only thing we will ever do with $\hat{H}_M$ is to take matrix elements between functions in the orbital product space,

$$\hat{H}_M = Z + \sum_i^N \sum_{tu}^m |\phi_t(i)\rangle\langle\phi_t(i)|\hat{h}(i)|\phi_u(i)\rangle\langle\phi_u(i)|$$

$$+ \sum_{i>j}^N \sum_{tuvw}^m |\phi_t(i)\rangle|\phi_v(j)\rangle\langle\phi_t(i)|\langle\phi_v(j)|r_{ij}^{-1}|\phi_u(i)\rangle|\phi_w(j)\rangle\langle\phi_u(i)|\langle\phi_w(j)| \tag{21}$$

$$= Z + \sum_{tu} h_{tu}\hat{E}_{tu} + \tfrac{1}{2}\sum_{tuvw}(tu|vw)\hat{E}_{tu,vw} \tag{22}$$

where we introduce the one and two electron *Hamiltonian integrals*

$$h_{tu} = \langle\phi_t|\hat{h}|\phi_u\rangle = \int d\tau_1 \phi_t^*(1)\hat{h}(1)\phi_u(1) \tag{23}$$

$$(tu|vw) = \langle\phi_t(1)|\langle\phi_v(2)|r_{12}^{-1}|\phi_u(1)\rangle|\phi_w(2)\rangle$$

$$= \int d\tau_1 \int d\tau_2 \phi_t^*(1)\phi_v^*(2)r_{12}^{-1}\phi_u(1)\phi_w(2) \tag{24}$$

For matrix elements between the N electron basis functions we then have

$$\langle\Phi_I|\hat{H}|\Phi_J\rangle = \langle\Phi_I|\hat{H}_M|\Phi_J\rangle \tag{25}$$

$$= Z\langle\Phi_I|\Phi_J\rangle + \sum_{tu} h_{tu}\langle\Phi_I|\hat{E}_{tu}|\Phi_J\rangle + \tfrac{1}{2}\sum_{tuvw}(tu|vw)\langle\Phi_I|\hat{E}_{tu,vw}|\Phi_J\rangle \tag{26}$$

In this way, we separate *integrals* $h_{tu}, (tu|vw)$ and *coupling coefficients* $\gamma_{tu}^{IJ} = \langle\Phi_I|\hat{E}_{tu}|\Phi_J\rangle$, $\Gamma_{tuvw}^{IJ} = \langle\Phi_I|\hat{E}_{tu,vw}|\Phi_J\rangle$. The coupling coefficients depend only on the algebraic structure of the N electron functions, and not on such factors as molecular geometry, external fields, etc..

For electronic systems, we may in fact reduce the basis set of orbital products by considering symmetry operations (those which commute with the Hamiltonian operator). In particular, because the wavefunction is antisymmetric with respect to electron coordinate exchange, we may replace the complete set of orbital products by the set of unique Slater determinants; furthermore, we need only include those Slater determinants with the same numbers of α and β spin orbitals, since others do not interact through the Hamiltonian operator. If the numbers of α and β spin orbitals in each determinant are $N_\alpha = \tfrac{1}{2}N + S$, $N_\beta = \tfrac{1}{2}N - S$, then the number of Slater determinants is obtained from simple combinatorial arguments as the number of ways of arranging N_α electrons in m positions, times the same for N_β,

$$M_D = \binom{m}{N_\alpha}\binom{m}{N_\beta} \tag{27}$$

Further reduction may follow on considering point group symmetry (only determinants belonging to the same irreducible representation in the (abelian) point group as the wavefunction need be considered) and spin symmetry; here, sets of spin coupled Slater determinants, configuration state functions (CSFs) can be used. The advantage of using CSFs as expansion functions is that there are fewer of them than determinants; the disadvantage is that they are more complicated in structure, being linear combinations of a few Slater determinants. As a simple example, for two electrons in two orbitals with $N_\alpha = N_\beta = 1$, the Slater determinants are $\phi_1^\alpha\phi_1^\beta$, $\phi_1^\alpha\phi_2^\beta$, $\phi_2^\alpha\phi_1^\beta$

and $\phi_2^\alpha \phi_2^\beta$; the CSFs with $S = 0$ are $\phi_1^\alpha \phi_1^\beta$, $\phi_2^\alpha \phi_2^\beta$ and $1/\sqrt{2}(\phi_1^\alpha \phi_2^\beta + \phi_2^\alpha \phi_1^\beta)$, and the CSF with $S = 1$ is $1/\sqrt{2}(\phi_1^\alpha \phi_2^\beta - \phi_2^\alpha \phi_1^\beta)$. Generally, the set of Slater determinants exactly spans the sets of CSFS with spin quantum numbers $S = N_\alpha - N_\beta, N_\alpha - N_\beta + 1, \ldots, \frac{1}{2}N$. Ignoring any point group symmetry, the number of CSFs with spin quantum number S is given by the Weyl formula (Paldus, 1974)

$$M_C = \frac{2S+1}{m+1}\binom{m+1}{\frac{1}{2}N - S}\binom{m+1}{m - \frac{1}{2}N - S} \quad , \tag{28}$$

$$= \frac{(N_\alpha - N_\beta + 1)(m+1)}{(m+1-N_\beta)(N_\alpha+1)}M_D \tag{29}$$

for the case that $S = N_\alpha - N_\beta$. So, for example, for $S = 0$ and large m, the number of CSFs is less than the number of Slater determinants by a factor of about $\frac{1}{2}N + 1$.

DIAGONALISATION OF THE HAMILTONIAN MATRIX

In the linear variational CI method, we aim to find the lowest (one or several) eigenvectors and eigenvalues of the Hamiltonian matrix in the basis of configurations selected for the problem of interest. The straightforward 'conventional' approach to this problem is to construct the M–dimensional matrix $\mathbf{H}$ in full, and then solve for all of the eigenvectors and eigenvalues using a standard method, e.g., the Givens–Householder algorithm (Wilkinson, 1965,Davidson, 1983). This requires the construction and storage of all M^2 elements of the $\mathbf{H}$ matrix, and the computation time varies as M^3. The very first molecular CI calculations followed this scheme (Foster and Boys, 1960), and it remained in use for some years. For small matrices, it is the method of choice, but it is easy to see that once M exceeds about 10^3 this approach becomes impossible, in terms of both storage and processing requirements.

In practice, we do not usually want all the eigenvectors of $\mathbf{H}$, only one or two of the lowest. Roos (1972) recognized that, given the existence of algorithms for the eigensolution of (10) using only the action of $\mathbf{H}$ on some trial vector

$$\mathbf{g} = \mathbf{H} \cdot \mathbf{c} \quad , \tag{30}$$

considerable enhancements in efficiency were possible for CI calculations. Depending on the particular kind of configuration expansion, evaluation of (30) can be considerably easier than evaluating all the individual non–zero H_{IJ}, since the additional summation introduced allows beneficial reordering of program logic; we consider an example in the next section. But the real advantage is that it is no longer necessary to store $\mathbf{H}$ in full, and also the computation time is reduced. Even if the cost of computing (30) scales as M^2, the overall cost will scale only as KM^2 where K is the number of evaluations of (30) required, which can be considerably less than M. Usually, also, $\mathbf{H}$ is extremely sparse, and the cost of evaluating (30) is sometimes barely more than linear in M.

Methods based on the use of (30) proceed (Davidson, 1983) by generating a sequence of vectors $\mathbf{b}_i, i = 1, 2, \ldots, K$, evaluating $\mathbf{g}_i = \mathbf{H}\mathbf{b}_i$ for each. The p'th eigenvector is approximated by a linear combination of the expansion vectors,

$$\mathbf{c}_p^{(K)} = \sum_i^K V_{ip}\mathbf{b}_i \quad . \tag{31}$$

Making the expectation value of $\hat{H}$ stationary with respect to variations in $\mathbf{V}_p$ gives the condition that $\mathbf{V}_p$ is an eigenvector of the projected eigenvalue equation

$$\mathbf{A}^{(K)}\mathbf{V}_p = \epsilon_p^{(K)}\mathbf{V}_p \quad , \tag{32}$$

with

$$A_{ij} = \mathbf{b}_i \cdot \mathbf{g}_j = \mathbf{b}_i^\dagger \mathbf{H}\mathbf{b}_j \quad , \tag{33}$$

and it is assumed that the $\mathbf{b}_i$ are orthogonal. MacDonald's theorem (MacDonald, 1933) guarantees that the p'th eigenvalue of the K–dimensional reduced problem, $\epsilon_p^{(K)}$, approaches E_p, the exact p'th eigenvalue of $\mathbf{H}$ from above as K is increased. When $K = M$, then the set $\mathbf{b}_i$ is nothing more than an orthogonal transformation of the original vector space, and $\epsilon_p^{(M)} = E_p$. There is value in adopting this approach only if it is possible to find a sequence of $\mathbf{b}_i$ vectors for which ϵ_p converges rather quickly towards E_p in a small number of iterations K.

The scheme most widely used in other areas of computational physics for generating a sequence of vectors is that of the Lanczos algorithm (Lanczos, 1950). The sequence is that obtained by Schmidt orthogonalisation of the Krylov sequence $\mathbf{H}^{(K-1)}\mathbf{b}_1, K = 1, 2, \ldots$, where $\mathbf{b}_1$ is a suitable starting vector, which in CI calculations will typically be the single Slater determinant with lowest energy. For full details of features of the Lanczos method, we refer to the discussion given by Davidson (1983).

Of wider use in quantum chemistry is the related method of Davidson (Davidson, 1975). Instead of taking the next expansion vector $\mathbf{b}_{K+1}$ as simply $\mathbf{H}\mathbf{b}_K$ (Schmidt orthogonalised to all previous vectors), it is chosen by perturbation theory. With the current approximate eigenvector given by (31), (32), the residual vector, measuring the remaining error of the eigensolution outside the $\mathbf{b}$ subspace, is

$$
\begin{aligned}
\mathbf{r}_p^{(K)} &= \left(\mathbf{H} - \epsilon_p^{(K)}\mathbf{1}\right)\mathbf{c}_p^{(K)} \\
&= \sum_i^K V_{ip}\left(\mathbf{g}_i - \epsilon_p^{(K)}\mathbf{b}_i\right) \quad .
\end{aligned}
\tag{34}
$$

We wish to change $\mathbf{c}$ to $\mathbf{c}+\Delta\mathbf{c}$, determining $\Delta\mathbf{c}$ so that the residual will vanish. Ignoring changes in ϵ (which will be second order in $\Delta\mathbf{c}$), insertion of $\mathbf{c} + \Delta\mathbf{c}$ into (34) gives the requirement

$$\Delta\mathbf{c} = (\epsilon\mathbf{1} - \mathbf{H})^{-1}\mathbf{r} \tag{35}$$

If this linear equation system were solved exactly, then iteration on (34), (35) would constitute a quadratically terminating Newton–Raphson procedure for the eigensolution. But solution of (35) would be as costly as the original matrix diagonalisation we are trying to perform, so it is more useful to approximate the inverse in (35) to give an approximate $\Delta\mathbf{c}$. The usual scheme is to ignore the off diagonal elements of $\mathbf{H}$, taking

$$\Delta c_I^{(K)} = r_I^{(K)}/(\epsilon_p^{(K)} - H_{II}) \tag{36}$$

Other choices of denominators are possible, for example energy differences from a zeroth order Hamiltonian such as a Fock operator (Seeger et al., 1978). $\Delta\mathbf{c}$ is then orthogonalised to

218

all previous b_i, normalised, and used as $b^{(K+1)}$. The next iteration then begins with the construction of $g^{(K+1)} = Hb^{(K+1)}$. Note that if H is approximated by a unit matrix in (35), the Lanczos method is obtained. The effect of the preconditioning energy denominators is to accelerate convergence toward the targeted p'th eigensolution, degrading the convergence of the other eigenvalues of the small matrix problem.

As convergence is reached, the construction of (34) and the orthogonalisation of Δc to previous b vectors becomes more and more subject to rounding errors, but this causes no numerical problems provided that the orthogonalisation is repeated as necessary to ensure that the set of b vectors is always accurately orthonormal. The algorithm is usually terminated when $|V_{Kp}|$, the contribution of the last expansion vector to the current eigenvector, becomes less than some predefined threshold, although other schemes are possible.

The use of the Davidson algorithm for one or more excited states is straightforward, and details can be found in the literature (Davidson, 1983, Liu, 1978). More recent generalisations (Werner and Knowles, 1985, Werner and Knowles, 1988) have improved efficiency in cases where the approximation of the inverse (36) begins to break down. This happens quite frequently in real CI calculations; for example, in the H_2 system considered in the previous section, as dissociation is reached, the two configurations σ_g^2 and σ_u^2 become degenerate, and (36) becomes less useful. Similar effects are observed in more complicated real problems. The solution involves augmenting the set of expansion vectors b_i by a small number of individual 'primary' configurations which are known to have energies close to that of the state of interest. Because they are simple configurations, it is easy to work out explicitly the Hamiltonian matrix elements between them, and these are then filled directly into A. That part of A which represent the coupling between the primary configurations and the b_i vectors is obtained simply as individual elements of the g_i vectors. For a small overhead, then, the number of b_i vectors required for convergence can be drastically reduced.

FULL CONFIGURATION INTERACTION

We now consider the possibilities and results of performing CI calculations in the full configuration space. Even with the reductions arising from symmetries discussed earlier, the size of the complete N electron basis can be exceedingly large; for a typical example with $m = 40$ orbitals, $N = 10$ electrons and $S = 0$, we obtain $M_D = 4.3 \times 10^{11}$ and $M_C = 8.2 \times 10^{10}$, and even the very latest techniques are unable to calculate eigenvectors of such huge matrices. So what is the point in pursuing full CI calculations? Firstly, they find an application in multiconfiguration SCF (MCSCF) calculations, to be described later. There it is found that it is useful to take a full CI expansion in a small subset of the orbitals. The development of efficient full CI algorithms is then central to solving the MCSCF problem. Secondly, if one can perform a full CI calculation in a small but still reasonable one particle basis set, then one has a "benchmark" by which the performance of all approximate quantum chemistry methods can be judged within the given basis set. Usually it is not possible to perform FCI in a basis which accurately reproduces experimental properties, however the small basis FCI calculation represents the exact answer of a model problem. The ability to do large full CI calculations has enabled over the last 5 years a number of important benchmarks (Bauschlicher et al., 1989, and references therein), which for the first time have given quantitative estimates of the accuracy of most quantum chemistry techniques. Thirdly, the techniques which have been perfected for FCI calculations over recent years have had an impact on the way other quantum chemistry methods are approached, and serve also as a good illustration of the advances that have been made in this subject.

In order to solve the FCI problem, we need an efficient algorithm to compute $g = Hc$ for the Davidson diagonalisation. The first generally applicable algorithm was that of Handy (1980), in which all the one and two particle coupling coefficients were computed in a 'brute force' approach, being multiplied by appropriate $(tu|vw)$ and c_J as they are formed. This allowed full CI matrices of dimension 5×10^5 to be diagonalised, but was extremely slow and not at all vectorisable. This method, however, made possible the first benchmark FCI calculation (Saxe et al., 1981), for H_2O in a double zeta basis set ($m = 13$ and $N = 8$).

Siegbahn (1984) recognized the value of using the completeness relation

$$\Gamma_{tuvw}^{IJ} = \sum_{K}^{M} \gamma_{tu}^{IK} \gamma_{vw}^{KJ} - \delta_{uv} \gamma_{tw}^{IJ} \tag{37}$$

in order to avoid direct computation of the very large number of two particle coupling coefficients. In (37) the sum is over the complete set of Slater determinants Φ_K. This insertion of a resolution of the identity leads to the algorithm for the the two electron part of $\mathbf{g} = \mathbf{Hc}$:

DO $K = 1, M$
    DO $t, u = 1, m$ such that $\gamma_{tu}^{KJ} \neq 0$
        $D_{tu}^{K} = D_{tu}^{K} + \gamma_{tu}^{KJ} c_J$
    END DO
END DO
$\tag{38}$

DO $v > w$
    DO $t > u$
        DO $K = 1, M$
            $E_{vw}^{K} = E_{vw}^{K} + D_{tu}^{K} (tu|vw)$
        END DO
    END DO
END DO
$\tag{39}$

DO $K = 1, M$
    DO $t, u = 1, m$ such that $\gamma_{tu}^{IK} \neq 0$
        $g_I = g_I + E_{tu}^{K} \gamma_{tu}^{IK}$
    END DO
END DO
$\tag{40}$

When there is insufficient storage to hold the complete matrices $\mathbf{D}$, $\mathbf{E}$, it is easy to split the above into batches, in which K extends over only a small range. For sufficiently large cases, the computation time is dominated by (39), requiring approximately $\frac{1}{2} M m^4$ floating point operations. This is to be compared with the conventional approach, where one would compute, or obtain from external storage, approximately $\frac{1}{8} M N^2 m^2$ two particle coupling coefficients Γ_{tuvw}^{IJ}, and then multiply with the appropriate coefficients c_J and integrals $(tu|vw)$. Computation of coupling coefficients is rather messy, requiring much logic, and in fact it proves best to compute them once, and read from disk when required. The whole of the computational effort in evaluating $\mathbf{g} = \mathbf{Hc}$ is then dominated by the disk access. In order to compare the two approaches, consider a typical case with $N = 8$, $m = 12$ and $S = 0$, giving $M_C = 70785$. The number of floating point operations for the Siegbahn algorithm is approximately 7.3×10^8; (39) is a matrix multiplication with long loop lengths, capable of driving a Cray–XMP at its peak performance of around 200 Mflop (million floating point operations per second), and so in this example would require about $3.7s$. The number of two particle coupling coefficients is estimated as 8.1×10^7, which would require around 900 Mbytes external storage. To read these once from the fastest Cray disk would take approximately $90s$. So although the algorithm takes considerably more floating point operations, optimum use of vector hardware results in a performance improvement of around a factor of 30. Furthermore, 900 Mbytes is probably near the limit of the disk availability of most computer systems, and so larger calculations would be impossible if one stores all Γ_{tuvw}^{IJ}. For the Siegbahn approach, one must store only the one particle coupling coefficients, of which there will be approximately $\frac{1}{2}MNm$.

Eventually, as the size of problem is increased, construction and storage of even the one particle coupling coefficients becomes troublesome. Knowles and Handy (1984) approached this problem by reverting to the use of Slater determinants as a basis, rather than the smaller number of CSFs. Although this increases the length of the K loop in (39), it becomes possible to obtain all the γ_{tu}^{IJ} when required, without any external storage. For Slater determinants, the one particle coupling coefficients take a rather simple form. Any determinant can be constructed as a product of a 'string' Φ^α of occupied α spin orbitals and a string Φ^β of occupied β spin orbitals. It is then helpful to think of the vector of coefficients c_J as a rectangular matrix $c(\Phi^\alpha, \Phi^\beta)$. The excitation operator $\hat{E}_{tu}$, as previously mentioned, is the sum of α, β spin operators $\hat{E}_{tu}^\alpha$, $\hat{E}_{tu}^\beta$, and so the effect of $\hat{E}_{tu}$ on a determinant is to produce two determinants,

$$
\begin{aligned}
\hat{E}_{tu}(\Phi^\alpha\Phi^\beta) &= \hat{E}_{tu}^\alpha(\Phi^\alpha\Phi^\beta) + \hat{E}_{tu}^\beta(\Phi^\alpha\Phi^\beta) \\
&= (\tilde{\Phi}^\alpha\Phi^\beta) + (\Phi^\alpha\tilde{\Phi}^\beta) \quad .
\end{aligned}
\tag{41}
$$

Note that the excitation $\hat{E}_{tu}^\alpha\Phi^\alpha \to \tilde{\Phi}^\alpha$ is completely independent of Φ^β, and so once the α spin excitation has been characterised, one can use the information found for all β strings. Furthermore, because $\tilde{\Phi}$ is just another Slater determinant, the numerical value of the coupling coefficient is ± 1, the possible sign flip arising from the antisymmetric properties of determinants. Hence the construction of $\mathbf{D}$ in (38) proceeds as

DO Φ^α
    DO $t, u = 1, m$ such that $\tilde{\Phi}^\alpha = \hat{E}_{tu}\Phi^\alpha$ exists
        Determine phase ± 1 of excitation
        DO Φ^β
            $D(\Phi^\alpha, \Phi^\beta, tu) \leftarrow \pm c(\tilde{\Phi}^\alpha, \Phi^\beta)$
        END DO
    END DO
END DO $\hspace{10cm}$ (42)

The innermost loop over Φ^β contains no logic or even multiplication and vectorises perfectly on all pipeline computers. A similar loop structure is required for the contributions from $\hat{E}_{tu}^\beta$, and the logic of (40) can be treated in a similar fashion. Because the number of α, β strings is rather small ($\sqrt{M_D}$), all the necessary single excitation information can be computed once and held in high speed storage. The result is a perfectly vectorized, disk free algorithm, where for reasonably sized problems at least, there is practically no overhead above the cost of the matrix multiplication (39). It is this method which has been used extensively in benchmark calculations with up to 3×10^7 Slater determinants (Bauschlicher et al., 1989), and the program is now publicly available (Knowles and Handy, 1989a).

There have been a number of recent algorithmic developments which have further enhanced the efficiency and applicability of the FCI method. Olsen et al. (1988) showed how it was possible to reduce the operation count to be proportional to N^2m^2 rather than m^4, with, however, some degradation of the vector performance; their method is particularly useful when the ration m/N is relatively large. Zarrabian et al. (1989) have used an alternative resolution of the identity to (37), with an intermediate summation over $N - 2$ electron (rather than N

electron) Slater determinants. Again, when m/N is large, there are many fewer of these, allowing for considerable enhancement in efficiency. This has made possible FCI calculations with up to 7.7×10^7 Slater determinants (Harrison and Zarrabian, 1989). When the CI expansion becomes so large, eventually the overriding computational problem is the storage of the vectors b_i, g_i in the Davidson procedure. The data compression techniques of Shepard (1989) prove useful in reducing the disk storage problem. However, order of magnitude increases in the maximum size of matrix have been achieved by exploiting the observation that the FCI eigenvector is extremely sparse (Knowles, 1989a, Knowles and Handy, 1989b). By dealing with only those configurations which make significant contributions, considerable reductions in both disk storage and CPU requirements are possible, even though there is then almost total loss of vectorisation, and it has proved possible to perform FCI calculations with more than 5×10^8 determinants (Knowles, 1989b). For full details of all these recent developments, the reader is referred to the literature.

THE MULTICONFIGURATION SELF CONSISTENT FIELD METHOD

In order to achieve chemical accuracy in quantum molecular calculations, it is generally necessary to use rather large one particle basis sets; typically, for triatomics, around 100 gaussian orbitals is common. With such large basis sets, FCI calculations are impossible, and one is faced with the problem of having to find approximate rather than exact eigenfunctions of the model Hamiltonian. Indeed, even in those cases where one can perform a FCI calculation with a reasonable basis set, it is found that much better results can be obtained for the same computational effort by using a more approximate technique in a bigger basis set. When looking for approximate methods, one might distinguish two levels of accuracy to consider. Firstly, we will want a method in which we ensure that all qualitative electron correlation effects are covered; these would include, for example, dissociation and reaction behaviour, interactions with low lying excited electronic states, etc.. This will be the problem on which we concentrate in this section. Secondly, having obtained a wavefunction with the correct qualitative features, we will wish to use it as a starting point for building an accurate function in which it is hoped to recover a large fraction of the remaining electron correlation energy. We will deal with the methods appropriate for this in the next section.

Under some circumstances, the SCF wavefunction already contains all the correct qualitative features, and one may then most efficiently proceed immediately to the use of methods to recover correlation effects based on the SCF function as a starting point. Falling into this category are closed shell atoms, and also many molecules when one is interested only in properties close to equilibrium geometry, for example vibrational frequencies. Many other problems can be described qualitatively by a spin unrestricted SCF wavefunction (UHF), where α and β spin orbitals are no longer constrained to be the same. For example, a wavefunction of this type allows for proper dissociation of the H_2 molecule. However there are problems associated with the fact that the UHF wavefunction is not a spin eigenfunction as it should be, and this can give rise to some spurious unphysical behaviour. SCF and UHF based methods form the backbone of the general quantum chemistry packages, such as GAUSSIAN and CADPAC, which have done much to further the application of theoretical methods to chemistry. However, there is a wider class of problems in which the electron correlation effects are too complicated for such treatment, and these are our concern now.

A more general qualitative wavefunction is built by selecting a number of configurations (determinants or CSFs) which are meant to describe all possible dissociation pathways, etc., and then writing the wavefunction as a linear CI expansion

$$\Psi = \sum_{I}^{M} c_I \Phi_I \quad . \tag{43}$$

The energy is then minimised with respect to not only the c_I (as in the CI method), but also to changes in the orbitals ϕ_t which are used to construct the Φ_I. This orbital optimisation is analogous to what is done in the SCF method, hence the name *multiconfiguration self consistent field* (MCSCF), which is given to this approach. Provided all the necessary configurations are included in the set Φ_I, then the method should give a qualitatively correct description of the electronic structure.

Nearly all molecules dissociate to valence states of their constituent atoms, in which only the valence orbitals (e.g., $2s, 2p$ in carbon) are occupied. So ignoring the complications which might occur for Rydberg molecular states, a good description can be obtained by including Φ_I which have only valence orbitals of the molecule occupied. This has important computational consequences, and we distinguish in a calculation the relatively small number of *internal* (or valence) orbitals $\phi_t, \phi_u, \phi_v, \ldots$ from the usually much larger number of *external* orbitals $\phi_a, \phi_b, \ldots$, which are unoccupied in all configurations, and so actually are not part of the wavefunction. The internal and external orbitals take the roles of the occupied and virtual orbitals in an SCF calculation; as the calculation proceeds, the internal and external orbitals are mixed amongst each other until the optimum internal orbitals are found. Taking these ideas to the extreme suggests the use of a CI expansion consisting of all possible configurations in the valence space, i.e., a FCI type of wavefunction. This approach (Ruedenberg et al., 1979, Roos et al., 1980) is often termed *complete active space SCF* (CASSCF) and has the feature that it is to some extent a 'black box'; the sometimes rather difficult problem of selecting suitable configurations Φ_I is replaced by the simpler identification of important orbitals. If the active orbital space coincides with the true valence space, then correct dissociation at all limits is automatically guaranteed, although there may be many configurations included which are completely unimportant. As a simple example, consider the ground state of N_2. The quartet spin N atom ground state is described by the configuration $2p_x^\alpha 2p_y^\alpha 2p_z^\alpha$. On bringing two N atoms together, one can make 20 CSFs with the correct spin (singlet) and space (A_g in D_{2h}), of which one is dominant near equilibrium bond length, but all of which are important at dissociation. The CASSCF wavefunction, a FCI expansion of 6 electrons in 6 orbitals, contains 32 CSFs. Although the ansatz may be wasteful in this way, we bear in mind that a complete CI expansion enables us to use the special efficient techniques described in the previous section, so a CASSCF calculation may actually be easier than a smaller more general MCSCF calculation with the same internal orbital space.

We have considered earlier how the matrix elements $H_{IJ} = \langle \Phi_I | \hat{H} | \Phi_J \rangle$ are obtained in terms of one and two electron integrals h_{tu}, $(tu|vw)$ and coupling coefficients γ_{tu}^{IJ}, Γ_{tuvw}^{IJ}:

$$\langle \Phi_I | \hat{H} | \Phi_J \rangle = \sum_{tu} \gamma_{tu}^{IJ} h_{tu} + \frac{1}{2} \sum_{tuvw} \Gamma_{tuvw}^{IJ} (tu|vw) \tag{44}$$

Thus the expression for the energy is

$$
\begin{aligned}
E &= \langle \sum_I c_I \Phi_I | \hat{H} | \sum_J c_J \Phi_J \rangle \\
&= \sum_{tu} \sum_{IJ} c_I c_J \gamma_{tu}^{IJ} h_{tu} + \frac{1}{2} \sum_{tuvw} \sum_{IJ} c_I c_J \Gamma_{tuvw}^{IJ} (tu|vw) \\
&= \sum_{tu} \gamma_{tu} h_{tu} + \frac{1}{2} \sum_{tuvw} \Gamma_{tuvw} (tu|vw)
\end{aligned} \tag{45}
$$

where we introduce the one and two electron *density matrices* γ_{tu}, Γ_{tuvw}, which can be viewed as expectation values of the coupling coefficients. This energy expression is the quantity which must be made stationary with respect to changes in the CI coefficients c_I and the orbitals ϕ_t, subject to the constraints

$$\sum_I c_I^2 = 1 \qquad \text{(normalisation)} \tag{46}$$

$$\langle \phi_t | \phi_u \rangle = \delta_{tu} \qquad \text{(orbital orthogonality)} \tag{47}$$

For the CI coefficients, introducing a Lagrange multiplier ϵ for the first constraint, and setting the differential with respect to c_I to zero, gives the stationary conditions

$$\sum_J \langle \Phi_I | \hat{H} | \Phi_J \rangle c_J - \epsilon c_I = 0 \tag{48}$$

i.e., the usual matrix eigenvalue equations obtained in regular CI theory. For the orbitals, the most straightforward approach is to parametrise orthogonal rotations $\mathbf{u}$ amongst the orbitals ($\phi_t \leftarrow \sum_p \phi_p u_{pt}$) by means of the matrix elements x_{tu} of an antisymmetric matrix. Any orthogonal matrix may be represented as

$$\mathbf{u} = \exp(\mathbf{x}) \qquad \text{where } \mathbf{x}^\dagger = -\mathbf{x} \tag{49}$$

The advantage of this formulation is that the $\frac{1}{2}m(m+1)$ orthogonality constraints are automatically satisfied, leaving $\frac{1}{2}m(m-1)$ free parameters which are contained in the lower triangle of $\mathbf{x}$. There is then no need for Lagrange multipliers, and numerical methods for unconstrained optimisation may be used.

To derive the variational conditions for orbital rotations, we note that the orbitals vary on $\mathbf{x}$ through (49) as

$$\left. \frac{\partial \phi_p}{\partial x_{rs}} \right|_{\mathbf{x}=0} = \delta_{sp}\phi_r - \delta_{rp}\phi_s \quad , \tag{50}$$

and that the integrals h_{tu}, $(tu|vw)$ given by (23), (24) are quadratic and quartic, respectively, in the orbitals. Then we obtain

$$\left. \frac{\partial}{\partial x_{rs}} h_{tu} \right|_{\mathbf{x}=0} = (1 - \tau_{rs})(1 + \tau_{tu})\delta_{st}h_{ru} \tag{51}$$

$$\left. \frac{\partial}{\partial x_{rs}} (tu|vw) \right|_{\mathbf{x}=0} = (1 - \tau_{rs})(1 + \tau_{tu})(1 + \tau_{tu,vw})\delta_{st}(ru|vw) \tag{52}$$

where τ_{ij} permutes the labels i, j in what follows it. Thus the derivative of the energy, which is zero for the converged wavefunction, is given by

$$0 = \frac{\partial E}{\partial x_{rs}} = 2(1 - \tau_{rs})F_{rs} \tag{53}$$

with

$$F_{rs} = \sum_u \gamma_{su} h_{ru} + \sum_{uvw} \Gamma_{suvw} (ru|vw) \tag{54}$$

(53), (48) constitute the equations which must be solved to obtain the MCSCF wavefunction. Note that for some orbital rotations x_{rs}, the variational condition (53) is always obeyed automatically; for example, if both r, s are external, then the density matrix elements are all zero. The same can occur in a more subtle way for certain internal–internal orbital rotations, e.g., for a CASSCF, all internal–internal rotations show this behaviour. When an x_{rs} behaves like this it is known as a redundant variable, and is best removed from the optimisation altogether. Note also that (53) is highly non–linear, in contrast to the linear eigenvalue problem which appears in the CI method; E is 4th order in the orbitals, and infinite order in $\mathbf{x}$, since the orbitals are in fact periodic functions because of the orthogonality constraint.

Standard numerical methods for unconstrained optimisation of non–linear functions are mostly based on the iterative non–linear Newton–Raphson approach (Fletcher, 1980). An iteration consists of approximating the energy E as a quadratic function $E^{(2)}$ of $\mathbf{x}$ and $\mathbf{c}$ (i.e. a Taylor expansion) about the current point, and then minimising the (simpler) $E^{(2)}$, to give a value of $\mathbf{x}$, $\Delta\mathbf{c}$; the wavefunction is then updated to incorporate this change, and a new iteration begins, with an expansion $E^{(2)}$ about the new point. Since $E^{(2)}$ is a quadratic function of the form

$$E^{(2)} = E_0 + \sum_i \left(\frac{\partial E}{\partial \lambda_i}\right)_0 \lambda_i + \tfrac{1}{2} \sum_{ij} \left(\frac{\partial^2 E}{\partial \lambda_i \partial \lambda_j}\right)_0 \lambda_i \lambda_j \tag{55}$$

its minimisation is nothing more than the solution of the linear equations

$$\sum_j \left(\frac{\partial^2 E}{\partial \lambda_i \partial \lambda_j}\right)_0 \lambda_j + \left(\frac{\partial E}{\partial \lambda_i}\right)_0 = 0 \quad . \tag{56}$$

In order to set up and solve these equations, we need not only the *gradient* vector $\partial E/\partial x_{rs}$, $\partial E/\partial c_I$, which is that which appears in the variational equations (48), (53), but also the *hessian* matrix, $\partial^2 E/\partial x_{rs} \partial x_{tu}$, $\partial^2 E/\partial x_{rs} \partial c_I$, $\partial^2 E/\partial c_I \partial c_J$. A typical example of a hessian matrix element is

$$\frac{\partial^2 E}{\partial x_{ta} \partial x_{ub}} = \gamma_{tu} h_{ab} - \tfrac{1}{2}\delta_{ab} \left(F_{tu} + F_{ut}\right)$$
$$+ \sum_{vw} \Gamma_{tuvw} J_{ab}^{vw} + \sum_{vw} \left(\Gamma_{tvwu} + \Gamma_{tvuw}\right) K_{ab}^{vw} \tag{57}$$

where t, u are internal orbitals and a, b are external orbitals. The matrices J^{vw}, K^{vw} consist of the two electron integrals, $J_{ab}^{vw} = (vw|ab)$ and $K_{ab}^{vw} = (va|bw)$, and the matrix formulation provides both conceptual and computational convenience.

Since in each iteration of the procedure, the orbitals change, then so also do the integrals, so they must be recalculated. Because the orbitals ϕ_t are linear combinations of the basis functions χ_α, then the two electron integrals are given by a four index transformation

$$J_{ab}^{vw} = \sum_{\alpha\beta\gamma\delta} (\alpha\beta|\gamma\delta) q_{\alpha a} q_{\beta b} q_{\gamma v} q_{\delta w} \tag{58}$$

with an analogous transformation for the exchange integrals $\mathbf{K}$. Note that for the hessian matrix, we require v, w to extend only over the m_{int} internal orbitals, but a, b run over the full set of m

orbitals. Straightforward implementation of (58) would require on the order of $m^6 m_{int}^2$ floating point operations, but it is easily recognised that this is unnecessarily wasteful; one can proceed most efficiently by performing each transformation sequentially, i.e.,

$$J_{\alpha\beta}^{\gamma w} = \sum_{\delta} (\alpha\beta|\gamma\delta) q_{\delta w} \tag{59}$$

$$J_{\alpha\beta}^{vw} = \sum_{\gamma} J_{\alpha\beta}^{\gamma w} q_{\gamma v} \tag{60}$$

$$J_{\alpha b}^{vw} = \sum_{\beta} J_{\alpha\beta}^{vw} q_{\beta b} \tag{61}$$

$$J_{ab}^{vw} = \sum_{\alpha} J_{\alpha b}^{vw} q_{\alpha a} \tag{62}$$

Note that greatest efficiency is achieved if the transformations to the internal indices v, w are performed first, and that then the dominant computational stage is (59), requiring approximately $2m^4 m_{int}$ floating point operations. Further reduction of the operation count to $\frac{3}{8} m^4 m_{int}$ is possible on using the index symmetry of the integrals (Werner and Meyer, 1980,Saunders, 1983). All these transformations can conveniently be arranged as matrix multiplications for optimum vector performance; with care, it is possible to arrange for the innermost loop to extend over two of the indices simultaneously, allowing very long loop lengths.

Early implementations of the integral transformation were troubled with the problem of getting the integrals in the correct order, given that they do not all fit in fast memory, and quite involved sorting operations (Yoshimine, 1973) were required. Nowadays, more memory is available (although not enough usually to hold all $(\alpha\beta|\gamma\delta)$, and the problems are somewhat simplified. Very often there is sufficient space to hold all $J_{\alpha\beta}^{vw}$; in that case, provided the integrals $(\alpha\beta|\gamma\delta)$ have been sorted into the correct order initially, such that all $(\alpha\beta|\gamma\delta)$ for a given α, β appear together, (59) and (60) can be processed through one sequential read of the $(\alpha\beta|\gamma\delta)$. It is then a simple matter to transform in memory $J_{\alpha\beta}^{vw}$ to J_{ab}^{vw} according to (61) and (62). If not all $J_{\alpha\beta}^{vw}$ can be held, then it is possible to perform this procedure in batches. The integral transformation usually represents the most costly part of an iteration in the MCSCF procedure, and the effective coupling of the design of efficient matrix algorithms with the advent of vector hardware and large high speed memories was an important breakthrough in this field.

Having obtained the integrals in this way, we must solve the linear Newton–Raphson equations. Since there may be several hundred orbital rotations x_{rs}, and anything up to 10^6 CI coefficients c_I, construction and storage of the hessian matrix is usually out of the question. The best approach is iterative solution of the linear equations (56) using a modified form of the Davidson diagonalisation method. In each iteration (which we term a *microiteration* to distinguish it from the *macroiterations* in which a new set of transformed integrals are produced) the significant step is the multiplication of the hessian matrix onto a trial vector. It is usually best to construct the orbital hessian in full initially, but for those parts involving CI coefficients, the action of the matrix on the vector is computed directly. In fact, the block of the hessian matrix coupling CI coefficients to CI coefficients is nothing more than the CI Hamiltonian matrix, and so all the techniques perfected for full CI calculations, for example, can be utilised as they stand. A further refinement (Knowles and Werner, 1985) has the effect of minimising the work in the CI–like operations, by choosing expansion vectors which are zero in the CI part for most microiterations; only in a few microiterations is an attempt made to improve the CI coefficients. In this way, it is possible to perform the whole of the MCSCF calculation with only about 25 microiterations which involve the CI coefficients. This is an important consideration when the CI expansion is large.

The Newton–Raphson method outlined above uses all the terms which are second order in wavefunction changes, and therefore it is expected to converge with quadratic termination.

However it is well known that for many functions, this quadratic convergence is seldom realised in practice. Usually, the starting approximate wavefunction is sufficiently far from the convergence point that the second order approximation is not good, with significant third and higher order terms appearing. In this case, the Newton–Raphson method can converge extremely slowly, and even diverge. In particular, if the hessian matrix has a negative eigenvalue, the Newton–Raphson step in the direction of the eigenvector will be in the wrong direction. This effect can be seen by considering a one dimensional example; if the second derivative is negative, then the solution of the Newton–Raphson equations is at a point with higher energy than the starting point. A simple and effective remedy for this problem is the replacement of the Newton–Raphson equations

$$h\lambda + g = 0 \tag{63}$$

(where h represents the hessian matrix, and g the gradient) by the eigenvalue equation

$$\begin{pmatrix} (h - \epsilon 1) & g \\ g^\dagger & -\epsilon \end{pmatrix} \begin{pmatrix} \lambda \\ 1 \end{pmatrix} = 0 \tag{64}$$

i.e.,

$$(h - \epsilon 1)\lambda + g = 0 \tag{65}$$

and

$$g^\dagger \lambda = \epsilon \tag{66}$$

The effect of this is to give a level shift $-\epsilon$ to the hessian matrix to force it to be positive definite, and to somewhat damp the procedure when far from convergence. The procedure is known as the Augmented Hessian method.

Further enhancements of convergence behaviour are possible by using the fact that the energy E is a periodic rather than polynomial function of x in reality. With little extra computational effort, it is possible to formulate an approximate energy expression which is correct to second order in the true orbital changes $u - 1$, rather than x, and thereby has the correct periodic behaviour built in. Implementation of this idea results in an MCSCF algorithm with optimum and reliable convergence, usually in about 3 macroiterations. The details of this approach are beyond the scope of these lectures, and we refer to the original literature for full details (Werner and Meyer, 1980, Werner and Knowles, 1985).

THE CONFIGURATION INTERACTION METHOD

The MCSCF approach described above gives a generally applicable scheme for finding qualitatively correct molecular wavefunctions. Typically, however, MCSCF recovers only about 20% to 50% of the electron correlation energy. To obtain most of the correlation energy in an accurate calculation, we begin with the MCSCF wavefunction Ψ_0, and write the exact wavefunction as $\Psi_{exact} = \Psi_0 + \lambda\Psi_1 + \lambda^2\Psi_2 + \ldots$, where λ is an ordering parameter which will eventually be set to 1. Suppose that we can find an operator $\hat{H}_0$ such that $\hat{H}_0\Psi_0 = E_0\Psi_0$. In the particular case where Ψ_0 is the solution of the SCF equations, an appropriate $\hat{H}_0$ is the Fock operator; in other cases it may not be possible to find a suitable operator, but the arguments we develop still hold. If we write $\hat{H} = \hat{H}_0 + \lambda\hat{H}_1$, and separate terms of different order in λ in the Schrödinger equation, at first order we obtain

$$\left(\hat{H}_0 - E_0\right)\Psi_1 = \hat{H}_1\Psi_0 - \langle\Psi_0|\hat{H}_1|\Psi_0\rangle\Psi_0 \tag{67}$$

Expand Ψ_1, the first order correction to the wavefunction, and also $\hat{H}\Psi_0$, the action of the full Hamiltonian on the approximate wavefunction, as linear combinations of symmetry adapted configurations:

$$\begin{aligned}
\Psi_1 &= \sum_I \phi_I C_I^{(1)} \\
\hat{H}\Psi_0 &= \sum_I \phi_I h_I
\end{aligned} \tag{68}$$

and assume (although again this is not critical) that $\hat{H}_0\psi_I = \epsilon_I\psi_I$. This will be true for the Fock $\hat{H}_0$, and approximately true for others. The first order equation then becomes

$$\sum_I C_I^{(1)}\phi_I(\epsilon_I - E_0) = \sum_I h_I\phi_I - \langle\Psi_0|\hat{H}|\Psi_0\rangle\Psi_0$$

This tells us that the functions which are required for Ψ_1 are exactly those which appear in the action of $\hat{H}$ on Ψ_0. This set of functions is often referred to as the *first order interacting space*. Recall that the Hamiltonian consists of single and double excitation operators; this means that in turn the first order space consists of all those configurations which are at most doubly excited with respect to the reference function Ψ_0. This is the physical justification for the commonly used 'singles plus doubles' configuration interaction calculation, which we consider in this section.

Since we are interested in singly and doubly excited configurations, it is fruitful to consider first of all a two electron problem. The full CI basis of normalised CSFs consists of the functions

$$\overline{\Phi}_p^{ab} = (2 + 2\delta_{ab})^{-\frac{1}{2}}\left(\mathcal{A}(\phi_a^\alpha\phi_b^\beta) + p\mathcal{A}(\phi_b^\alpha\phi_a^\beta)\right) \qquad, a \geq b \tag{69}$$

where $p = +1$ for spin $S = 0$ (singlet) and $p = -1$ for $S = 1$ (triplet). It is easily verified that these functions $\overline{\Phi}_p^{ab}, a \geq b$ are orthogonal and normalised, since

$$\langle\overline{\Phi}_p^{ab}|\overline{\Phi}_q^{cd}\rangle = (1 + \delta_{ab})^{-\frac{1}{2}}(1 + \delta_{cd})^{-\frac{1}{2}}(\delta_{ac}\delta_{bd} + p\delta_{ad}\delta_{bc})\delta_{pq} \tag{70}$$

We may thus write the wavefunction as

$$\begin{aligned}
\Psi &= \sum_{a \geq b}\overline{C}_{ab}\overline{\Phi}_p^{ab} \\
&= \sum_{ab}\overline{C}_{ab}(\tfrac{1}{2} + \tfrac{1}{2}\delta_{ab})\overline{\Phi}_p^{ab} \qquad, \text{with } \overline{C}_{ba} = p\overline{C}_{ab}
\end{aligned} \tag{71}$$

The action of a single particle excitation operator on $\overline{\Phi}_p^{ab}$ is then

$$\begin{aligned}
\hat{E}_{tu}\overline{\Phi}_p^{ab} &= (2 + 2\delta_{ab})^{-\frac{1}{2}}(1 + p\tau_{ab})\left(\delta_{ua}\mathcal{A}(\phi_t^\alpha\phi_b^\beta) + \delta_{ub}p\mathcal{A}(\phi_a^\alpha\phi_t^\beta)\right) \\
&= (2 + 2\delta_{ab})^{-\frac{1}{2}}(1 + p\tau_{ab})\delta_{ub}(2 + 2\delta_{at})^{\frac{1}{2}}\overline{\Phi}_p^{at}
\end{aligned} \tag{72}$$

It is then clear that it is in fact much simpler to work with the unnormalised functions

$$
\begin{aligned}
\Phi_p^{ab} &= \mathcal{A}(\phi_a^\alpha \phi_b^\beta) + p\mathcal{A}(\phi_b^\alpha \phi_a^\beta) \\
&= (2 + 2\delta_{ab})^{\frac{1}{2}} \overline{\Phi}_p^{ab}
\end{aligned}
\tag{73}
$$

and write the wavefunction as

$$
\begin{aligned}
\Psi &= \sum_{a \geq b} C_{ab}(1 + p\delta_{ab})\Phi_p^{ab} \\
&= \sum_{ab} C_{ab}\Phi_p^{ab}
\end{aligned}
\tag{74}
$$

This formalism will eventually allow a completely matrix oriented computation, and the inconvenience introduced by having non–normalised functions is not a serious practical problem.

With these functions,

$$
\hat{E}_{tu}\Phi_p^{ab} = (1 + p\tau_{ab})\delta_{ub}\Phi_p^{at}
\tag{75}
$$

and

$$
\hat{E}_{tu,vw}\Phi_p^{ab} = (1 + p\tau_{ab})\delta_{ua}\delta_{wb}\Phi_p^{tv} \quad ,
\tag{76}
$$

and so the action of the Hamiltonian operator is

$$
\hat{H}\Phi_p^{ab} = (1 + p\tau_{ab})\left(\sum_v h_{vb}\Phi_p^{av} + \tfrac{1}{2}\sum_{tv}(ta|bv)\Phi_p^{tv}\right) \quad ,
\tag{77}
$$

i.e.,

$$
\begin{aligned}
\hat{H}\Psi &= \sum_{ab} C_{ab}^p \hat{H}\Phi_p^{ab} \\
&= \sum_{tv} \Phi_p^{tv}\left(K(\mathbf{C}^p)_{tv} + 2(\mathbf{h}\mathbf{C}^p)_{tv}\right) \quad .
\end{aligned}
\tag{78}
$$

Here, we have defined a generalised exchange matrix $K(\mathbf{C})$, which for any given coefficient matrix $\mathbf{C}$ is

$$
K(\mathbf{C})_{tv} = \sum_{ab} C_{ab}(ta|bv) \quad .
\tag{79}
$$

In (78), all two electron integrals in the basis of orthogonal orbitals are seen to be required. Usually, these orbitals are obtained from, e.g., an MCSCF calculation as a linear combination of (non-orthogonal) atomic orbitals, and so a full transformation of the original atomic orbital integrals appears to be required. The cost of such a transformation necessarily scales as the fifth power of the basis set size, and so for large basis sets this represents a substantial computational step. However, as recognised by Meyer (1976), the transformation is easily avoided since the integrals are required only once in each iteration of the Davidson diagonalisation procedure, through (79). This can easily be formulated in the atomic orbital basis as

$$C_{\alpha\beta}^p = \sum_{ab} C_{ab}^p q_{\alpha a} q_{\beta b}$$

$$K(\mathbf{C}^p)_{\alpha\beta} = \sum_{\gamma\delta} (\alpha\gamma|\delta\beta) C_{\gamma\delta}^p$$

$$K(\mathbf{C}^p)_{ab} = \sum_{\alpha\beta} K(\mathbf{C}^p)_{\alpha\beta} q_{\alpha a} q_{\beta b} \tag{80}$$

Thus $K(\mathbf{C}^p)$ is formed rather like a Fock matrix, in one sequential read of the atomic orbital integrals. The cost of the additional transformations introduced scales as m^3, and is in most cases negligible. The whole calculation of $\hat{H}\Psi$, (78), is a series of matrix products, capable of optimal performance on most vector computers.

Returning to the N electron problem, these ideas are easily generalised. Since the first order interacting space consists only of singly and doubly excited configurations, it is convenient to partition the wavefunction, a linear combination of CSFs, as

$$\Psi = \sum_I c_I \Phi_I + \sum_{Sa} c_a^S \Phi_S^a + \sum_{Pab} C_{ab}^P \Phi_P^{ab} \tag{81}$$

where the three types of CSF Φ_I, Φ_S^a, Φ_P^{ab} contain respectively 0, 1, 2 occupied external orbitals. In order to span the first order internal space, this set of configurations must be the union of the sets of CSFs obtained by making all possible single and double excitations on each reference configuration in turn. Because none of the reference configurations contains occupied external orbitals, CSFs with 3 or more external orbitals do not appear in Ψ. We also note that since there are usually many more external orbitals than internal orbitals, the configurations Φ_P^{ab} are expected to be by far the most numerous. For the case that Ψ_0 consists of a single closed shell configuration, (81) is the single reference 'CISD' wavefunction; when Ψ_0 contains more than one configuration, variational treatment of (81) is usually referred to as *multireference CI* (MRCI or MRCISD).

For the closed shell single reference problem, it is convenient to formulate the CSFs Φ_P^{ab} directly in terms of two electron excitations, analogous to the two electron problem:

$$\Psi = c_0 \Phi_0 + \sum_{ia} c_a^i \hat{E}_{ai} \Phi_0 + \sum_{i \geq j, p} \sum_{a \geq b} C_{ab}^{ijp} \tfrac{1}{2} (\hat{E}_{ai,bj} + p\hat{E}_{aj,bi}) \Phi_0 \tag{82}$$

In the configuration $\Phi_{ijp}^{ab} \equiv \tfrac{1}{2}(\hat{E}_{ai,bj} + p\hat{E}_{aj,bi})\Phi_0$, orbitals ϕ_i, ϕ_j in the reference are replaced by ϕ_a, ϕ_b. Note that for given $i \neq j$ and $a \neq b$, there are two possible CSFs Φ_{ij1}^{ab}, Φ_{ij-1}^{ab} which correspond exactly to the singlet and triplet two electron wavefunctions. Note also that the configurations are only partially normalised in the same sense as for the two electron problem. Formulae for the Hamiltonian matrix elements are easily derived, and can be found in full in the literature (Ahlrichs, 1983, Saunders, 1983, Meyer, 1976, Werner and Reinsch, 1982). We note here that the whole problem can be formulated as a series of matrix operations; for example, that part of $\hat{H}\Psi$ which arises from all external integrals occurs simply as

$$\langle \Phi_{ijp}^{ab} | \hat{H} | \Psi \rangle = K(\mathbf{C}^{ijp})_{ab} \tag{83}$$

which can be performed in the atomic orbital basis if required. Other terms introduce matrix products involving the generalised Coulomb and exchange operators met already in MCSCF theory.

The multireference problem is far less straightforward. Similar matrix elements occur, with the additional complication that non–trivial coupling coefficients appear; for example, the Coulomb integrals J_{ab}^{ij} are multiplied by

$$\alpha_{ij}(P,Q) = \langle \Phi_P^{ab} | \hat{E}_{ij} | \Phi_Q^{ab} \rangle \tag{84}$$

for the interaction of configurations Φ_P^{ab}, Φ_Q^{cd}. These coupling coefficients are usually generated by group theoretical methods (Shavitt, 1978, Kotani et al., 1963, Knowles and Werner, 1988). No coupling coefficients involving external orbitals are required, but even so, the number of coupling coefficients makes their generation and possible storage a severe bottleneck. The other main problem with MRCI wavefunctions is that the number of configurations quickly grows to be unmanageable, since (81) contains double excitations for each reference configuration. Despite these drawbacks, efficient matrix oriented MRCI procedures (Lischka et al., 1981, Saunders, 1983) (Siegbahn, 1980) are in widespread general use and have been shown to give reliable results for most systems which can be treated (Bauschlicher et al., 1989).

An alternative formulation which avoids the rapid increase in basis size with the number of reference configurations is possible (Meyer, 1977). Instead of selecting singly and doubly excited CSFs from each reference configuration, we can construct configurations by applying excitation operators to the reference wavefunction as a single entity:

$$\Psi = \sum_{ijkl} C^{ijkl} \hat{E}_{ij,kl} \Phi_0 + \sum_{ijka} C_a^{ijk} \hat{E}_{ai,jk} \Phi_0 + \sum_{ijab} C_{ab}^{ij} \hat{E}_{ai,jb} \Phi_0 \tag{85}$$

This is the *internally contracted* MRCI wavefunction, and it is obvious that the number of configurations is now independent of the number of reference functions, depending only on the numbers of internal and external orbitals. In this way, the size of CI expansion is reduced typically by one or two orders of magnitude; the configuration set, however, still spans the first order interacting space. The price that is paid is that the configurations are now much more complicated, being in fact linear contractions of CSFs according to the values of the reference coefficients. This means that coupling coefficient evaluation is now a formidable problem; the simple CSF coupling coefficients are replaced by reduced density matrices of high order. An additional problem is that the configurations are non–orthogonal in a non–trivial way, and their orthogonalisation can be a computational bottleneck. These two difficulties which trouble the original implementation of this approach (Werner and Reinsch, 1982) have now been mostly overcome through new symmetric group techniques for the coupling coefficients (Knowles and Werner, 1988), and a hybrid approach which combines the best features of uncontracted and contracted wavefunctions (Werner and Knowles, 1988). It has then been possible to perform calculations with thousands of reference configurations, equivalent to uncontracted MRCI expansions with nearly 10^8 CSFs.

REFERENCES

Ahlrichs, R., 1983, Pair Correlation Theories, *in*: "Methods in Computational Molecular Physics," G. H. F. Diercksen and S. Wilson, ed., Reidel, Dordrecht.

Bauschlicher, C. W., Langhoff, S. R., and Taylor, P. R., 1989, *Adv. Chem. Phys.*, in press.

Davidson, E. R., 1975, *J. Comput. Phys.*, 17:87.

Davidson, E. R., 1983, Matrix Eigenvector Methods, *in*: "Methods in Computational Molecular Physics," G. H. F. Diercksen and S. Wilson, ed., Reidel, Dordrecht.

Fletcher, R., 1980, "Practical Methods of Optimization, volume 1," Wiley, Chichester.

Foster, J. M., and Boys, S. F., 1960,*Rev. Mod. Phys.* 32:305.

Handy, N. C., 1980, *Chem. Phys. Letters*, 74:280.

Harrison, R. J., and Zarrabian, S., 1989, *Chem. Phys. Letters*, in press.

Jeffreys, H. and Jeffreys, B., 1956,"Methods of Mathematical Physics," Cambridge University Press, Cambridge.

Jørgensen, P., and Simons, J., 1981, "Second Quantization–Based Methods in Quantum Chemistry," Academic Press, New York.

Knowles, P. J. and Handy, N. C., 1984, *Chem. Phys. Letters*, 111:315.

Knowles, P. J. and Handy, N. C., 1989, *Comp. Phys. Commun.*, 54:75.

Knowles, P. J. and Handy, N. C., 1989, *J. Chem. Phys.*, 91:2396.

Knowles, P. J., and Werner, H.-J., 1985, *Chem. Phys. Letters*, 115:259.

Knowles, P. J., and Werner, H.-J., 1988, *Chem. Phys. Letters*, 145:514.

Knowles, P. J., 1989, *Chem. Phys. Letters*, 155:513.

Knowles, P. J., 1989, *J. Chem. Phys.*, in preparation.

Kotani, M., Amemiya, A., Ishiguro, E., and Kimura, T., 1963, "Tables of molecular integrals," Maruzen, Tokyo.

Lanczos, C., 1950, *J. Res. Natl. Bur. Stand.*, 45:255.

Lischka, H., Shepard, R., Brown, F. B., and Shavitt, I., 1981, *Int. J. Quantum Chem. Symp.*, 15:91.

Liu, B., 1978, *in*: "Numerical Algorithms in Chemistry: Algebraic Methods," C. Moler and I. Shavitt, ed., LBL-8158 Lawrence Berkeley Laboratory.

MacDonald, J. K. L., 1933, *Phys. Rev.*, 43:830.

McWeeny, R., and Sutcliffe, B. T., 1969, "Methods of Molecular Quantum Mechanics," Academic Press, London.

Meyer, W., 1976, *J. Chem. Phys.*, 64:2901.

Meyer, W., 1977, *in*: "Modern Theoretical Chemistry," vol. 3, H.F. Schaefer, ed., Plenum, New York.

Olsen, J., Roos, B. O., Jørgensen, P., and Jensen, H. J. Aa., 1988, *J. Chem. Phys.*, 89:2185.

Pack, R. T. and Byers Brown, W., 1966, *J. Chem. Phys.*, 45:556.

Paldus, J., 1974, *J. Chem. Phys.*, 61:5321.

Roos, B., Taylor, P., and Siegbahn, P. E. M., 1980, *Chem. Phys.*, 48:157.

Roos, B. O., 1972, *Chem. Phys. Letters*, 15:153.

Roothaan, C. C. J., 1951, *Rev. Mod. Phys.*, 23:69.

Ruedenberg, K., Cheung, L. M., and Elbert, S. T., 1979, *Intern. J. Quantum Chem.*, 16:1069.

Saunders, V. R., and van Lenthe, J. H., 1983, *Mol. Phys.*, 48:923.

Saxe, P., Schaefer, H. F., and Handy, N. C., 1981, *Chem. Phys. Letters*, 79:202.

Seeger, R., Krishnan, R., and Pople, J. A., 1978, *J. Chem. Phys.*, 68:2519.

Shavitt, I., 1978, *Int. J. Quantum Chem. Symp.*, 12:5.

Shepard, R., 1989, *J. Comp. Chem.*, in press.

Siegbahn, P. E. M., 1984, *Chem. Phys. Letters*, 109:417.

Siegbahn, P. E. M., 1980, *J. Chem. Phys.*, 72:1647.

Werner, H.-J., and Knowles, P. J., 1985, *J. Chem. Phys.*, 82:5053.

Werner, H.-J., and Knowles, P. J., 1988, *J. Chem. Phys.*, 89:5803.

Werner, H.-J., and Meyer, W., 1980, *J. Chem. Phys.*, 73:2342.

Werner, H.-J., and Reinsch, E.-A., 1982, *J. Chem. Phys.*, 76:3144.

Wilkinson, J. H., 1965, "The Algebraic Eigenvalue Problem", Oxford University Press, New York.

Yoshimine, M., 1973, *J. Comp. Phys.*, 11:449.

Zarrabian, S., Sarma, C. R., and Paldus, J., 1989, *Chem. Phys. Letters*, 155:183.

ENERGY MINIMISATION AND

STRUCTURE FACTOR REFINEMENT METHODS

I. Haneef

Astbury Department of Biophysics, University of Leeds, Leeds LS2 9JT, U.K.

INTRODUCTION

From a computational viewpoint, energy minimization and structure factor refinements of molecules fall into the general area of nonlinear optimization problems. Given a set of independent variables x and a specified objective function $F = F(x)$, the task is to find the set of variables $x^\star$ for which the function F has its minimum value $F(x^\star) = min(F(x))$. Clearly, one is interested in a method that delivers the minimum of F with the least amount of computational cost. However, there are often many other factors that can determine the method one uses - e.g. the amount of computer memory required, whether or not the derivatives of the function can be easily obtained or even if they exist, and indeed also whether the human resources exist to set up and implement the most efficient method.

The field of function minimization is vast and varied, and is ubiquitous in many branches of social sciences, economics, science and engineering. In these lecture notes we shall concentrate on the techniques that are commonly employed in the field of energy minimization and structure factor refinement of macromolecules. This narrows down the field considerably, and hopefully can be fitted adequately into a single lecture.

In this lecture we are concerned with finding the set of parameters defining the conformation of macromolecules that minimize a given objective function. A complete description of the conformation of a molecule is given by the $3N$ atomic coordinates of the system. The objective functions in terms of these coordinates represent very complicated surfaces, and in general have very many minima. Clearly, one would like to determine the variables x that give the global minimum for the function F. Little or no theory exists for finding the global minimum of a general function; further, there is no method for distinguishing the global minimum from the many local minima. The classical methods for searching for the global minimum are variants of the multi-start method. This involves starting minimizations from a large number of starting points and selecting the set of parameters which deliver the least value of F. Each such minimization delivers a local minimum, and since for a large system the number of minimizations is necessarily limited to a finite number, there is no guarantee that such a method will deliver the global minimum. We shall later mention one particular technique, the simulated annealing method, which holds considerable promise for important progress in global minimization.

For the most part, we shall not be concerned with the global minimization problem. For macromolecules, we assume that we have an approximate solution to the correct conformation

Supercomputational Science
Edited by R.G. Evans and S. Wilson
Plenum Press, New York, 1990

of the molecule. Using this conformation as our starting structure, we may improve upon it using a number of minimization methods to obtain a structure with lower energy (in the case of energy minimization) or better fit to x-ray diffraction data (in the case of structure factor refinement), or both.

ENERGY MINIMISATION

Energy minimization is perhaps the simplest of all computer simulation techniques for studying theoretically the energetics of macromolecules. The objective function in this case is the potential function describing in detail the interactions between the atoms of the system. The function describing the total energy of the system is assumed to be solely dependent on the coordinates of the atomic nuclei within the molecule, a model justified by the Born-Oppenheimer approximation. Therefore, no explicit account is taken of the electron distributions or energies. For macromolecules, the potential function comprises of energy terms representing bonds, bond angles, torsion angles, van der Waals interaction, and electrostatic interactions. A typical potential function has the form

$$V(R) = \frac{1}{2} \sum_{bonds} k_b(b - b_0)^2 + \frac{1}{2} \sum_{angles} k_\theta(\theta - \theta_0)^2 + \frac{1}{2} \sum_{torsions} k_\phi(1 + cos(n\phi + \delta)) + \tag{1}$$

$$\sum_i \sum_{j>i} \frac{A_{ij}}{r_{ij}^{12}} - \frac{B_{ij}}{r_{ij}^6} + \frac{q_i q_j}{D r_{ij}} \tag{2}$$

The total energy of the system is a function of the positions R of all the atoms involved; the energy of the system for any given set of coordinates R is calculated by first determining the internal coordinates for bonds (b), bond angles (θ), torsion angles (ϕ) and the interatomic distances (r), and then determining their contributions to the total energy using the above equation. These contributions are dependent on the valence energy parameters k_b, k_θ, k_ϕ, Lennard-Jones parameters A and B, and partial atomic charges q_i and the 'dielectric' constant D.

Any continuous, differentiable function of independent variables x can be expanded as a Taylor series about a point $x + \Delta x$,

$$V(x + \Delta x) = V(x) + g^T \Delta x + \frac{1}{2} \Delta x^T H \Delta x \quad .... \tag{3}$$

where g is the vector of first derivatives and H is the second derivative matrix of the function. The various minimization methods can be classified by their order, which is defined by the highest order derivatives used in the method.

1. ZEROTH ORDER METHODS

The conceptually simplest way of locating the minimum of $V(x)$ is to scan the space defined by x in regular increments of x_1, x_2, etc., and choosing that point x^* at which $V(x)$ is a minimum. Clearly, the ability of such grid search methods to locate the minimum depends on the fineness of the grid and the roughness of the surface. Iterative methods can be established by beginning with a relatively coarse grid and using successively finer grids to isolate the true minimum.

One method in this class worthy of particular mention is the simplex method of Nelder and Mead (1965). Although the method is not very efficient in terms of number of function evaluations, it may often be the *best* method to use if one is simply interested in quickly getting a method that works. Such situations do often arise. For example, when testing different potential functions which may contain cross terms of complex nature, it is very expensive in human resources to implement and debug methods that require derivatives.

In an n-dimensional problem $n+1$ points define a simplex. In two dimensions, a simplex is a triangle. In three dimensions it is a tetrahedron. In general, one is only interested in simplexes that are nondegenerate, *i.e.* which enclose a finite inner n-dimensional volume. If any one point of a nondegenerate simplex is taken as the origin, then the n other points define vector directions that span the n-dimensional vector space.

The simplex method is started by defining an initial simplex, each vertex corresponding to one particular value of $V(x)$. The simplest method of generating an initial simplex is to take some point x_0 and then define n other points as

$$x_i = x_0 + \lambda e_i \tag{4}$$

where the e's are n unit vectors, and λ is a constant determining the problem's characteristic length scale. Minimization is achieved by successively inverting the vertex with the maximum function value through the midpoint of the remaining vertices to a lower function value. The basic procedure can be improved by expansion and contraction of the simplex, thus allowing the method to pass through valley-like regions of the potential energy surface. The minimization is terminated when the drop in function value is smaller than some predefined tolerance.

2. FIRST ORDER METHODS

First order methods truncate the Taylor series after the second term, making use of information about the local slope of the potential energy surface. The first derivatives of the potential energy with respects to atomic coordinates yield the force upon any particular atom. The minimum energy structure is then clearly that in which there is no force on any atom in the structure.

We shall describe the first order methods that fall into the general class of iterative descents methods. Each, say k-th, iteration consists of three parts.

First, a descent direction s_k of unit length is chosen; second a descent step size λ_k is determined which gives the least value of the function in the direction s_k. Third, the new set of coordinates x_k for the molecule are set to $x_k = x_{k-1} + \lambda_k s_k$.

Steepest Descent Method. In the Taylor expansion of $V(x + \Delta x)$, the terms after $V(x)$ on the right hand side provide a correction to the function value at x to give an approximation to the function at $x + \Delta x$. Taking only two terms in the series

$$\Delta V = g^T \Delta x = \mid g \mid\mid \Delta x \mid \cos\theta \tag{5}$$

Clearly, ΔV takes its maximum negative value when Δx is in the direction of $-g$. Thus the coordinates at iteration k are given by $x_k = x_{k-1} + \lambda_k g_k$. The step size λ_k is obtained from a separate iterative process. Typically, an initial step size is chosen and the first step is taken. If the energy is reduced by this step, the step size is increased by some multiplicative factor for the next step, a process which is repeated as long as each iteration reduces the energy. Whenever an iteration produces an increase in energy, it is assumed that the step size was too large, resulting in a leap across the valley containing the minimum and up the slope on the opposite side, so the multiplicative factor is reduced for the next iteration. This process is continued until a step size is obtained that minimizes the energy along the direction g.

Since the direction of the gradient is determined by the largest interatomic forces, steepest descent can eliminate the worst steric conflicts and bring bond lengths and bond angles close to their reference values, but will not produce the collective motions that are necessary to generate optimum overall stereochemical structures. The method, although excellent for initially optimizing bad starting local geometries, has poor convergence properties.

Conjugate Gradients Method. A generally more efficient technique is the conjugate gradient method. Steepest descents performs many small steps down a long, narrow valley, even if the valley is a perfect quadratic form due to the fact that each successive step is perpendicular to the direction just traversed. Such perpendicular steps do not in general lead to the minimum.

In conjugate gradients method, each search direction is chosen to be conjugate to the previous gradient, and, insofar as possible, to all previous directions traversed. The algorithm that achieves this can be described thus:

$$x_k = x_{k-1} + \alpha p_k \tag{6}$$
$$p_k = -g_k + \beta p_{k-1} \tag{7}$$
$$\beta = \frac{|g_k|^2}{|g_{k-1}|^2} \tag{8}$$

where $p_0 = -g_0$, and α is chose to give minimum in the direction p_k. It can be proven that, for a quadratic surface, this algorithm will deliver the minimum within n steps for an n-dimensional surface.

3. SECOND ORDER METHODS

The Taylor expansion for the function $V(x)$ upto the second order derivatives can be re-written as

$$0 = g + H\Delta x \tag{9}$$

which immediately leads to the solution for the shifts required in the coordinates to achieve the minimum:

$$\Delta x = -H^{-1}g \tag{10}$$

For a quadratic function, H is a constant; thus, the second order methods deliver the minimum of the function in one step. However, for non-quadratic functions, many iterations may be required to achieve the minimum using the following iteration scheme.

$$x_{k+1} = x_k - H_k^{-1}g_k \tag{11}$$

For macromolecules, the amount of storage required is $O(n^2)$; a further problem with these methods is that the solution for atomic shifts requires the inversion of the Hessian matrix, a task that requires $O(n^3)$ computer time. For these reasons, second order minimization methods are not frequently used for macromolecular systems.

STRUCTURE FACTOR REFINEMENT

Structure factor refinement refers to optimizing the agreement between the observed and calculated structure factor amplitudes. The observed structure factors are measured in an x-ray (or neutron) diffraction experiment. Very considerable effort is required to obtain an approximate structure of the macromolecule that is the solution to all known experimental constraints. Once this approximate structure has been obtained, further improvements are required to give conformational details of the structure at the atomic level. The ultimate test of how good the structure determination is the agreement between the calculated structure factor amplitudes, from the model structure, and the observed structure factor amplitudes. The most commonly used measure of this agreement is the R-factor

$$ R = \frac{\sum_h || F_{obs}(h) | - | F_{calc}(h) ||}{\sum_h | F_{obs}(h) |} \tag{12}$$

where $| F_{obs} |$ is observed structure factor amplitude and F_{calc} is the calculated structure factor. The summations are over all observed reflections. F_{calc} is obtained from the model of the structure, and is a function of the atom scattering factor, atomic positions, atomic temperature factors and atomic occupancies. During the refinement, the task is to find the atomic positions, temperature factors and occupancies that minimize the error function

$$ E = \sum_h w_f(| F_{obs}(h) | - G | F_{calc}(h) |)^2 \tag{13}$$

where w_f is a weight applied to a given reflection and G is a scale factor.

A function of the form r^2 has first and second derivatives

$$ g_i(p) = 2r\frac{\partial r}{\partial p_j} \tag{14}$$

$$ H_{ij}(p) = 2(\frac{\partial r}{\partial p_i}\frac{\partial r}{\partial p_j} + r\frac{\partial^2 r}{\partial p_i \partial p_j}) \tag{15}$$

If the second derivatives of r are ignored one arrives at an approximation to the Hessian (the normal matrix of least-squares theory). In this approximation only the first derivatives need be evaluated. The computational effort required to compute all elements of the normal matrix is very large for macromolecules; for macromolecules, therefore, most refinement programs compute only the diagonal elements of the matrix.

The solution for the atomic shifts is obtained in the manner described above. However, due to the Taylor series approximation and the diagonal nature of the matrix, many iterative cycles are required to obtain the minimum for the error function.

To obtain an accurate and realistic solution for the structure from least-squares refinement generally requires approximately ten observations for each parameter to be refined. Macromolecules seldom diffract to a sufficiently high resolution for such situations to arise. Therefore, supplementary experimental data are incorporated into refinement programs. Such data consist of stereochemical information to give refined structures with reasonable molecular geometry.

ENERGY MINIMISATION AND STRUCTURE FACTOR REFINEMENT

Most refinement programs impose molecular geometry on the structure using pseudo-energy terms. These terms consist of interatomic distances for local geometry of the molecule, planarity restraints and chiral volumes. Jack and Levitt (1978) incorporated energy functions into a refinement procedure to carry out simultaneous energy minimization and structure factor refinement. In this method, the objective function is a weighted sum of the crystallographic residual and the potential energy:

$$T = E + \lambda V \qquad (16)$$

where E is the crystallographic objective function, V is the energy term, and λ is a scaling factor for weighting the two terms together. Since the calculation of the structure factors and their derivatives is very demanding computationally, an assumption is made that calculated structure factors are a linear function of atomic positions: Thus, on each iteration of minimization, E and its first derivatives are updated according to

$$E = E_0 + \sum_i \frac{\partial E}{\partial x_i} \delta x_i + \frac{1}{2} \sum_i \sum_j \frac{\partial^2 E}{\partial x_i \partial x_j} \delta x_i \delta x_j \qquad (17)$$

$$\frac{\partial E}{\partial x_i} = \left(\frac{\partial E}{\partial x_i} \right)_0 + \sum_j \frac{\partial^2 E}{\partial x_i \partial x_j} \delta x_j \qquad (18)$$

Exact values for the structure factors or their derivatives can be calculated at the end of each iteration. Fewer rounds of recalculations of these quantities

can be achieved by requiring that these be calculated only when the atomic shifts have occurred over and above some tolerance value.

1. SIMULATED ANNEALING

Conventional structure factor refinement of macromolecules is an iterative process, requiring several rounds of automated refinement followed by manual rebuilding of the structure. Manual rebuilding is required due to the fact that automated refinement methods lead only to a local minimum. As described earlier, there are no mathematical techniques for locating the global minimum for a general function. In this section we give a brief discussion of a powerful technique that holds considerable promise towards solving some problems.

Classical techniques generate a sequence of function values $\{F\}$ such that each successive value is strictly lower than the previous values. Such a method can be thought of a 'greedy' method that delivers the nearest local minimum. In the simulated annealing method (Kirkpatrick *et al*, 1983), there is no such requirement to generate a strictly monotonically decreasing sequence. Instead, there is a finite probability that the computed value of the function may be larger than the previous function value. A physical analogy is attached to this technique. At high temperatures, the molecules of a liquid move freely with respect to one another. If the liquid is cooled slowly, thermal mobility is lost. Slow cooling allows the atoms of the liquid to line up and form a pure crystal that is completely ordered in all directions. This crystal is the state of lowest energy. The formation of a crystalline state happens when the liquid is cooled slowly; if the liquid is cooled rapidly it does not achieve a crystalline state, but rather forms a polycrystalline or amorphous state which has higher energy. The essential requirement for crystal formation is slow cooling which allows the atoms ample time to redistribute as they lose their kinetic energy.

In analogy with the physical process, the annealing method generates a sequence of configurations of the system at a high 'temperature' - the temperature being controlled by a probability distribution function

$$P(F) = e^{-\frac{F}{kT}} \tag{19}$$

The temperature of the system is then slowly reduced to a low value. Even at low temperature, there is a chance, albeit it small, that the system will be in a state of high energy. Therefore, there is a corresponding chance for the system to get out of a local minimum in favour of a better, more global, one. Thus, in the method of simulated annealing the sequence of function values generated go up as well as down - but lower the temperature, the less likely the chance of increase in function value.

The simulated annealing has found applications in a number of diverse fields. Currently, it is being used extensively at early stages of refinement of macromolecules.

A complete description of the method requires some knowledge of molecular dynamics simulation. Here we have given a qualitative description; in another lecture in this series we shall see how to carry out molecular dynamics simulations.

REFERENCES AND FURTHER READING

Nelder J A and Mead R (1965), Computer Journal **7**, 308
Jack A and Levitt M (1978), Acta Cryst **A34**, 931
Kirkpatrick S, Gellat C D and Vecchi M P (1983), Science **220**, 671

Chapter 10 on Minimization and Maximization of Functions: Press W H, Flannery B P, Teukolsky S A and Vetterling W T, 'Numerical Recipes' (Cambridge Uni Press), 1987

The Refinement of Macromolecules. Isaacs N (1982), 'Computational Crystallography', Ed. Sayre D, pp 381-397
Refinement Techniques: Use of the FFT. Isaacs N (1982), 'Computational Crystallography', Ed. Sayre D, pp 397-408

MOLECULAR DYNAMICS METHODS

I. Haneef

Astbury Department of Biophysics, University of Leeds, Leeds LS2 9JT, U.K.

INTRODUCTION

Although macromolecules have been traditionally described in terms of rigid and unique three-dimensional structures, the dynamics of these molecules have become increasingly important in the understanding the relationships between structure and mechanism. It has been suggested that vibrational modes in macromolecules may act, for example, to channel energy from the solvent to the active site of an enzyme to enable the reaction pathway to proceed through the transition state. It has also been shown that the dynamics of a protein may be important in allowing the access of the substrate to enzyme and that changes in the vibrational modes may contribute to entropic terms affecting the free energy interactions.

In this lecture we shall give an overview of the technique of molecular dynamics for studying the dynamics of macromolecules. However, the technique is far more powerful - it is not simply confined to providing a description of the motion of atoms in a molecule, but can be used to determine thermodynamic quantities for the system under study.

THEORETICAL CALCULATIONS

Statistical mechanics is the central discipline for analyzing the aggregate properties of a many particle system subject to some interaction potential $V(r)$. The most important statistical thermodynamic quantity is the partition function Q_N:

$$Q_N = \int e^{\frac{-E_N}{kT}} dr \tag{1}$$

where E_N is the configurational energy, k the Boltzmann constant, and T the absolute temperature; the integration is carried out over whole of the configurational space of the N particle system. Other statistical thermodynamic quantities can be expressed in terms of the partition function using the well-known results of statistical mechanics (McQuarrie, 1976).

Central to the calculation of the properties of any given system is the knowledge of the interaction potential for that system. Thus, given a potential function $V(r)$ for any system, statistical mechanical results provide a mechanism by which we can calculate the properties of that system. These properties can then be compared with experimental data. Any discrepancy between the calculated and observed properties can be ascribed to errors in the potential function $V(r)$.

Supercomputational Science
Edited by R.G. Evans and S. Wilson
Plenum Press, New York, 1990

Unfortunately, the picture of theoretical calculations presented so far is very limited. In practice, the direct calculation of the properties of a system from the potential function is not possible for realistic systems due to the very complex nature of statistical mechanical expressions that relate $V(r)$ to the properties of the system. Indeed, we find ourself in a situation similar to that exemplified by the famous statement of Dirac for quantum mechanical studies of molecules:

'The underlying physical laws necessary for the mathematical theory of a large part of physics and the whole of chemistry are thus completely known, and the difficulty is only that the exact application of these laws leads to equations much too complicated to be soluble'.

Statistical mechanical methods are essentially analytical and can only be applied in an exact form for extremely simple systems. In particular, for systems with very large number of degrees of freedom, the exact analytical approach is impossible and one has to resort to using numerical methods (computer simulations) to solve statistical mechanical equations. The essential problem in computer simulations can be appreciated simply from the expression for the partition function. The integration over whole of the configurational space for a realistic many particle system is simply impractical. In computer simulations, therefore, one attempts to restrict the integration over those parts of configurational space which make the most significant contribution to the integrand. For most practical applications, this is done by starting the simulations from a configuration of the system that is reasonably close to the real system being studied. Even in such studies, the computational cost of such simulations is prohibitive and only a partial sampling of the configurational space is possible (typically $O(10^4)$-$O(10^6)$ configurations).

A number of computational techniques are used to derive the properties of a system from its potential function. Various simulation methods can often be grouped into one of the four techniques: energy minimization, normal mode analysis, Monte Carlo, and molecular dynamics. Of these, energy minimization (EM) and molecular dynamics (md) are by far the most commonly employed techniques for studying protein molecules.

The technique of energy minimization is described in another lecture in this series. Specific examples of what one can achieve using EM will be described in that lecture. In this lecture we describe the technique of molecular dynamics. Md simulations generate a trajectory (configurations as a function of time) of the system by numerically integrating Newton's equations of motion. The advantage of md over EM is that it provides a Boltzmann weighted ensemble of configurations for the system and, thus, permits the calculation of aggregate properties of the system. However, in order to obtain accurate trajectories it is necessary to employ (integration) time step of the order of femto-seconds. For typical protein molecules (*ca.* 2000 atoms), the computational cost effectively limits such md simulations to few tens of pico-seconds and at best to a few hundred pico-seconds.

The accuracy of the results obtained from statistical mechanics depends solely on the accuracy of the potential functions *i.e.* if one feeds in a lousy potential into statistical mechanics, one obtains lousy results; conversely, lousy results necessarily imply a lousy potential. This simple concept ('lousy results imply lousy potentials') plays an important role in theoretical calculations of macromolecules. For protein molecules, it provides the only means for designing accurate potential functions for these important molecules. (For small molecules, the potential functions can be obtained from detailed quantum mechanical studies; for macromolecules, however, empirical energy functions of the molecular mechanics (Boyd and Lipkowitz, 1982) type are the only possible source of such information.)

The results obtained from computer simulations are also affected by the accuracy of the potential functions; here, however, there exists another major problem - namely the inability of simulations to sample the configurational space adequately. The results from simulations will necessarily have some error due to incomplete sampling of configurational space. This point must always be kept in mind when interpreting the results from any md simulation. As we shall point out later, there are also many problems of deriving thermodynamic properties of the system which are sensitive to the way in which the simulations are carried out.

MOLECULAR DYNAMICS

From the theoretical point of view, the description of the dynamics of a macromolecules is a classical many-particle problem. In a system where the forces between the particle cannot be adequately described by harmonic forces, the method of molecular dynamics provides the most appropriate methodology for extracting the dynamics of the system.

The technique itself consists of a procedure for numerical integration of Newton's equations of motion for the interacting particles of the system. In general the calculation starts by defining the initial coordinates r and velocities v of the particles, and an interaction potential $V(r)$, function of the positions of all the particles. Since the number of particles is still small on the macroscopic scale, in most cases periodic boundary conditions are imposed where the macroscopic system is represented by an infinite number of identical cells each containing an equal number of particles at positions related by translational symmetry.

1. MATHEMATICAL MODEL

Assuming that the dynamics of the system of N particles, with masses m_i and position vectors r_i, is governed by an interaction potential $V(r)$ which depends on the positions of all the particles, md sets up Newton's equations of motion

$$F_i = m_i \frac{d^2 r_i}{dt^2} \tag{2}$$

subject to the initial conditions

$$r(0) = r_0 \tag{3}$$
$$v(0) = v_0 \tag{4}$$

where F_i is obtained from the potential energy of the system

$$F_i = -\frac{\partial V(r)}{\partial r_i} \tag{5}$$

This procedure, therefore, constitutes an initial boundary value problem subject to $3N$ coupled differential equations. The simultaneous integration of $3N$ differential equations yields a time trajectory for all N particles of the system.

INTEGRATION PROCEDURES

Due to the many-particle nature of the problem, the only method for obtaining a solution of the differential equations is by a numerical integration procedure. In such a procedure, a new configuration of the system is calculated from the previous one by assuming that the forces F_i are constant over a small time step Δt. The choice of the time step Δt is governed by

245

the accuracy and the length of the trajectory required - very small time step will yield a very accurate simulation but will be limited in its duration due to the computational cost.

There are very many numerical methods for solving a set of differential equations. All methods are based on finite differences and solve the equations step by step in time. Often the step size is kept constant. One requirement of md immediately rules out a number of methods. The computation of the forces on the particles is a very computationally demanding task compared to the manipulation of the various coordinates to take one step forward in time. This, therefore, immediately rules out any method requiring more than one force evaluation per time step. For example, the well-known Runge-Kutta method and its variants require 4 force evaluations per step in its usual version, and cannot therefore be a method of choice for md simulations. Another requirement is that an algorithm should behave well for the type of force that one encounters in md of macromolecules. Normally md simulations produce trajectories in the valley regions of the potential energy surface. In the valley regions the second derivatives of the potential with respect to the coordinates is positive. This means that the second spatial derivatives of the potential have a systematic sign and the algorithm should at least incorporate the proper treatment of the first derivatives of the forces to avoid accumulating errors and instabilities of the solution. This means that the order of the algorithm, defined as the highest order of the time step Δt in the equation for the solution of the coordinates, should be at least 3. Higher orders correspond to higher than first derivatives of the forces. It is expected that these have a more erratic and nonsystematic character.

We shall describe three algorithms for calculating the trajectories in md simulations. Two of these are second order methods (Verlet and Beeman algorithms) and one is fifth order (the Gear method). Which of these methods is used depends on a number of factors: If we are confined by the physics of the problem to use a very small time step, then the method of choice is the Gear method; where larger time steps can be used, then Verlet and Beeman algorithms may be used.

The accuracy of an md simulation is most commonly determined by taking the ratio of the rms's of the total and kinetic energy. If this ratio is less than 1%, the simulation is said to be accurate. The time step used in simulation for any given method is chosen to satisfy this criterion.

1. VERLET METHOD

Verlet algorithm (Verlet, 1967) generates the new configuration $r_i(t + \Delta t)$ from the previous one $r_i(t)$ using the equation

$$r_i(t + \Delta t) = 2r_i(t) - r_i(t - \Delta t) + \frac{F_i(t)}{m_i}\Delta t^2 \qquad (6)$$

where m_i is the mass of the particle i and F_i is the force acting on that particle.

In many instances, we are also interested in either monitoring or altering the temperature of the system. To do this we need to know the velocities of the particles during the simulation. One method for calculating the velocities is to use the equation

$$v_i = \frac{(r_i(t + \Delta t) - r_i(t - \Delta t))}{2\Delta t} \qquad (7)$$

There are two disadvantages in using this equation. First, the velocities are obtained as difference of two quantities. If this is a small difference between two large numbers, substantial numerical errors can arise. This can lead to errors in the kinetic energy and temperature. Second, we may also like to control the temperature of the system, therefore the calculation of the positions of the particles should be made a function of the velocities. These disadvantages may be removed by using the following, so called, leap-frog formulation.

If w_i is the average velocity over the time interval t and $t + \Delta t$, then the position at the end of the interval is exactly

$$r_i(t + \Delta t) = r_i(t) + w_i \Delta t \tag{8}$$

Assuming that the forces acting on the particles are constant over the time step Δt, then the average velocity is equal to the instantaneous velocity at time $t + \frac{\Delta t}{2}$ and can be calculated from

$$v_i(t + \frac{\Delta t}{2}) = v_i(t - \frac{\Delta t}{2}) + \frac{F_i(t)}{m_i} \Delta t \tag{9}$$

leading to the equation for updating the positions of the particles

$$r_i(t + \Delta t) = r_i(t) + v_i(t + \frac{\Delta t}{2}) \Delta t \tag{10}$$

2. BEEMAN METHOD

The Beeman method (Beeman, 1976) assumes that, during the time interval Δt, the force varies linearly with time according to the relation

$$F_i(t_0 + t) = \frac{(F_i(t_0) - F_i(t_0 - \Delta t))}{\Delta t} t \tag{11}$$

By integrating this expression we may obtain the expression for the velocities

$$v_i(t_0 + t) = v_i(t_0) + \frac{(3F_i(t_0) - F_i(t_0 - \Delta t))}{m_i} t \tag{12}$$

Integrating again leads to the expression for the positions

$$r_i(t_0 + t) = r_i(t_0) + v_i(t_0)t + \frac{(4F_i(t_0) - F_i(t_0 - \Delta t))}{6m_i} t^2 \tag{13}$$

This, in the notation used above, is

$$r_i(t + \Delta t) = r_i(t) + v_i(t)\Delta t + \frac{(4F_i(t) - F_i(t - \Delta t))}{6m_i} \Delta t^2 \tag{14}$$

247

After some manipulation, the expression for the velocities may be shown to be

$$v_i(t + \Delta t) = v_i(t) + \frac{(2F_i(t + \Delta t) + 5F_i(t) - F_i(t - \Delta t))}{6m_i} \Delta t \tag{15}$$

The principal advantage of the Beeman algorithm lies in the its efficiency. Since it treats the first-order treatment of the forces during the time interval, it is effectively a third-order method. This allows the use of larger time steps than possible with Verlet method.

3. GEAR METHOD

A class of algorithms for numerically solving differential equations is the predictor-corrector method. These methods first predict the values of various quantities with a predictor formula and then use a further formula to correct the predicted values. The prediction-correction procedure can be repeated and iterated until the correction becomes as small as desired. However, such an iterative scheme requires more than one evaluation of the forces per step in md simulations. Here we describe the method due to Gear (1971) where only one force evaluation is required.

In the 5-level Gear method, derivatives of r upto fifth order are used. The predictor expressions (indicated here with superscript p) used in this 5-level method are

$$x_0^p = x_0 + x_1 + x_2 + x_3 + x_4 + x_5 \tag{16}$$
$$x_1^p = x_1 + 2x_2 + 3x_3 + 4x_4 + 5x_5 \tag{17}$$
$$x_2^p = x_2 + 3x_3 + 6x_4 + 10x_5 \tag{18}$$
$$x_3^p = x_3 + 4x_4 + 10x_5 \tag{19}$$
$$x_4^p = x_4 + 5x_5 \tag{20}$$
$$x_5^p = x_5 \tag{21}$$

where we use the notation $x_n = n!\Delta t^n \frac{d^n r}{dt^n}$ and variables with superscript p are the predicted values. We now use the predicted forces to obtain the correction factor

$$\Delta F = \frac{F_i}{m_i} - x_2^p \tag{22}$$

where F_i is the force on the particles in their predicted configuration. This correction factor may be used to give corrected values at time $t + \Delta t$

$$x_0 = x_0^p + \frac{3}{16}\Delta F \tag{23}$$

$$x_1 = x_1^p + \frac{251}{360}\Delta F \tag{24}$$

$$x_2 = x_2^p + \Delta F \tag{25}$$

$$x_3 = x_3^p + \frac{11}{18}\Delta F \tag{26}$$

$$x_4 = x_4^p + \frac{1}{6}\Delta F \tag{27}$$

$$x_5 = x_5^p + \frac{1}{60}\Delta F \tag{28}$$

PROTOCOL

The molecular dynamics simulation starts by first defining the initial conditions for the system. There are total of $6N$ conditions to be defined for a system of N particles. $3N$ of these are the coordinates of the initial configuration from which the simulation is to start. Another $3N$ conditions are supplied in the form of the components of the velocities for the particles. The positions of the atoms may be obtained experimentally (e.g. from crystal structure). However, we have no way of assigning the velocities in a realistic fashion. In md simulations, the velocities are initially randomly assigned. This is done by assigning velocities taken from a Gaussian distribution corresponding to some specific temperature, where the temperature is defined by

$$3NkT = \sum_i^N m_i v_i^2 \tag{29}$$

Since the velocities are assigned in a random fashion, initially they may not correspond to the equilibrated set for the system (we know from the equipartition theorem that each degree of freedom of the system must have the same amount of energy; a random assignment of velocities is unlikely to impart such a situation). It is, therefore, necessary to run the simulation for some time and allow it find an equilibrated state where energy is equally distributed to all modes of vibration of the system. Once the system has converged to an equilibrated state, we may calculate various (thermodynamic) properties of the system.

Herein lies a problem. How long do we need to run a simulation before it converges to an equilibrated state? Consider carrying out an md simulation for a perfect harmonic system with, say, just two degrees of freedom. If we assign the velocities in a random fashion, we may, for example, impart 30% kinetic energy to one degree of freedom, and 70% to the other. If we now proceed with our simulation, the two degrees of freedom will retain their respective amounts of kinetic energies (since the system is perfectly harmonic, the two degrees of freedom are totally independent of each other and therefore cannot exchange energy). Thus, for a perfectly harmonic system the simulation will never converge to an equilibrated state. Although this situation arises only for a perfectly harmonic system, approach to an equilibrated state will depend on how quickly energy can be redistributed between the various modes of the system. There are, however, no hard and fast rules which can be applied to determine the length of the equilibration stage, nor any hard and fast indicators for determining the onset of equilibration.

THERMODYNAMIC PERTURBATION METHOD

Computational methods that can predict the relative stabilities of related molecules would be of tremendous value. In pharmacology, for example, one is often concerned with binding of a number of drugs that differ only in one substituent. Similar problems may now also be found in protein engineering where one is interested in the relative stability of a number of site-specific mutants differing by a single amino acid.

Md simulations provide methods for calculating free energy differences, using a relatively new technique, the thermodynamic perturbation method. This method makes use of the fact that the free energy difference between two states of a system, A and B, can be described by the statistical mechanical relation

$$\Delta G = -kT \ln \left\langle e^{\frac{-H_{AB}}{kT}} \right\rangle_A \tag{30}$$

where H_{AB} is the difference in the Hamiltonian of states A and B, ΔG is the free energy difference between these states, k the Boltzmann constant, T the absolute temperature, and $\langle\rangle_A$ indicates an ensemble average over the reference state A. The two systems cannot be radically different since the average will then be too slowly converging. Where the differences between the two states is large, the problem can be overcome by considering a number of intermediate states. Thus, defining a coupling parameter λ, the intermediate states between A and B are defined by

$$H_\lambda = \lambda H_A + (1 - \lambda) H_B \tag{31}$$

The free energy difference between two states defined by λ and λ' is

$$\Delta G_\lambda = -kT \ln \left\langle e^{\frac{H_\lambda - H_{\lambda'}}{kT}} \right\rangle_\lambda \tag{32}$$

The total free energy change is obtained from the sum of the free energy changes over the various intermediate states

$$\Delta G_{AB} = \sum_{\lambda=0}^{\lambda=1} \Delta G_\lambda \tag{33}$$

An equivalent formulation is to describe the total change as an integration for the free energy difference ΔG:

$$\Delta G = \int_0^1 \left\langle \frac{\partial H}{\partial \lambda} \right\rangle_\lambda d\lambda \tag{34}$$

This formulation is particularly useful for molecular dynamics simulations. If λ is changed very slowly from 0 to 1 during an md simulation, the integration can be carried out in the course of the simulation. As long as the change in λ is carried out slowly such that the system remains essentially in equilibrium for each intermediate value of λ, ΔG_{AB} can be obtained for rather different states A and B.

REFERENCES AND FURTHER READING

Verlet L (1967), Phys Rev **159**, 98
Gear C W (1971), 'Numerical Initial Value Problems in Ordinary Differential Equations', Prentice-Hall
Beeman D (1976), J Comp Phys **20**, 130

MOLECULAR DYNAMICS OF PROTEIN MOLECULES

D.S. Moss and T.P. Flores

Birkbeck College, Malet St., London WC1E 7HX

INTRODUCTION

The dynamics of protein molecules are fundamental to the behaviour of all biological systems. Almost all chemical reactions in living organisms are catalysed by proteins called enzymes and the catalytic processes are dependent on the conformations and mobility of the enzyme molecules. The transport of ions and small molecules by proteins (eg. oxygen by haemoglobin) also depends on the conformational rearrangements possible in the protein molecule.

An understanding of these dynamic processes is the basis for understanding the effect of engineering modified proteins. Techniques such as site directed mutagenesis enable changes to be made to the amino acid composition of an enzyme which may lead to a modified rate of catalysis. Similarly chemical modifications of inhibitors (molecules which inhibit enzyme activity by binding to protein molecules) will lead to changed binding constants. By predicting these states, molecular dynamics is playing an increasing role in the molecular design of drug molecules.

Protein molecules consist of one or more polymer chains built up of amino acid residues. Each chain consists of between 1,000 and 20,000 atoms and *in vivo* adopts a single fairly well defined conformation. This biologically active conformation is dependent on its environment for its existence which is often aqueous but may also be in cell membranes which consist of lipid molecules. Computer simulation of protein systems must take into account the dynamic properties of this environment.

Motions in protein molecules cover a wide range of time scales. Vibrations of covalent bonds take place in $10^{-14}s$, whereas, large scale conformational changes may take more than $10^2 s$. It is this range of characteristic times that presents molecular simulation with one of its greatest challenges. The types of motion which are exhibited in protein molecules has been the subject of several reviews. Karplus and McCammon (1986) have given an overview of the different simulation techniques and their application to the different types of dynamic processes in protein molecules.

Most molecular dynamics studies of protein molecules have been based on classical equations of motion. The position and velocity of each atom have been assumed to be simultaneously defined. This assumption is reasonable for carbon atoms but a quantum mechanical treatment becomes necessary for lighter particles such as electrons and possibly protons. A path integral method of treating the quantum mechanical problem has been developed (Kuki and Wolynes, 1987 and Zheng *et al.*, 1988) but this chapter will concentrate on the classical methods which can be applied to protein dynamics as long as proton and electron transfer are not relevant.

Supercomputational Science
Edited by R.G. Evans and S. Wilson
Plenum Press, New York, 1990

1. MOLECULAR DYNAMICS

The essential principle of MD is the numerical integration of the classical equations of motion for a system of interacting particles over a certain period of time. The trajectories and velocities of the atoms are followed over this time period which is often limited by the computing resources available. One hour of processor time on a CRAY X-MP is required for the simulation of one picosecond $(10^{-12}s)$ of a small protein in its aqueous environment. The folding of a protein molecule into its native conformation may take several seconds and such studies are therefore not practicable. Most studies are restricted to time periods of less than one nanosecond $(10^{-9}s)$. The atoms are usually assigned initial velocities corresponding to a Maxwellian distribution at a given temperature. The simulation proceeds in a series of small time increments and, after each time step the force on each atom is evaluated.

The force $F_i(t)$ on an atom i is obtained by taking the derivative of the potential energy function with respect to its position $r_i(t)$:

$$F_i(t) = -\frac{\delta}{\delta r_i} \mathcal{V}(\vec{r}_1, \vec{r}_2, \ldots, \vec{r}_{3N_{at}}) \tag{1}$$

The acceleration $a_i(t)$ of this atom with mass, m_i, is found by:

$$a_i(t) = \frac{F_i(t)}{m_i} \tag{2}$$

and hence the atomic position:

$$\frac{d^2 r_i}{dt^2}(t) = \frac{F_i(t)}{m_i} \tag{3}$$

It follows that for each atom there are three scalar equations which can be written in component form as:

$$m_i a_i = \sum_j f_{ij} \tag{4}$$

The summation on the right hand side is over all atoms j exerting forces on atom i which have to be evaluated. The computer solution of the differential equations (4) is by replacing them with difference equations which are successively solved for small time steps, Δt. Consider the x co-ordinate of atom i in the following two difference equations, which are Taylor series approximations:

$$x_i(t + \Delta t) = x_i(t) + v_i \Delta t + a_i \frac{\Delta t^2}{2} \tag{5}$$

$$x_i(t - \Delta t) = x_i(t) - v_i \Delta t + a_i \frac{\Delta^2 t}{2} \tag{6}$$

Adding equations (5) and (6) gives:

$$x_i(t + \Delta t) = 2x_i(t) - x_i(t - \Delta t) + a_i(t)\Delta t^2 \tag{7}$$

Substituting from equation (4) then gives:

$$x_i(t + \Delta t) = 2x_i(t) - x_i(t - \Delta t) + \sum_j \frac{f_{ij}(t)}{m_i} \tag{8}$$

Equation (8) gives us a way of predicting the position of atom i at time $t + \Delta t$ if we are given its positions at time t and $t - \Delta t$. Similarly by subtracting equations (5) and (6) we obtain:

$$v_i(t) = \frac{x_i(t + \Delta t) - x_i(t - \Delta t)}{2\Delta t} \tag{9}$$

which gives the velocity at time t.

The equation (8) is known as the Verlet algorithm and is used to track the position of each atom at succeeding time steps (Verlet, 1967). Numerous other integration algorithms have been used, such as Gear, Leapfrog and Beeman. Some techniques, such as the Runge-Kutta methods, require several force evaluations per time step. These are unsuitable for molecular dynamics of proteins, where force evaluation is the most time consuming part of the dynamics calculation.

2. POTENTIAL ENERGY FUNCTIONS

For two reasons, the potential energy (PE) plays a central role in molecular dynamics simulation. Firstly, according to equation (1), the force acting on an atom is related to the first derivative of the potential energy function. Secondly, during a molecular dynamics simulation, the total energy (E) must be carefully monitored. This is the sum of the kinetic and potential energies:

$$E = \frac{1}{2} \sum_{i=1}^{N_{df}} m_i v_i^2 + \mathcal{V}(\vec{r}) \tag{10}$$

where N_{df} is the number of degrees of freedom. The kinetic energy is simple to calculate but the PE is a complicated function of atomic positions. This function must be able to predict molecular properties that are measurable by experiment before being applied to situations that are inaccessible to any experimental probes. An excellent review of PE functions has been carried out by Lifson (1981) and recently in several papers (Maple et al, 1988, Hagler et al., 1989, Burt et al, 1989).

The PE function contains many parameters. Ideally, these would be determined by solving the Schrödinger equation, but this is still only possible for a few simple models. The Born-Oppenheimer approximation, which seperates the Schrödinger equation into two parts - electronic and nuclear, can be used to obtain a detailed picture of the PE surface for systems of up to 10–20 atoms, but such calculations are not yet feasible for large molecules (McCammon, 1984). Instead an empirical PE function is used, consisting of terms that account for covalent bond stretching, bond angle bending, harmonic dihedral bending, sinusoidal dihedral torsions and non-bonded (van der Waals and Coulombic) interations[1]. This energy function can be considered as an approximation of the Born-Oppenheimer aimed at representing the surface at the second level (ie. nuclear)(Lifson, 1981). This approximation can be understood as applicable when we consider that during a small displacement of the nucleus the electrons that surround it will have circled it many thousands of times and that therefore their effect can be considered as an average shell. The parameters in empirical PE functions are obtained from experimental

---

[1] Quantum corrections to this classical approach have been shown to be very small, being significant for local vibrations with frequencies above 300cm^{-1} (Karplus & McCammon, 1981)

and quantum-mechanical studies. One computer program that is widely used for molecular dynamics of macromolecules is *GROMOS87*. The *GROMOS87* PE function has the form (Aqvist et al., 1985):

$$
\begin{aligned}
\mathcal{V}(\vec{r}) &= \mathcal{V}(\vec{r}_1, \vec{r}_2, \ldots, \vec{r}_{N_{at}}) \qquad (11) \\
&= \underbrace{\sum_{n=1}^{N_b} \frac{1}{2} K_{b_n} [b_n - b_{0_n}]^2}_{bonds} + \underbrace{\sum_{n=1}^{N_\theta} \frac{1}{2} K_{\theta_n} [\theta_n - \theta_{0_n}]^2}_{angles} \\
&\quad + \underbrace{\sum_{n=1}^{N_\xi} \frac{1}{2} K_{\xi_n} [\xi_n - \xi_{0_n}]^2}_{improper\ torsions} + \underbrace{\sum_{n'=1}^{N_\phi} K_{\phi_{n'}} [1 + \cos(n_{n'}\phi_{n'} - \delta_{n'})]}_{proper\ torsions} \\
&\quad + \sum_{i<j}^{N_{at}} \left[\underbrace{A_{i,j}/r_{ij}^{12} - C_{i,j}/r_{ij}^6}_{van\ der\ Waals} + \underbrace{q_i q_j / (4\pi\varepsilon_0\varepsilon_r r_{ij})}_{electrostatic} \right] \\
&\quad + additional\ terms \qquad (12)
\end{aligned}
$$

where $\vec{r}_1, \vec{r}_2, \ldots, \vec{r}_{N_{at}}$ represents the coordinates of the system that is to be investigated. These may be the explicit atomic cartesian coordinates or the internal coordinates (bond lengths, bond angles and torsional angles) from which all interatomic distances can be calculated. Work is currently in progress to determine better parameters and potential energy functions (Palca, 1986).

2.1 BOND POTENTIAL

It is possible to obtain a good fit to the second level of the Born-Oppenheimer approximation for bonds using the Morse potential (Morse, 1929):

$$
\mathcal{V}_{bonds} = \sum_{n=1}^{N_b} \left\{ D_{b_n} [1 - e^{-\alpha_n (b_n - b_{0_n})}]^2 - D_{b_n} \right\} \qquad (13)
$$

where $-D_{b_n}$ is the energy at the equilibrium bond length b_{0_n} and α_n is used to adjust the potential so that it is able to produce the molecular vibration spectrum of diatomic molecules. For general situations where the fluctuations of bond lengths are close to the equilibrium value, a simple harmonic approximation is sufficient, as in equation (12), where $K_{b_n} = 2D_{b_n}\alpha_n^2$. These two curves are shown in figure 1.

2.2 BOND ANGLES

Bonds angles are understood principally from a qualitative point of view and therefore the derivation of a PE function describing bonds angles is not so simple. For small deviations, treating them as quadratic is a reasonable approximation and, as no better function has been identified, this has become the function of choice for peptides and proteins. This potential is not very accurate for large deviations and this fact should be borne in mind. In equation (12) K_{θ_n}, θ_n and θ_{0_n} correspond to the equivalent bond parameters.

2.3 PROPER TORSIONS

Proper torsions (or dihedral rotations) describe the rotation around a given bond (see figure 2). The most commonly used form of potential function using torsion angles is known as the Pitzer potential after the first person to describe it (Pitzer, 1951). In equation (12), $K_{\phi_{n'}}$ is the force constant, $\delta_{n'}$ is the reference angle where the potential energy is a maximum and $n_{n'}$ is multiplicity, that is, the number of potential minima in one full rotation. The peptide bond has a partial double bond character with a torsional energy barrier of around 20kcal/mol. All peptide bonds are usually found as *trans* in proteins except prolines which occasionally occur as *cis* isomer. The boundaries for the ϕ, ψ and χ torsional angles are much lower. The nature of torsional potentials are not fully understood and there is even some dispute of the periodicity and location of the energy minima of these functions (Lifson, 1981).

Improper torsions are the out of plane bending of a central atom with the three surrounding atoms to which it is bonded (see figure 2). These are particularly important when the united atom approach is used (described later). As with bond angles the theoretical basis is not strong, but deviations from the equilibrium value are small in proteins and the quadratic form is sufficient. In equation (12) K_{ξ_n}, ξ_n and ξ_{0_n} correspond to the equivalent bond parameters.

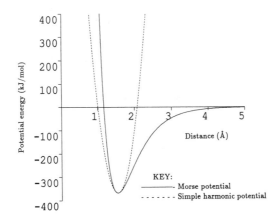

Figure 1. Comparison of the Morse and simple harmonic bond potentials.

2.4 CROSS TERMS

Some force fields contain additional potential terms that account for coupling of interactions. These are known as cross terms and may take the form:

$$
\begin{aligned}
\mathcal{V}_{ct} \;=\; & \underbrace{\sum_{n=1}^{N_{bb'}} F_{bb'}(b_n - b_{0_n})(b'_n - b'_{0_n})}_{bond-bond} + \underbrace{\sum_{n=1}^{N_{b\theta}} F_{b\theta}(b_n - b_{0_n})(\theta_n - \theta_{0_n})}_{bond-angle} \\[2mm]
& + \underbrace{\sum_{n=1}^{N_{\theta\theta'}} F_{\theta\theta'}(\theta_n - \theta_{0_n})(\theta'_n - \theta'_{0_n})}_{angle-angle} + \underbrace{\sum_{n=1}^{N_{\xi\xi'}} F_{\xi\xi'}(\xi_n - \xi_{0_n})(\xi'_n - \xi'_{0_n})}_{improper\ torsion-improper\ torsion} \\[2mm]
& + \underbrace{\sum_{n=1}^{N_{\phi\theta\theta'}} F_{\phi\theta\theta'}\cos\phi_n(\theta_n - \theta_{0_n})(\theta'_n - \theta'_{0_n})}_{proper\ torsion-angle-angle}
\end{aligned}
\tag{14}
$$

Previously these terms have often been neglected and only included when calculating vibrational spectra. The importance of these terms has been recently investigated and the results would suggest that the use of cross terms is important for properly evaluating energetics and geometry (Hagler *et al*, 1989).

2.5 NONBONDED INTERACTIONS

Nonbonded interations are split into three parts:

- Dispersion (attractive) term

- Repulsion term

- Coulombic (electrostatic) term

Calculation of long range interaction could be carried out by a variety of methods, such as Ewald summation (Hansen, 1973). Unfortunately these are computationally very expensive and generally only applicable to infinitely periodic systems (eg. crystals). It is not possible to get exact solutions to the interactions between two atoms. Generally, information has been obtained by extensive quantum mechanical calculations and crystal packing data. The first two terms account for the van der Waals interaction and all take a similar form. These interactions are not calculated for atoms separated by two consecutive bonds as they would be very large. The nonbonded interactions for these are effectively supplied by the first four terms in equation (12). The interaction with the third neighbour is adjusted so that its contribution to the torsional barrier is taken into account.

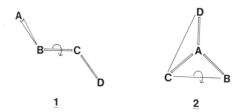

1 **2**

Figure 2. Definitions of (1) Proper torsion and (2) Improper torsion angles. Open bars show the connecting bonds between atoms A, B, C & D. The thin lines represent connections defined purely for calculation purposes. In both cases the angle is defined as that between the planes ABC and BCD, as shown.

2.6 DISPERSION TERMS

At distances where the electron clouds do not overlap, the atoms will experience a net attractive force. This is because at any given moment there are instantaneous dipoles created due to the nuclear and electronic fluctuations. Dipoles are induced in other atoms by this producing a dispersive force. The work in this area is mainly due to that of London (1930) where the attraction force has the form of a power series:

$$\mathcal{V}_{disp} = -\frac{C_{ij}}{r_{ij}^6} - \frac{C'_{ij}}{r_{ij}^8} - \frac{C''_{ij}}{r_{ij}^{10}} - \cdots \qquad (15)$$

as $-\frac{C_{ij}}{r_{ij}^6}$ is the dominating term at long distances the remainder is neglected. It is important to remember this an approximation and that at closer distances the remaining terms may be significant. Slater and Kirkwood derived a theoretical relationship for C_{ij} by finding the best fit using experimental data from work on noble gases. This takes the form:

$$C_{ij} = \frac{3e\hbar}{2M_e^{\frac{1}{2}}} \frac{\alpha_i \alpha_j}{(\frac{\alpha_i}{N_i})^{\frac{1}{2}} + (\frac{\alpha_j}{N_j})^{\frac{1}{2}}} \qquad (16)$$

where α and N are the polarisabilities and number of electrons in the outer shell for atoms of the type i and j, respectively. As mentioned earlier this equation is derived from work on the noble gases and has been assumed to be applicable to polyatomic molecules but never proved. Although there are only a limited set of atoms that occur in macromolecules, we would require $\frac{N(1+N)}{2}$ non independant parameters, most of which are can not be determined by empirical methods. It is therefore beneficial to determine a combination rule which enables the calculation of these coefficients from those parameters that are obtainable from empirical methods, ie. from C_{ii}. From equation (16) we note that the coefficients C_{ij} relate to C_{ii} and C_{jj} by the following rule:

$$2\frac{\alpha_i \alpha_j}{C_{ij}} = \frac{\alpha_i^2}{C_{ii}} + \frac{\alpha_j^2}{C_{jj}} \qquad (17)$$

It is now possible to calculate all of these coefficients from N empirical parameters. This is usually taken one step further using the geometric mean:

$$C_{ij}^2 = C_{ii}C_{jj} \qquad (18)$$

Although this has the advantage of avoiding the use of polarisabilities it is exceptionally inaccurate. Using equation (17) the RMS deviation from experiment was 3.3% as opposed to 73.5% when using equation (18) (Kramer and Herschbach, 1970).

2.7 REPULSIVE TERMS

When atoms come close to each other their electron clouds overlap and produce a repulsive force. This force rapidly increases the closer the two atoms become and the nature of this force is considered to be exponential. In simple terms this may be expressed as:

$$\mathcal{V}_{rep} = Ae^{-br_{ij}} \qquad (19)$$

Determination of A and b is not a trivial matter and in any case this form of the repulsion term is not computationally efficient. As the nature of this function is to create a steep repulsive force as two atoms become close, this term can be replaced by one relying on high powers of r_{ij}^n. The work in this area was principly carried out by Lennard-Jones (1924), who found that this power was arbitrary as long as it was sufficiently steep. Often $n = 9$ is used but more commonly $n = 12$, as this is computationally more convenient. Once again the geometric mean is used to produce all of the coefficients. The resultant potential is that shown in equation (12).

2.8 ELECTROSTATIC TERMS

The electrostatic interactions are an important part of the force field that is used for macro-molecular calculations as these systems contain many highly polar groups. The electrostatic PE function in equation (12) is that given by Coulombs law, where q_i and q_j are the partial charges and ε_r is the relative dielectric permittivity. This potential can be extended to include higher order terms that account for dipole moments, quadrupole moments, etc.

The choice of a value for the relative dielectric permittivity has in the past been the cause of some dispute. In general, values of $\varepsilon = 1 \rightarrow 8$ (in one case $\varepsilon = 20$, Rees, 1980) have been used depending on the method by which the atomic charges have been calculated (Burt *et al.*, 1989). In some recent work, the use of a distance-dependent dielectric has been incorporated (Brooks *et al*, 1983), thereby damping the long-range interactions more than those at shorter ranges. The meaning of the relative dielectric constant is very complex and it is reasonable to set it to unity for most applications (Lifson, 1981). Partial atomic charges are usually calculated using Mulliken population analysis (Mulliken, 1955) or derived from fitting to crystal geometries and parameters.

2.9 HYDROGEN BONDS

The nature of the origin of hydrogen bonds has been a matter of some debate since first being recognised some eighty years ago. As they are one of the most prominent features and strongest nonbonded interaction found in biological systems it is important that any PE function must be able to reproduce them.

In some potential energy functions an explicit term for hydrogen bonding is introduced to obtain reasonable equilibrium hydrogen bond distances (Brooks *et al.*, 1983), especially if the coulombic term is neglected (Levitt, 1983). In these terms the hydrogen bond is given a distance and angular dependence.

Other groups have not found this extra term to be necessary, accounting for the hydrogen bond as a function of van der Waals and electrostatic interactions. In these cases the usual parameters are use with the exception of the nonbonded parameters of polar hydrogens which are set to zero. The suitability of this assumption has been elegantly demonstrated by Hagler and coworkers (1989) by examining the spatial electron densities.

3. TREATMENT OF BOUNDARIES

Most of the early simulations were carried out in vacuo. That is, the isolated molecule was simulated without any boundary conditions. This makes molecules become distorted, particularly if they are not spherical, as they tend to minimise their surface area. The outermost atoms become unrealistic as they lack any interaction with surrounding atoms. This has a further effect of removing any shielding by the solvent with high dielectric constant on electric interactions. The most recent vacuo simulation has been of the largest protein molecule yet simulated and analysis of the results was limited to the interior of the protein.

To overcome this an effectively infinite system can be produced by introducing periodic boundary conditions. The molecules are confined within a cell which is surrounded by periodic replicas of itself. This means that whenever a particle leaves the cell through one of its faces, its image in the neighbouring cell on the opposite face takes its place (figure 3). Most simulations employ cubic boundary conditions. However, the most suitable shape, in terms of computational efficiency, is the truncated octahedron (figure 4), which is obtained by symmetrically cutting off the corners of a cube until the volume is reduced by almost half (Fincham & Heyes, 1985). As crystals contain a natural periodic structure, they offer a natural choice for simulations.

During simulations of molecules in solvent, particularly with proteins, much of the time is

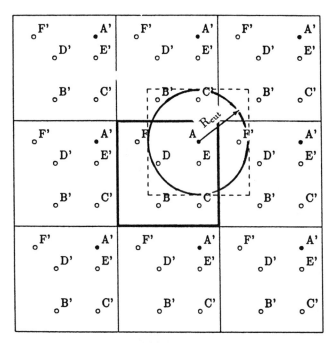

Figure 3. Simple periodic boundary conditions. The central box (dark boarders) contains the *real* atoms while the surrounding boxes contain calculated replicas. Atom A interacts with *real* atoms D & E and with images of C & F, as these lie within the cutoff radius R_{cut}, which must be less than half the box length.

spent simulating bulk water. To reduce this expense, the use of stochastic boundary conditions may be employed. This method can be used to avoid explicit treatment of part of the system whilst maintaining its influence on the remainder. The motion in this region is determined primarily by the time dependant variations of its nonbonded interactions with neighbouring atoms (figure 5). These interactions produce randomly varying forces which can be approximated by a stochastic force. Stochastic dynamics is simulated by integrating a set of langevin equations of motion containing a stochastic R_i and frictional force proportional to a frictional coefficient γ_i:

$$\frac{d^2 r_i}{dt^2} = \frac{F_i + R_i}{m_i} - \gamma_i \frac{dr_i}{dt} \tag{20}$$

This method has been used to simulate the active site dynamics of ribonuclease (Brünger *et al.*, 1985).

4. CALCULATION OF NONBONDED INTERACTIONS

It is computationally far too expensive to calculate nonbonded interactions between all pairs of atoms as the increase in computing time is of the order of N^2. To reduce computing time, a cut of radius R_{cut} is used, outside of which interactions are considered to be negligible and therefore not included. It is generally accepted that R_{cut} should not be lower than 8Å. As the electrostatic interaction has a $\frac{1}{r_{ij}}$ dependence, its effect at these distances are not negligible. Longer distances of over 15Å would be required to reduce these errors. To overcome this, local atoms can be treated as charge groups and, if their centroid lies within R_{cut} of the charge group whose interactions are being calculated, then the whole group is considered. If the atomic charges

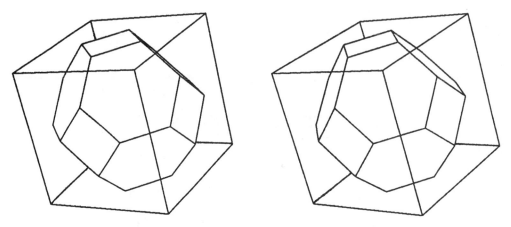

Figure 4. Stereo drawing of the truncated octahedron inside the equivalent cube.

in these groups add up to exactly zero, then the electrostatic interaction of two such groups can be considered to be dipolar in character and to demonstrate a $\frac{1}{r_{ij}^3}$ distance dependence (van Gunsteren & Berendsen, 1987).

As mentioned, calculation of the nonbonded interaction requires a considerable amount of computing time. This requirement can be further reduced by calculating and updating the neighbour list after several steps, typically 10. Furthermore, this list can be split into two parts, one accounting for local interactions and the other for long range interactions. The long range interactions list can be updated less frequently. Both these methods effectively discount the high frequency fluctuations in nonbonded interactions.

A further saving of computing time can be achieved by using a united atom approach for hydrogen atoms that are bonded to carbon atoms. Their influence is maintained by increasing the van der Walls radii of the carbon atoms that they are bonded to. As there are almost as many of these hydrogens as there are other atoms, a significant reduction in computing time is achieved.

5. CONSTRAINED DYNAMICS

Another method for saving computer time is to constrain the degrees of freedom that have the highest frequency. This then allows a larger integration step Δt to be taken and thereby achieves a simulation of longer length for the equivalent number of iterations. It is important that those degrees of freedom that are removed are only weakly coupled to the remaining ones and are separable from other modes so as not to perturb longer scale motions.

This principle has been applied sucessfully to bond lengths, but has been found to be inappropriate for constraining angles both from a physical and computational point of view. The numerical algorithm has been incorporated into MD simulations as the *SHAKE* procedure (van Gunsteren & Berendsen, 1977) and allows several fold increase in step size (up to 2fs). Effectively an additional zero term is added to the potential that does not contain the term whose force is to be removed. This extra term is the constraint force which compensates for the components of the potential that act along the direction of the constraint.

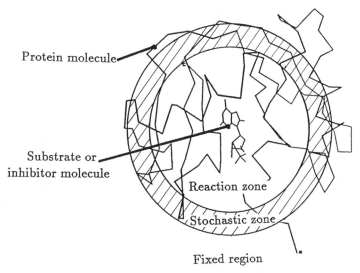

Figure 5. Diagram showing the use of stochastic boundary conditions. All atoms in the reaction zone are treated with pure MD while atoms in the stochastic zone are treated with SD.

6. CONSTANT TEMPERATURE AND PRESSURE

The temperature T is defined by kinetic energy of a system (Brooks *et al.*, 1983):

$$\sum_{i=1}^{N_{df}} \frac{m_i v_i^2}{2} = \frac{N_{df} K_B T}{2} \tag{21}$$

where m_i is the mass of atom i with velocity v_i and N_{df} is the number of degrees of freedom and K_B is Boltzmann's constant. The temperature T can be kept constant during a molecular dynamics simulation by a variety of methods. Probably the most simple is method is that derived by Woodcock (1971). The temperature at each step is calculated and a position increment scaling factor is determined. This can be incorporated into the Verlet leapfrog procedure. If T_0 is the prespecified temperature and $T(t)$ is calculated from equation (21), then the scaling factor f can be obtained from:

$$f = \sqrt{\frac{T_0}{T(t)}} \tag{22}$$

The current atomic positions are then scaled by this factor when predicting the next positions.

Another approach to keeping temperature constant is to weakly couple the system to an external bath (Berendsen *et al.*, 1984 and van Gunsteren *et al.*, 1983). This thermal bath is used to scale the velocities at each step by the relation:

$$\frac{dT(t)}{dt} = \tau^{-1}[T_0 - T(t)] \tag{23}$$

The strength of this coupling is determined by τ the temperature relaxation time. The velocities are then scaled by a temperature scaling factor:

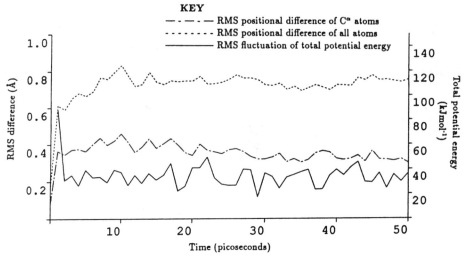

Figure 6. Diagram of the RMS fluctuations of potential energy and RMS positional differences between the crystal structure and the MD simulation plotted against simulated time.

$$\lambda \;=\; \sqrt{1 + t/(T_0/T(t - \tfrac{1}{2}\Delta t) - 1)} \tag{24}$$

$$V_i(t + \tfrac{1}{2}\Delta t) \;=\; V_i(t - \tfrac{1}{2}\Delta t)\lambda \tag{25}$$

Pressure can also be calculated from MD (van der Ploeg, 1982). This can be kept constant in a similar manner by adjusting the volume of the cell (Fincham & Heyes, 1985 and Berendsen et al., 1984).

7. MOLECULAR DYNAMIC SIMULATIONS

An example of output from a constant temperature MD simulation of deamino oxytocin is shown (figure 6). In this case, two unit cells of the crystal structure was simulated and the structure naturally provided the periodic boundaries. The root-mean square (RMS) positional differences are between the crystal structure atomic positions and those of the MD simulation. The potential energy is also shown and it can be noted that during the first few picoseconds the RMS fluctuations in the PE and the positional differences have not stabilised, indicating that equilibrium was not reached until around $10ps$ after the simulation began. Figure 7 shows equiprobability ellipsoids drawn about the mean atomic positions. Their size and shape indicate the motion of the atoms and its anisotropy.

Figure 8 shows the RMS deviations from the crystal structure of the enzyme ribonuclease-A (data from Haneef, 1986). The larger peaks generally correspond to regions of the protein exposed to the solvent where the X-ray structure can not model the full flexibility of the protein.

8. SOLUTION OF NMR STRUCTURES

With the advent of two-dimensional nuclear magnetic resonance (NMR), significant progress has been made towards the determination of macromolecules with molecular weights of up to 10,000 daltons (Wagner, G & Wüthrich, 1982). This has meant that the three-dimensional structure of macromolecules can be illucidated in different solutions without the need to crystallise them first. By identification of nuclear proton–proton distances from nuclear enhancement spectra, it is possible to predict the three-dimensional structure by distance geometry. Such a procedure has been applied to lipid bound glucagon (Braun et al., 1983), insectotoxin I_5A

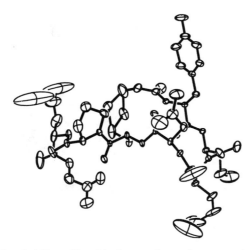

Figure 7. Equiprobability ellipsoids drawn about the mean atomic positions.

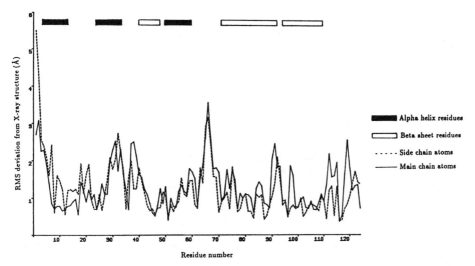

Figure 8. RMS deviations of the average MD structure from the crystal structure.

(Arseniev *et al.*, 1984), proteinase IIA (Williamson *et al* 1985) and bovine pancreatic trypsin inhibitor (Havel & Wüthrich, 1985). To further improve the quality of the final structures, the inter proton distances can be incorporated into molecular dynamics simulations by using a pseudo-potential term introduced into the potential energy function. This additional term takes the form of a skewed biharmonic effective potential (Clore *et al.*, 1985, figure 9). This term is incorporated as a restraint term:

$$
\mathcal{V}_{res}(r_{ij}) = \begin{cases} \frac{1}{2}K_{res}^{u}(r_{ij} - r_{ij}^{u})^{2} & \text{if } r_{ij} > r_{ij}^{u} \\ 0 & \text{if } r_{ij}^{l} \leq r_{ij} \leq r_{ij}^{u} \\ \frac{1}{2}K_{res}^{l}(r_{ij} - r_{ij}^{l})^{2} & \text{if } r_{ij} < r_{ij}^{l} \end{cases} \tag{26}
$$

where r_{ij}^{u} and r_{ij}^{l} are the upper and lower distances respectively. K_{res}^{u} and K_{res}^{l} are upper and lower restraint force constants respectively. The magnitude of this parameter must be chosen carefully so that the restraining term is balanced and will lead to the best sampling of conformations. The value can be coupled to the error within the NMR experiments as:

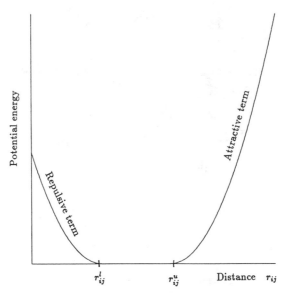

Figure 9. Graphical representation of the skewed biharmonic effective potential used as NOE restraint.

$$K_{res} = \frac{k_B T S}{2(\Delta_{ij})^2} \tag{27}$$

where S is a scaling factor and Δ_{ij} is the positive and negative error estimates of r_{ij} for the upper and lower values respectively. The use of this restraining term is not restricted to NMR. Any modelling that requires restraining of atomic distances can utilise this force.

As the only possible conformations that satisfy a set of given restraints are being searched for, it is not necessary to enforce the whole force field exactly. Infact, it is often advantageous to alter many of the parameters, in particular nonbonded interactions, in order to allow the atoms to pass each other. After this the full force field is slowly built up again. When using a united atom approach, it is necessary to use pseudo-atoms to represent those hydrogens that are not included in the calculation, but are identified to be within NOE distances found by in NMR experiments.

9. REFINEMENT OF X-RAY CRYSTALLOGRAPHIC DATA WITH MD

In a similar way to NMR refinement, it possible to include an energy function that can aid the refinement of X-ray structures (Fujinaga et al, 1989, Brünger, 1988). The aim is to minimise the difference between calculated X-ray diffraction structure factor amplitudes $(F_{calc}(h, k, l)$, h, k and l are the reciprocal lattice points of the crystal) and the observed ones $(F_{obs}(h, k, l))$, where the structure factor is related to the X-ray reflection intensities, $|F(h, k, l)|^2 \propto I(h, k, l)$. When the sum of weighted residuals is a minimum, the quality of this difference is generally quoted by its R-factor:

$$R = \frac{\sum_{h,k,l} ||F_{obs}(h, k, l)| - |F_{calc}(h, k, l)||}{\sum_{h,k,l} |F_{obs}(h, k, l)|} \tag{28}$$

The structure factor is defined as the Fourier transform of the electron density, $\varrho(x, y, z)$,

$$F(h,k,l) \propto \int \int \int \varrho(x,y,z)e^{2\pi i(hx+ky+lz)}dx\,dy\,dz \qquad (29)$$

Traditionally a least-squares refinement method is employed to minimise this difference. However, this procedure becomes trapped local minima requiring human intervention to rebuild regions in the current model which poorly fit the observed electron density. To increase the radius of convergence of the refinement, the following PE term can be included in the standard empirical PE function:

$$\mathcal{V}_{X-ray} = K_{X-ray} \sum_{h,k,l} \{|F_{obs}(h,k,l)| - |F_{calc}(h,k,l)|\}^2 \qquad (30)$$

In a similar way to NMR it is recommended that initial calculations start with low resolution intensities which slowly increase during the simulation.

10. CALCULATION OF FREE ENERGIES OF PERTURBATION

In recent years, calculation of free energies of perturbation has become one of the most important applications of MD simulation (Beveridge & DiCapua, 1989, van Gunsteren, 1989, Singh et al., 1987, and Warshel et al., 1988). Free energy differences are related to the equilibrium constant K by the equation:

$$\Delta G = -RT \ln K \qquad (31)$$

and hence protein-ligand binding equilibria can be studied by MD simulations. The most commonly used approach in conjunction with MD is that of thermodynamic integration, whereby the difference in free energy of two states is calculated. This can be achieved by either simulating a number of intermediate steps between the two states, or by slowly changing the parameters of one state into the other state. These methods are called *windowing* and *slow growth* respectively, and are described below.

If we have two physical states, a and b, that are slightly different in character, they will have an difference in free energy ΔG. Between these two states we can consider many intermediate states that are separated by very small spaces λ, the sum of which add up to the free energy difference between a and b: that is;

$$\Delta G = G_b - G_a = \sum_{i=1}^{N_s} \Delta G_i \qquad (32)$$

From basic statistical mechanics it can be shown that:

$$\Delta G_i = -RT \ln \left\langle e^{-\frac{\mathcal{V}(\lambda_i) - \mathcal{V}(\lambda_{i-1})}{RT}} \right\rangle_{\lambda_{i-1}} \qquad (33)$$

where $<>$ denotes the average of the equilibrium ensemble of states corresponding to λ_{i-1}. At each value λ_{i-1} an MD simulation is carried out and the average in equation (33) is evaluated. λ is altered in steps from zero to one by spacings of $\delta\lambda_i$. These spacings do not need to be equal and it may be more efficient to vary this value. This method is known as *windowing*.

In the *slow growth* method, $\delta\lambda_i$ is taken as exceedingly small so that we can equate ΔG_i with a single instantaneous value:

$$\Delta G_i \approx -RT \ln e^{-\frac{\mathcal{V}(\lambda_i) - \mathcal{V}(\lambda_{i-1})}{RT}} \tag{34}$$

$$= \mathcal{V}(\lambda_i) - \mathcal{V}(\lambda_{i-1}) \tag{35}$$

and therefore the overall difference in free energy can be expressed:

$$\Delta G = \sum_{i=1}^{N_s} \mathcal{V}(\lambda_i) - \mathcal{V}(\lambda_{i-1}) \tag{36}$$

This is easily incorporated into the PE function where each term is coupled to the spacing parameter λ. For instance, for bonds the potential term is:

$$\mathcal{V}_{bonds} = \sum_{n=1}^{N_b} \frac{1}{2}((1-\lambda)K_{b_n}^a + \lambda K_{b_n}^b)(b_n - ((1-\lambda)b_{0_n}^a + \lambda b_{0_n}^b)^2 \tag{37}$$

Setting $\lambda = 0$, equation (37) gives the contribution to the PE for a bond of equilibrium length $b_{0_n}^a$ and force constant $K_{b_n}^a$. When $\lambda = 1$, the equation gives the PE for a bond with parameters $b_{0_n}^b$ and $K_{b_n}^b$. By carrying out the MD while gradually varying λ and evaluating the equation (35) at each step, the free energy difference between the system with bond a and that with bond b can be evaluated. The fact that intermediate values of λ do not correspond to chemically realistic molecules is irrelevant, because ΔG is independent of the path that is taken between the two states.

In practice, this procedure is usually used to evaluate ΔG values in a thermodynamic cycle and yields the changes in the free energy of binding when engineered changes to a protein or ligand are carried out. This method may be extended to the calculation of the changes in enzyme rate constants by using MD simulations of transistion state complexes.

REFERENCES

Aqvist, J., van Gunsteren, W. F., Leijonmarck, M. & Tapia, O. (1985). *J. Mol. Biol.* **183**, 461-477

Arseniev, S. A., Kondakov, V. I., Maiorov, V. N. & Brystrov, V. F. (1984), *FEBS lett.* **165**, 57-62

Berendsen, H. J. C., Postma, J. P. M., van Gunsteren, W. F., DiNola, A. & Hack, J. R. (1984). *J. Chem. Phys.* **81**, 3684-3690

Beveridge, D. L. & DiCapua, F. M. (1989) *Computer simulation of biomolecular systems. Theoretical and experimental applications* (van Gunsteren, W. F. & Weiner, P. K., ed.), pp.1-27, Escom Leiden.

Braun, W., Wider, G., Lee, K. M. & Wuthrich, K. (1983). *J. Mol. Biol.* **169**, 921-948

Brooks, B. R., Bruccoleri, R. E., Olafson, B. D., States, D. J., Swaminathan, S. & Karplus, M. (1983). *J. Comp. Chem.* **4**, 187-217

Brünger, A. T., Brooks *III*, C. L. & Karplus, M. (1985). *Proc. Nat. Acad. Sci. USA* **82**, 8458-8462

Brünger, A. T. (1988). *J. Mol. Biol.* **203**, 803-816

Burt, S. K., Mackay, D. & Hagler, A. T. (1989). *Computer-Aided Drug Design. Methods and applications* (Penn, T. J. ed.), pp.55-91, DEKKER

Clore, G. M., Gronenborn, A. M., Brünger, A. T. & Karplus, M. (1985). *J. Mol. Biol.* **186**, 435-455

Fincham, D. & Heyes, D. M. (1985). *Adv. Chem. Phys.* **63**,493-575

Fujinaga, M., Gros, P., & van Gunsteren, W. F. (1989). *J. Appl. Cryst.* **22**, 1-8

van Gunsteren, W. F. (1989). *Computer simulation of biomolecular systems. Theoretical and experimental applications* (van Gunsteren, W. F. & Weiner, P. K., ed.), pp.27-59, Escom Leiden.

van Gunsteren W. F. & Berendsen, H. J. C. (1977). *Mol. Phys.* **34**, 1311-1327

van Gunsteren, W. F. & Berendsen, H. J. C. (1987). *Groningen Molecular Simulation (GROMOS) Library Manual* pp 1-229 BIOMOS, Nijenborgh 16, Groningen, The Netherlands.

van Gunsteren, W. F., Berendsen, H. J. C., Hermans, J., Hol, W. G. J. and Postma, J. P. M. (1983). *Proc. Natl. Acad. Sci.* **80**, 4315-4319

Hagler, A. T., Maple, J. R., Thacher, T. S., Fitzgerald, G. B. & Dinur, U. (1989). *Computer simulation of biomolecular systems. Theoretical and experimental applications* (van Gunsteren, W. F. & Weiner, P. K., ed.), pp.149-167, Escom Leiden.

Haneef, I. (1986). *PhD Thesis, London*

Hansen, J. P. (1973). *Phys. Rev.* **A8**, 3096-3109

Havel, T. F. & Wuthrich, K. (1985). *J. Mol. Biol.* **182**, 281-294

Karplus, M. & McCammon, J. A. (1986) *Sci.Amer.* **254**, 42-51

Kramer, H. L. & Herschbach, D. R. (1970). *J. Chem. Phys.* **53**, 2792

Kuki, A. & Wolynes, P. G. (1987). *Science* **236**, 1647-1652

Lifson, S. (1981). *NATO Advanced Study Institute / FEBS Advanced Course No.78. Current Methods in Structural Molecular Biology*, pp.1-27

Lennard-Jones, J. E. (1924). *Proc. Roy. Soc. London A* **106**, 463

Levitt, M. (1983). *J. Mol. Biol.* **168**, 595-620

London, F. (1930). *Z. Physik. Chem. B* **11**, 222

Maple, J. R., Dinur, U. & Hagler, A. T. (1988). *Proc. Nat. Acad. Sci. USA* **85**, 5350-5354

McCammon, J. A. (1984) *Rep. Prog. Phys.* **47**, 1-46

Morse, P. M. (1929). *Phys. Rev.* **34**, 57

Mulliken, R. S. (1955). *J. Chem. Phys.* **23**, 1833

Palca, J. (1986). *Nature* **322**, p586

Pitzer, K. S. (1951). *Disc Faraday Soc.* **10**, 66

van der Ploeg, P. (1982). *PhD Thesis, Groningen*

Rees, D. C. (1980). *J. Mol. Biol.* **141**, 323-326

Singh, U. C., Brown, F. K., Bash, P. A. & Kollman, P. A. (1987). *J. Am. Chem. Soc.* **109**, 1607-1614

Verlet, L. (1967). *Phys. Rev.* **159**, 98-103

Warshel, A., Sussman, F. & Hwang, J-K. (1988). *J. Mol. Biol.* **201**, 139-159

Williamson, M. P., Havel, T. F. & Wuthrich, K. (1985). *J. Mol. Biol.* **182**, 295-315

Woodcock, L. V. (1971). *Chem. Phys. Lett.* **10**, 257

Zheng, C., Wong, C. F., M[c]Cammon, J. A. & Wolynes, P. G. (1988), *Nature* **334**, 726-728

SUPERCOMPUTERS IN DRUG DESIGN

W. Graham Richards

Oxford Centre for Molecular Sciences and Physical Chemistry Laboratory,
South Parks Road,
Oxford OX1 3QZ

INTRODUCTION

Supercomputers are having a real impact in drug design. The irrefutable evidence for this is that a number of the leading pharmaceutical companies have purchased their own supercomputers. They are not merely using time bought from bureaux, nor relying on academic collaborations with access to national facilities. My own group in Oxford used approximately 1800 hours of supercomputer time last year, again indicating that this is a major undertaking, not a peripheral area of research. What is more, the techniques being used are eminently suitable for parallelisation so the field is one where academic, commercial and computational interests are all in harmony.

In this short article we will describe the computational methods rather briefly and then concentrate on some of the applications to the design of drugs.

COMPUTATIONAL METHODS

There are two major uses of supercomputers at present; quantum mechanical calculations and statistical mechanical calculations and simulations. The former are used to provide gas phase energy differences between molecular species and also energies and structures of transition states. The statistical mechanical methods are based on molecular mechanics potentials and typically include solvent interactions.

1. Quantum Mechanical Calculations

In general, in the application of computational methods to drug design the quantum mechanical methods are used to generate optimized geometries of molecules and charge distributions. For such work semi–empirical methods derived from the Dewar school are preferred and can be used on mini–computers or workstations. Apart from increasing the size of molecule which is tractable, supercomputers have little to offer in those cases. Where, however, *ab initio* methods are necessary, progress is only possible with the power of supercomputers.

In these increasingly important problems, programs such as GAMESS, CADPAC and GAUSSIAN'88 are the tools of choice. They need to be applied with large basis sets and correlation effects have to be considered; again typically Moller–Plesset perturbation methods are favoured. The requirement is to compute energy differences between two species to an accuracy of about 1 kcal mol^{-1}. This level of precision is essential if the results are to be of use in thermodynamic cycles where limits of 1 kcal mol^{-1} can be achieved in statistical mechanical calculations.

2. Statistical Mechanical Calculations

The quantum chemical methods are very familiar and have evolved over a thirty–year period. The statistical mechanical methods by contrast have almost burst onto the scene in the past three years and have only been useful since supercomputers have been available.

Currently the variant which is attracting most attention is the free energy perturbation technique (Richards et al. 1989, van Gunsteren 1988, Zwanzig 1954), its importance lying in the fact that experimentalists tend inevitably to measure free energies or differences in free energy.

In any equlibrium $A = B$, the equilibrium constant is

$$K_{eq} = \frac{Q_b}{Q_a}$$

with Q being the partition function, which classically is defined as an integral over phase space.

$$Q = (N!\, h^{3N})^{-1} \int ... \int \exp[-H(p,q)/kT]\, dp\, dq$$

Here H is the classical Hamiltonian. If the Hamiltonian for B is $H_a + \Delta H$ then the difference in Helmholtz free energies is given by

$$\Delta F = -kT\, n <\exp[-\Delta H/kT]>_a$$

so that the free energy difference can be obtained without evaluating the partition functions; $< >_a$ indicating an average taken over system A, and obtainable either using Monte Carlo techniques or by running molecular dynamics simulations.

The key equation above requires ΔH to be small; experience suggests less than kT. This is very important, so in practice the free energy difference between A and B is found from a number of simulations in which the potential energy functions used to compute H gradually change from being those appropriate for A to those appropriate for B. This may be done either by continuous change during the simulation (thermodynamic integration) or in discrete steps or "windows". The simulation usually takes place in a box of molecules surrounded by images with periodic boundary conditions to emulate an infinite system. If the box contains a fixed number of molecules at constant pressure and temperature then it will be the Gibbs free energy, ΔG, which emerges rather than ΔF,

$$\Delta G = \sum_{i=0}^{i=n} \Delta G(\lambda_i)$$

with i labelling the steps or windows and λ being a dimensionless coupling parameter which indicates how far the system has moved from state A to state B. During the course of a simulation all the molecular mechanics parameters are changed according to

Parameter at $\lambda = (1 - \lambda)$ (Parameter for A) $+ \lambda$ (Parameter for B)

The power of the technique lies in the fact that changes need not be physically realisable. Thus for two combinations

we may be interested in $\Delta G_1 - \Delta G_2$ but this can be equated to $\Delta G_3 - \Delta G_4$ which is far easier to simulate.

In this general scheme A could be a biological receptor or macro–molecule with B_1 and B_2 being different drugs; A could be an inhibitor and B_1 and B_2 mutations of an enzyme; A could be solvent and B_1 and B_2 different solutes.

The technique has been used in a number of drug design problems some of which will now be illustrated, but in cell biology the essential feature consists of having a small molecule (drug inhibitor, hormone etc) binding to a macromolecular species (DNA, protein, receptor). The different applications in large part vary in just how much is known about the macromolecular target.

DEFINED TARGETS

Nucleic Acids

We have recently completed an application of the thermodynamic cycle methods where a drug netropsin is bound to two different DNA molecules (Gago and Richards, 1990). A simulation was run for the binding of the drug to a length of DNA containing inosine residues. These residues were then gradually "mutated" into guanosines. The figure shows how in the simulation a hydrogen atom is perturbed into an amino group with the aid of two dummy (Dm) atoms.

The difference in binding free energy computed was 4.13 kcal mol^{-1} which compares with an experimental value of 4.0 kcal mol^{-1}: the sort of accuracy of which this technique seems capable if sufficient care is employed.

Enzymes

An exactly parallel application, where in our general scheme A is an enzyme and B_1 and B_2 different inhibitors, is the example of computing the differences in free energies of binding of sulphonamide inhibitors to carbonic anhydrase (Menziani, Reynolds and Richards, 1989). For such a calculation one starts with the enzyme crystal structure but incorporates solvent water into the system by placing a sphere of water molecules of about 15–20 Å radius around the binding site. These water molecules are allowed to move in the energy minimizations and in the molecular dynamics. Again in this example, differences in binding free energies of about 1 kcal mol^{-1} accuracy were obtained both when running the simulations in a forward and in the reverse directions.

We have had a long interest in designing inhibitors of the enzyme dihydrofolate reductase as candidates for anti–cancer drugs. In particular we are attempting to design bioreductive inhibitors which will inbibit the enzyme when they are in a reduced form but not when oxidized (Reynolds, Richards and Goodford, 1987). The logic behind this is the notion that tumours are less well furnished with blood and hence oxygen than are normal cells. A vital part of this design strategy then is the computation of redox potentials for compounds which can bind suitably to DHFR. The free energy perturbation method yet again permits this to be done but an essential feature of the thermo–dynamic cycle includes a gas–phase energy difference which requires ab initio calculations including correlation energy (Reynolds, King and Richards 1988). Accuracies of about 1 kcal mol^{-1} in these calculations translate into redox potentials within a few millivolts of experiment, comparable with experimental accuracy (Compton et al. 1989).

If we were to be restricted to problems where we can start with an X–ray crystal structure of an enzyme, there would be a very constricting limitation of work of this kind. However it is increasingly possible to produce an enzyme structure starting with the primary sequence providing there are homologies with proteins of known structure. These homologies need not be very high. For example we have produced the structure of a cytochrome P450 target which has only about 20% homology with another cytochrome by using novel graphics software (Morris, 1988). The supercomputer is used to mimimize the energy of the modelled enzyme before any inhibitor design is contemplated.

UNDEFINED TARGETS

Even with homology modelling, problems where the structure of the macromolecule is known only represent perhaps five per cent of the problems of the pharmaceutical and agrochemical industries. For many of the others the problem presents itself in the form of a biochemical transformation catalysed by an unknown enzyme whose blockade would have therapeutic benefit. In such cases there is a logical strategy. If we compute a reaction profile for the reaction and then characterize the transition state, a stable transition state mimic should inhibit the enzyme. Penicillin operates in this way. Computationally the problem is then in two stages: (a) find the transition state structure; (b) design a stable mimic. We have produced similarity techniques which go some way towards acheiving the second step (Richards and Hodgkin, 1988), but finding transition state structures remains formidable and certainly needs ab initio methods. For this work supercomputers are mandatory.

GENE SEQUENCES

No form of information is entering the literature faster than are gene sequences, to the extent that there are well–developed plans to sequence the entire human genome. These data present another challenge for the supercomputer in its application to drug design. As has been mentioned above, it may be possible to model and build the protein structures which are targets, based on sequence homologies. The problem is the vast amount of data to be searched and the time taken to do this. Only with supercomputers can this be contemplated. However with these machines the scope to exploit the knowledge of gene sequences makes the future of computer–aided drug design very rosy indeed.

ACKNOWLEDGEMENT

This work was conducted in part pursuant to a contract with the National Foundation for Cancer Research.

REFERENCES

Compton, R.G., King, P.M., Reynolds, C.A., Richards, W.G., and Waller, A.M., 1989, J Electronal Chem **258** 79

Gago, F., and Richards, W.G., 1990, Mol Pharmacol (in press)

Menziani, M.C., Reynolds, C.A., and Richards, W.G., 1989, J Chem Soc Chem Commun 853

Morris, G.M., 1988, J Molec Graphics **6** 135

Reynolds, C.A., King P.M., and Richards, W.G., 1988, Nature **334** 80

Reynolds, C.A., Richards, W.G., and Goodford, P.J., 1987, Anti–Cancer Drug Design **1** 291

Richards, W.G., and Hogkins, E.E., 1988, Chem. in Britain **24** 1141

Richards, W.G., King, P.M., and Reynolds, C.A., 1989, Protein Eng. **2** 319

van Gunsteren, W.F., 1988, Protein Eng **2** 5

Zwanzig, R.W., 1954, J Chem Phys **22** 1420

PATH INTEGRAL SIMULATIONS OF

EXCESS ELECTRONS IN CONDENSED MATTER

J.O. Baum
Rutherford Appleton Laboratory, Chilton, Didcot, Oxon, OX11 0QX

and L. Cruzeiro-Hansson
Birkbeck College, Malet St., London WC1E 7HX

INTRODUCTION

Numerical methods constitute a powerful way of simulating and having insight into systems which are too complex to be dealt with analytically. Some of the numerical methods used in classical systems are described in this volume (see chapters by Haneef). Such methods are applicable provided that quantum effects such as tunnelling (i. e. the penetration of particles into classically forbidden regions) or exchange between the different particles can be neglected.

When quantum effects cannot be neglected, the classical simulation techniques break down and it is necessary to resort to quantum mechanical descriptions. Examples of such systems are liquid helium and systems in which there is an unbound electron. Examples of quantum mechanical treatments are the standard methods of quantum chemistry to calculate the wave-function (see the chapters by Knowles and Wilson) or of solid state physics (see the chapter by Temmerman). However, particularly in the case of disordered condensed phase systems, the latter methods are often impractical.

In recent years, a new method of quantum simulation has been proposed which is well suited to study the statistical thermodynamical properties of quantum systems, and been applied with notable success, especially in the case of systems with excess electrons in condensed matter. It is referred to as path integral simulation, because it is based on Feynman's path integral theory of quantum mechanics (Feynman & Hibbs, 1965).

In this chapter, we will firstly present the derivation of a formula for the quantum mechanical partition function based on path integral theory, and show its relationship to 'classical' configurational integrals. Then, we will discuss some practical aspects of sampling the partition function via Monte Carlo simulations. Finally some results will be shown for selected systems.

1. A BRIEF INTRODUCTION TO PATH INTEGRAL QUANTUM MECHANICS

According to the Principle of Least Action (Goldstein, 1950) of classical mechanics a system evolves from one initial state to a final state via the path which minimises the action. In quantum systems on the other hand, because of Heisenberg's Uncertainty Principle, an infinite number of paths are possible. All these paths have the same probability amplitude (Feynman & Hibbs, 1965) but different phases, given by $iS/\hbar$, where S is the action of the path and $2\pi\hbar$ is Planck's constant. The probability amplitude of the final state is the sum over all the paths.

Supercomputational Science
Edited by R.G. Evans and S. Wilson
Plenum Press, New York, 1990

The correspondence between quantum and classical mechanics can be seen by noting that in the classical limit, the action S and changes in S which are small on a classical scale are very much larger than $\hbar$. Thus in general a set of closely related paths will have very different phases, and cancel each other. The only paths for which this will not happen are those very close to a path for which S is an extremum (the classical path).

Let us consider a particle moving in three-dimensional space under the influence of an external potential $U(\mathbf{r})$, where $\mathbf{r}$ denotes the particle position vector. The probability amplitude for moving from $\mathbf{r}_a$ at time t_a to $\mathbf{r}_b$ at time t_b is then given by

$$K(\mathbf{r}_b, t_b, \mathbf{r}_a, t_a) = \int_{\mathbf{r}_a}^{\mathbf{r}_b} e^{(i/\hbar)S[\mathbf{r}_b, \mathbf{r}_a]} \mathcal{D}\mathbf{r}(t) \tag{1}$$

where the integral over $\mathcal{D}\mathbf{r}(t)$ is over all paths which have the correct end-points, and is suitably normalised, and $S[\mathbf{r}_b, \mathbf{r}_a]$ is the action given by

$$S[\mathbf{r}_b, \mathbf{r}_a] = \int_{t_a}^{t_b} L(\mathbf{p}, \mathbf{r}, t)dt \tag{2}$$

where L is the Lagrangian of the system, here given by $L = \frac{\mathbf{p}^2}{2\mathbf{m}}$, where $\mathbf{p}$ is the momentum.

For a free particle, $U(\mathbf{r}) = 0$, and one obtains (without approximations) (Feynman & Hibbs, 1965)

$$
\begin{aligned}
K(\mathbf{r}_b, t_b, \mathbf{r}_a, t_a) &= \left(\frac{m}{2\pi i\hbar(t_b - t_a)}\right)^{\frac{3}{2}} \exp\left[\frac{im}{2\hbar(t_b - t_a)}\left((x_b - x_a)^2 + (y_b - y_a)^2 + (z_b - z_a)^2\right)\right] \\
&= \left(\frac{m}{2\pi i\hbar(t_b - t_a)}\right)^{\frac{3}{2}} \exp\left[\frac{im}{2\hbar(t_b - t_a)}(\mathbf{r}_b - \mathbf{r}_a)^2\right]
\end{aligned}
\tag{3}
$$

where $\mathbf{r}_a = (x_a, y_a, z_a)$ and $\mathbf{r}_b = (x_b, y_b, z_b)$.

For a particle in a time-independent field, an approximation valid at short times and for smooth potentials gives

$$K(\mathbf{r}_b, t_b, \mathbf{r}_a, t_a) = \left(\frac{m}{2\pi i\hbar(t_b - t_a)}\right)^{\frac{3}{2}} \exp\left[\frac{im}{2\hbar(t_b - t_a)}(\mathbf{r}_b - \mathbf{r}_a)^2 - \frac{i(t_b - t_a)}{2\hbar}\left(U(\mathbf{r}_a) + U(\mathbf{r}_b)\right)\right] \tag{4}$$

The probability amplitude K, which is also known as a propagator, is more commonly written using Dirac notation, in the Schrödinger picture, as

$$K(\mathbf{r}_b, \mathbf{r}_a; t) = \langle \mathbf{r}_b \mid e^{iHt/\hbar} \mid \mathbf{r}_a \rangle \tag{5}$$

where $t = t_b - t_a$, and H is the Hamiltonian of the system.

2. THE DENSITY MATRIX AND STATISTICAL MECHANICS

We are interested here in properties of systems at thermal equilibrium and thus need to discuss the statistical mechanics of these systems. A measured value of a property A of the system arises from the arithmetic average of the value of A for the system in different states, weighted by the probability of the system being in the particular state.

This probability is proportional to the Boltzmann factor. For a canonical ensemble the probability of occupancy of an energy level E is proportional to e^{-E/k_BT}, where k_B is the Boltzmann constant, and T is the absolute temperature. The constant of proportionality is Z^{-1} where

$$Z = \int e^{-E(r,p)/k_BT} dr\,dp \tag{6}$$

and the integration is carried out over all of phase space.

In quantum mechanics the probability of occupancy of a state is the density matrix ρ, which in its unnormalised form can be written in a way formally very similar to that of the propagator K in equation 5 above. For a given inverse temperature $\beta = 1/k_B T$ the density matrix in the coordinate representation is

$$\rho(\mathbf{r}_b, \mathbf{r}_a; \beta) = \langle \mathbf{r}_b \mid e^{-\beta H} \mid \mathbf{r}_a \rangle \tag{7}$$

The trace of this density matrix is the partition function

$$Z = \int d\mathbf{r} \rho(\mathbf{r}, \mathbf{r}; \beta) \tag{8}$$

which is the missing normalisation factor from the definition of ρ.

By replacing $(t_b - t_a)$, in equation 4, with $-i\beta\hbar$, we can obtain an approximation to the density matrix valid at high temperatures, which here is the equivalent of short times.

$$\rho(\mathbf{r}_b, \mathbf{r}_a; \beta) = \left(\frac{m}{2\pi\beta\hbar^2} \right)^{\frac{3}{2}} \exp\left[-\frac{m}{2\beta\hbar^2} (\mathbf{r}_b - \mathbf{r}_a)^2 \right] \exp\left[-\frac{\beta}{2} \left(U(\mathbf{r}_a) + U(\mathbf{r}_b) \right) \right] \tag{9}$$

In general equation 9 will not be valid at temperatures of interest (a few hundred Kelvin). We therefore manipulate the equation for the partition function, making use of the identity

$$1 = \int \mid \mathbf{r}_i \rangle \langle \mathbf{r}_i \mid d\mathbf{r}_i \tag{10}$$

where the integration is over all possible states $\mid \mathbf{r}_i \rangle$, here all possible coordinate values $\mathbf{r}_i$.

If we insert $P - 1$ intermediate states between $\mathbf{r}_a$ and $\mathbf{r}_b$, which we will name $\mathbf{r}_1$ to $\mathbf{r}_{P-1}$, and integrate over all possible values of these intermediate states, using the above identity, we get

$$
\begin{aligned}
\rho(\mathbf{r}_b, \mathbf{r}_a; \beta) &= \langle \mathbf{r}_b \mid (e^{-\beta H/P})^P \mid \mathbf{r}_a \rangle \\[2mm]
&= \int \langle \mathbf{r}_b \mid e^{-\beta H/P} \mid \mathbf{r}_1 \rangle \langle \mathbf{r}_1 \mid e^{-\beta H/P} \mid \mathbf{r}_2 \rangle \cdots \langle \mathbf{r}_{P-1} \mid e^{-\beta H/P} \mid \mathbf{r}_a \rangle d\mathbf{r}_1 d\mathbf{r}_2 \ldots d\mathbf{r}_{P-1} \\[2mm]
&= \int \rho(\mathbf{r}_b, \mathbf{r}_1; \beta/P) \rho(\mathbf{r}_1, \mathbf{r}_2; \beta/P) \ldots \rho(\mathbf{r}_{P-1}, \mathbf{r}_a; \beta/P) d\mathbf{r}_1 d\mathbf{r}_2 \ldots d\mathbf{r}_{P-1} \tag{11}
\end{aligned}
$$

This can be viewed as the explicit discretisation of the 'path' taken by the quantum particle in steps of β/P in negative imaginary time. The density matrix elements are now at temperature PT, which for large enough values of P will be sufficiently high for the approximation given above to be valid.

For the partition function, the density matrix elements of interest have $\mathbf{r}_a = \mathbf{r}_b$, which we relabel $\mathbf{r}_0$ or $\mathbf{r}_P$. The 'paths' now repeat themselves after a 'time' $-i\beta\hbar$ and thus are closed. Substitution of the high temperature approximation to the density matrix into the above expression gives for the partition function of a single particle of mass m in three dimensional space at an inverse temperature β

$$Z_P = \int dr_1 dr_2 \ldots dr_P \left(\frac{mP}{2\pi\beta\hbar^2}\right)^{\frac{3P}{2}} \exp\left[-\frac{mP}{2\beta\hbar^2}\sum_{i=1}^{P}(\mathbf{r}_i - \mathbf{r}_{i+1})^2 - \frac{\beta}{P}\sum_{i=1}^{P}U(\mathbf{r}_i)\right] \quad (12)$$

This is exactly equal to the true partition function Z in the limit of P infinite. For a system of N particles of mass m, ignoring exchange, we get

$$Z_P = \frac{1}{N!}\int dr_{1_1} dr_{1_2} \ldots dr_{N_P} \left(\frac{P}{2\pi\lambda^2}\right)^{\frac{3NP}{2}} \exp\left[-\frac{P}{2\lambda^2}\sum_{n=1}^{N}\sum_{i=1}^{P}(\mathbf{r}_{n_i} - \mathbf{r}_{n_{i+1}})^2 - \frac{\beta}{P}\sum_{n=1}^{N}\sum_{i=1}^{P}U(\mathbf{r}_{n_i})\right]$$
(13)

where the de Broglie wavelength λ is defined by $\lambda^2 = \hbar^2\beta/m$.

3. THE ISOMORPHISM OF THE QUANTUM AND CLASSICAL SYSTEMS

Equation 13 for the partition function of a quantum system has been recognised to be closely related to that of a classical system, following reinterpretation of the terms. (Chandler & Wolynes, 1981). The exponential is seen to be of the form $\exp[-\beta\mathcal{E}]$, where $\mathcal{E}$ is the 'energy' of the isomorphous classical system.

Each particle in the quantum system is replaced in the classical system by a ring polymer of P monomers. The monomers, which we shall refer to as 'beads', are structureless and of mass m. They interact within their own polymer only with their nearest neighbour beads, the interaction being that of a harmonic spring of zero equilibrium length. This is seen by equating the first term in the previous equation with the '$\frac{1}{2}kx^2$' energy term of a spring. Thus the 'spring constant' is given by $P/\beta\lambda^2$.

The potential term in equation 13 should for clarity be written as $U(|\mathbf{r}_{n_i} - \mathbf{r}_{m_i}|)$, where n and m are particle labels. Thus, interactions between polymers occur only between beads with the same discretisation index i. Using the imaginary time analogy, only beads at the same 'time' interact. The division by P means that the classical potential is merely replaced by its average over the particle density function, as represented by the bead positions.

Finally, we note that we have found an equivalence between a *partition function* of a quantum system, and a *configurational integral* of a classical system. There are a number of simulation techniques available for evaluating properties of classical systems with such configurational integrals. Thus, possibilities suggest themselves for evaluating the properties of the quantum system.

Two basic methods exist: the Monte Carlo and the molecular dynamics techniques. The former explicitly use the configurational integral. The latter use the momenta of the system as well. To use molecular dynamics techniques here requires the introduction of artificial momenta (Berne & Thirumalai, 1986). It should be noted that although such simulations will have apparent dynamics, such dynamics is quite artificial, and in this instance, molecular dynamics is only being used as a means of sampling configuration space. We will not consider molecular dynamics further here, but instead concentrate on path integral Monte Carlo simulation techniques.

SAMPLING THE PARTITION FUNCTION IN PRACTICE

We are interested in evaluating properties of the system such as the total energy, and the kinetic and potential components, and also in determining structural features. Other properties such as the free energy are of interest, but require more sophisticated simulation techniques than will be discussed here. For further details on free energy simulation methods, see the book by Allen and Tildesley (1987).

278

1. IMPORTANCE SAMPLING AND METROPOLIS MONTE CARLO

Using the isomorphism, the partition function has now become the configurational integral

$$Q = C \int \exp\left[-\beta\mathcal{E}\right] d\mathbf{R}^N \tag{14}$$

where C is a constant, $\mathbf{R}^N$ represents the system coordinates, and $\mathcal{E}$ the system energy, all of which are defined by comparison with equation 13.

The expectation value of a property F is given by

$$\langle F \rangle = \frac{\int F \exp\left[-\beta\mathcal{E}\right] d\mathbf{R}^N}{Q} \tag{15}$$

Because of the large number of dimensions of the system $(3N)$, analytical evaluation or explicit numerical evaluation by quadrature of the integral is impractical.

The Monte Carlo method was devised with this kind of integral in mind, and involves direct random sampling of points in the integration region. However, this approach will not work here for two reasons. Firstly, the Boltzmann weighting factor ensures that only a very small number of states (configuration points) contribute much, as it is the nature of condensed systems that most points in phase space have severely overlapping atoms, with concomitant highly repulsive energies. Secondly, there are severe difficulties in evaluating Q.

To get around these problems one uses the method of importance sampling in which a Markov chain of configuration is built with the limiting distribution required, i. e. one samples phase space from the distribution $\pi(\mathbf{R}^N) = \exp[-\beta\mathcal{E}(\mathbf{R}^N)]$, suitably normalised, and the ensemble average value of property F is given by

$$
\begin{aligned}
\langle F \rangle &= \frac{\int [F(\mathbf{R}^N)]\pi(\mathbf{R}^N)d\mathbf{R}^N}{[1]\pi(\mathbf{R}^N)d\mathbf{R}^N} \\
&= \frac{\langle F \rangle_\pi}{\langle 1 \rangle_\pi} \\
&= \langle F \rangle_\pi
\end{aligned}
\tag{16}
$$

where $\langle\rangle_\pi$ signifies an average over the distribution function π.

In practice, a new configuration is obtained by making limited random changes to the current configuration following well defined transition probabilities. New configurations will not necessarily be included in the averaging, as they can be rejected. However, the acceptance/rejection of a new configuration depends only on the *ratio* of $\pi(\mathbf{R}^N)$ for the old and new configurations, and thus there is no need for the normalisation constant.

If the changes made to one configuration labelled $\mathbf{R}$ to generate the next one labelled $\mathbf{R}'$ are made according to the transition probability $\mathcal{T}(\mathbf{R}'/\mathbf{R})$ then the acceptance criterion for the move $\mathbf{R} \to \mathbf{R}'$ is given by

$$\mathcal{A}(\mathbf{R}', \mathbf{R}) = \min\left[1, \frac{\mathcal{T}(\mathbf{R}/\mathbf{R}')\pi(\mathbf{R}')}{\mathcal{T}(\mathbf{R}'/\mathbf{R})\pi(\mathbf{R})}\right] \tag{17}$$

Frequently in standard Monte Carlo simulations of condensed systems, $\mathcal{T}(\mathbf{R}'/\mathbf{R})$ is a move of a single particle a random displacement with uniform probability anywhere inside a small cube centred on its old position. Thus, this prescription, which is called Metropolis Monte Carlo

(Metropolis *et. al.*, 1953) consists of the selection of a particle, randomly shifting it within a limiting cube, followed by acceptance based on the Boltzmann weighting factors. If the new configuration energy is lower than the old, the new configuration is automatically accepted. If the energy has increased, the configuration is accepted if a random number chosen between 0 and 1 does not exceed the ratio of the new to the old Boltzmann factors.

2. THE PRIMITIVE ALGORITHM

The most straightforward way of sampling the integral of equation 13, and that used in most early path integral work, is referred to as the primitive algorithm. In this, the quantum 'beads' are moved individually, moving just one to make a new configuration. The moves are made using the transition probability $\mathcal{T}$ described above, and accepted as described above, using the Boltzmann factor given by the isomorphic classical system.

Because there is no *a priori* way of determining the number of discretisations needed (P), several simulations must be performed, using different numbers of beads, in order to find the point at which increasing P has no effect on the calculated properties.

It transpires that for the excess electron systems considered here, a large value of P (often several thousand) is required to get converged values of properties. These simulations not only become rather expensive, but also suffer from ergodicity problems.

In the first place, Monte Carlo codes are only vectorisable / parallelisable in their energy calculation routines, because each generated configuration must be generated from that directly preceding it. The energy routines calculate the energy change on moving just one 'bead', and can be vectorised over all the other particles. However, this will have to be done many millions of times, and is almost always too small a task to be worth parallelising. Hence, these codes become computer time eaters.

Furthermore, because of the dependence of the 'spring constants' on the discretisation P, as P increases, the 'springs' become harder, and increasingly restrict the movement of 'beads' away from each other. This can make it extremely difficult for the 'polymer' to move any considerable distance during the simulation, so that phase space is inadequately sampled.

Two possible remedies exist for these problems. Firstly, if the approximation used for the density matrix is more accurate, then the number of 'beads' needed will be reduced. This has been the approach principally of Pollock & Ceperley (1984). Secondly, one can design sampling algorithms which allow many 'beads' to move simultaneously. The first multi-bead algorithm suggested was that of Sprik *et al.* (1985) which was termed 'staging'. These approaches can even be combined, to be even more efficient.

Improving the approximations hopefully results in reducing the work actually done, but apart from altering the isomorphic classical system and thus using a different energy expression $\mathcal{E}$, the algorithm is the same as before. Multi-bead moves, however, result in some or all of the energy calculation routines doing much more work than previously, improving the possibilities for optimisation, particularly at the level of the second inner loop. The increased task size may well make parallel running of the code more desirable.

For reasons of space, we will not discuss in any further detail the improved algorithms of Pollock & Ceperley (1984) or Sprik *et al.* (1985), nor that of Coker *et al.* (1987) which goes some way towards combining the two. Instead, we will discuss a version of staging which we believe to be the most efficient yet proposed (Cruzeiro-Hansson *et al.*, 1990).

3. A STAGING ALGORITHM

The basic idea of staging is that the cyclic polymer is split in some specified way into groups of beads which are subsequently treated as a unit and moved *en masse.*

Perhaps the simplest implementation of the idea is that used by Coker and his co-workers (1987), where in each move a fixed length of the polymer is picked at random. The chain has none of the organisational structure which will be mentioned shortly.

Whilst this method does indeed improve the sampling efficiency, it can be difficult to generate acceptable moves for a large number of beads at a time. The problem of a priori generation of configurations mentioned above can return with a vengeance to severely reduce the efficiency.

For this reason, other staging schemes have been proposed where some form of initial screening of the moves is carried out. In these schemes, the chain is divided into two levels or stages. The first of these, the A-chain, is a cyclic polymer with P_A beads , where P_A is chosen sufficiently small that large moves of individual A-chain beads are possible. The second level is that of B-chains which span between the A-chain beads .

The concept of 'large moves' needs further elaboration. Frequently in condensed systems, excess electrons have many minima available, often in the interstices between atoms, usually many of similar energy, but separated by quite large barriers. In particular, the interiors of the atoms are highly repulsive. To properly sample the available minima, an electron polymer chain must be able to cross these barriers efficiently, which means that moves of the order of an atomic diameter are desirable. These are the moves which can be made by the A-chain beads.

The version of staging which will be described below is that of Cruzeiro-Hansson *et al.* (1990) which, as shown in the final section of this article, is efficient in the simulation of both hard sphere and smoother potential forms.

As before, the ring polymer of P beads is redefined in terms of an A-chain of P_A beads with B-chains of P_B beads linking the A-beads, so that $P = P_A P_B$. This form, and the nomenclature are taken substantially intact from the paper of Sprik *et al.* (1985).

The A-beads are labelled

$$\mathbf{r}_i^a \text{ with } i = 0, 1, \ldots, P_A \text{ and } \mathbf{r}_0^a \equiv \mathbf{r}_{P_A}^a \tag{18}$$

and the B-chain beads, defined with reference to the A-beads joined are labelled

$$\mathbf{r}_{ij}^b \text{ with } i = 1, 2, \ldots, P_A; j = 0, 1, \ldots, P_B \tag{19}$$

The B-chains start and end on A-beads, so that

$$\mathbf{r}_{i0}^b \equiv \mathbf{r}_{i-1}^a \text{ and } \mathbf{r}_{iP_B}^b \equiv \mathbf{r}_i^a \tag{20}$$

and are defined by displacements $\boldsymbol{\Delta}_{ij}$ from the straight line joining the two A-beads

$$\mathbf{r}_{ij}^b = \mathbf{R}_{ij}^b + \boldsymbol{\Delta}_{ij} \quad \text{with} \quad \boldsymbol{\Delta}_{i0} = \boldsymbol{\Delta}_{iP_B} = 0 \tag{21}$$

$$\text{and} \quad \mathbf{R}_{ij}^b = \mathbf{r}_{i-1}^a + \frac{j}{P_B}(\mathbf{r}_i^a - \mathbf{r}_{i-1}^a) \tag{22}$$

Equation 12 can then be transformed, as shown by Sprik *et al.* (1985) into

$$Z_{P_A P_B} = \int \prod_{i=1}^{P_A} \mathbf{r}_i^a \prod_{i=1}^{P_A} \prod_{j=1}^{P_B} \boldsymbol{\Delta}_{ij} \left(\frac{P_A P_B}{2\pi\lambda^2}\right)^{\frac{3NP_A P_B}{2}} \exp\left[-\frac{P_A}{2\lambda^2}\sum_{i=1}^{P_A}(\mathbf{r}_i^a - \mathbf{r}_{i-1}^a)^2\right]$$

$$\exp\left[-\frac{P_A P_B}{2\lambda^2}\sum_{i=1}^{P_A}\sum_{j=1}^{P_B}(\boldsymbol{\Delta}_{ij} - \boldsymbol{\Delta}_{ij-1})^2\right] \exp\left[-\frac{\beta}{P_A P_B}\sum_{i=1}^{P_A}\sum_{j=1}^{P_B} U(\mathbf{r}_i^a, \boldsymbol{\Delta}_{ij})\right]$$

$$\tag{23}$$

in which the kinetic energy term has been separated into components solely dependent on the A-bead coordinates, and terms solely dependent on the B-bead Δ coordinates. Thus, the exponential can be seen as $\exp[A - chain]\exp[B - chains]$.

From equation 17, it can be seen that the generation of new configurations $\mathbf{R}'$ from $\mathbf{R}$ requires the calculation of the ratio

$$\frac{\mathcal{T}(\mathbf{R}/\mathbf{R}')\pi(\mathbf{R}')}{\mathcal{T}(\mathbf{R}'/\mathbf{R})\pi(\mathbf{R})}$$

We wish to generate new configurations in such a way as to explore phase space efficiently, but also wish to generate them as efficiently as possible. If we generate particle moves within a cube of equal probability density, the ratio of transition probabilities is always unity, so that only the ratio $\pi(\mathbf{R}')/\pi(\mathbf{R})$ is required. We use

$$\pi(\mathbf{R}) = \exp\left[-P_A T^a - P_A P_B T^\Delta - \frac{U}{P_A P_B}\right] \tag{24}$$

where

$$T^a = \frac{1}{2\lambda^2}\sum_{i=1}^{P_A}(\mathbf{r}_i^a - \mathbf{r}_{i-1}^a)^2 \tag{25}$$

$$T^\Delta = \frac{1}{2\lambda^2}\sum_{i=1}^{P_A}\sum_{j=1}^{P_B}(\Delta_{ij}^a - \Delta_{ij-1}^a)^2 \tag{26}$$

$$V = \beta\sum_{i=1}^{P_A}\sum_{j=1}^{P_B}V(\mathbf{r}_i^a, \Delta_{ij}) \tag{27}$$

The terms T^a and T^Δ are related to the free particle motion, a system which has been solved analytically. Lévy (1954) derived a formula for interpolating a Brownian motion between two given endpoints. This formula, originally employed on similar problems by Jordan & Fosdick (1968), is especially beneficial in generating moves efficiently, compared to random moves in a cube, as will be shown.

Two types of bead moves are made — one A-chain bead is moved first, and if this move is accepted, then a trial move is made for the two B-chains attached to this moved A-bead. If the B-chain moves are accepted, then the new configuration properties are accumulated. However, if the B-chain move is rejected, they and the A-bead are returned to their old positions, and the old configuration properties accumulated.

If a move of the uth A-bead is generated using the Lévy formula for a Brownian path conditioned to start and finish at $\mathbf{r}_0^a$, such that the bead moves from $\mathbf{r}_u^a$ to $\mathbf{r}_u^{a'}$, then the ratio of transition probabilities is given by

$$\frac{\mathcal{T}(\mathbf{r}_u^a/\mathbf{r}_u^{a'})}{\mathcal{T}(\mathbf{r}_u^{a'}/\mathbf{r}_u^a)} = \exp(+P_A\Delta T_u^a) \tag{28}$$

where

$$\begin{aligned}\Delta T_u^a &= T^a(\mathbf{r}_u^{a'}) - T^a(\mathbf{r}_u^a) \\ &= \frac{1}{2\lambda^2}\left[(\mathbf{r}_u^{a'} - \mathbf{r}_{u-1}^a)^2 + (\mathbf{r}_{u+1}^a - \mathbf{r}_u^{a'})^2 - (\mathbf{r}_u^a - \mathbf{r}_{u-1}^a)^2 - (\mathbf{r}_{u+1}^a - \mathbf{r}_u^a)^2\right]\end{aligned} \tag{29}$$

(Note the ordering of $\mathbf{R}$ and $\mathbf{R}'$ in equation 17.)

This exactly cancels the terms in T^a from the π terms, so that, as there is no change in T^Δ only the change in the potential energy term, ΔV_u^a appears in the acceptance criterion for this A-bead move:

$$A(\mathbf{r}_u^{a'} / \mathbf{r}_u^a) = \min\left[1, \exp\left(-\frac{\Delta V_u^a}{P_A P_B}\right)\right] \qquad (30)$$

where

$$\Delta V_u^a = V(\mathbf{r}_u^{a'}) - V(\mathbf{r}_u^a) \qquad (31)$$

By sampling the moves from the free particle distribution, we should be sampling phase space more efficiently. The extra effort involved in generating the moves is not wasted, as it reduces the calcuation necessary to determine the move acceptance. Depending on the form used for the Lévy interpolation formula, it may be desirable to move one of the A-beads uniformly in a cube (Cruzeiro-Hansson et al., 1990). All the other A-beads would be moved according to the above scheme.

We now turn to the B-chain moves, which we note will only be made after the acceptance of an A-bead move. The two B-chains to be moved after moving the uth A-bead are the (u)th and $(u + 1)$th. New $\mathbf{\Delta}_{uj}$ coordinates for the uth B-chain are generated using the Lévy formula for a Brownian walk with constrained endpoints $\mathbf{r}_{u-1}^a$ and $\mathbf{r}_u^a$.

Ignoring for a moment the dependence on accepting an A-bead move, the transition probability ratio for generating the two B-chains is given by

$$\frac{T(\{\mathbf{r}_{uj}^b, \mathbf{r}_{u+1j}^b\} / \{\mathbf{r}_{uj}^{b'}, \mathbf{r}_{u+1j}^{b'}\})}{T(\{\mathbf{r}_{uj}^{b'}, \mathbf{r}_{u+1j}^{b'}\} / \{\mathbf{r}_{uj}^b, \mathbf{r}_{u+1j}^b\})} = \exp(+P_A P_B \Delta T_u^\Delta) \qquad (32)$$

where

$$
\begin{aligned}
\Delta T_u^\Delta &= T^\Delta(\{\mathbf{\Delta}_{uj}', \mathbf{\Delta}_{u+1j}'\}) - T^\Delta(\{\mathbf{\Delta}_{uj}, \mathbf{\Delta}_{u+1j}\}) \\
&= \frac{1}{2\lambda^2} \sum_{j=1}^{P_B} \left[(\mathbf{\Delta}_{uj}' - \mathbf{\Delta}_{uj-1}')^2 + (\mathbf{\Delta}_{u+1j}' - \mathbf{\Delta}_{u+1j-1}')^2 - \right. \\
&\qquad \left. (\mathbf{\Delta}_{uj} - \mathbf{\Delta}_{uj-1})^2 - (\mathbf{\Delta}_{u+1j} - \mathbf{\Delta}_{u+1j-1})^2 \right]
\end{aligned}
\qquad (33)
$$

and the notation $\{\cdots\}$ signifies all the coordinates of a B-chain, i.e. all possible values of the second subscript are implied.

The extra factor to be added to the above to account for the dependance on a successful A-bead move is

$$\frac{\min\left[1, \exp\left(+\frac{\Delta V_u^a}{P_A P_B}\right)\right]}{\min\left[1, \exp\left(-\frac{\Delta V_u^a}{P_A P_B}\right)\right]} = \exp\left(+\frac{\Delta V_u^a}{P_A P_B}\right)$$

so that the final B-chain move acceptance criterion is

$$A(\{\mathbf{r}_{uj}^{b'}, \mathbf{r}_{u+1j}^{b'}\} / \{\mathbf{r}_{uj}^b, \mathbf{r}_{u+1j}^b\}) = \min\left[1, \exp\left(-P_A \Delta T_u^a + \frac{\Delta V_u^a}{P_A P_B} - \frac{\Delta V_u^b}{P_A P_B}\right)\right] \qquad (34)$$

where

$$\Delta V_u^b = V(\{\mathbf{r}_{uj}^{b'}, \mathbf{r}_{u+1j}^{b'}\}) - V(\{\mathbf{r}_{uj}^b, \mathbf{r}_{u+1j}^b\}) \qquad (35)$$

Typical numbers of beads are $P_A = 64$ and $P_B = 16$ i. e. $P = 1024$ for a hard sphere liquid with an excess electron at $\beta = 36$. As mentioned above, several simulations have to be performed, in order to verify that the resultant system properties are independent of the value of P.

AN EXCESS ELECTRON IN HARD SPHERES

As mentioned in the introduction, one important quantum effect which can be modelled with path integral techniques is the penetration or tunneling of a particle through an energy barrier. In a system with an excess electron, there will in reality be both attractive and repulsive forces. Nevertheless, much can be learned of the possible electron states from studies of systems that are purely repulsive. We have simulated a variety of hard sphere condensed phase systems containing an excess electron. Both crystal and fluid hard sphere phases have been investigated.

The possible electron states can be crudely divided into localised and delocalised. The latter are states in which the electron density extends over the de Broglie thermal wavelength λ and is approximately isotropic. Delocalised states are more compact than this, but may nevertheless extend over several hard spheres.

In real systems the occupied states determine the conductivity properties, as the localised states will be of negligible mobility compared with the delocalised states. When localised states exist, they are in equilibrium with higher-energy delocalised states. The results quoted below are part of a study in progress with the aim of improving understanding of these states in repulsive systems.

In the following work, systems of 432 hard spheres were used, and all the data are for simulations in which the electron was represented by 1024 beads with $P_A = 64$ and $P_B = 16$. The temperature was $\beta = 36$, so the de Broglie wavelength of the electron is 6 bohrs. It can be shown that the average distance between beads at a labelling $P/2$ apart in a free electron will be $\sqrt{3}\lambda/2 = 5.2$ bohrs (Nicholls et al., 1984). The density of hard spheres, is expressed as $\rho\sigma^3$ where σ (the hard sphere diameter) is 1 bohr and was 0.201 or 0.500. The electron interacted with the hard spheres via a 'hard sphere' potential, where the electron - hard sphere diameter d was either taken to be equal to or smaller than σ. The latter allowed penetration of the electron into the hard spheres.

Figure 1 shows the radial distribution function (rdf) for the electron centre-of-mass to hard sphere distances. The hard sphere crystal simulation, in which no movement of the hard spheres was allowed, shows that the electron does not 'sit' on a hard sphere, but as expected remains in the interstices. There are no preferable sites, so that the rdf is almost featureless. (The small oscillations are statistically of no meaning.) The two fluid simulations show that the electron forms a cavity for itself. At higher hard sphere densities, the cavity is smaller, and much better defined. Not surprisingly, as the electron is allowed to penetrate the hard spheres, this cavity in the fluid disappears, and the rdf begins to look like that of the crystal.

Figure 2 shows the electron density from the electron centre-of-mass. In the crystal, the electron is quite delocalised, whereas in the fluid at the same density it is significantly localised. At the higher density, the localisation is even greater. This corresponds with the cavity sizes shown in figure 1. The average distance between beads at labels $P/2$ apart in the crystal simulation is 3.8 bohr, whereas for the fluid, at the lower density the average distance is 2.7 bohr, and at the higher density 1.5 bohr. When the electron can penetrate to within 0.27 bohr of the hard sphere centre, at both densities the fluid simulations give the same average distance as quoted above for the crystal.

Further work is in progress to gain a better understanding of the nature of electron solvation in such hard sphere systems. Simulations are also in progress using more realistic potentials to model organic and biological systems.

We wish to acknowledge the support of the Science and Engineering Research Council and the Medical Research Council.

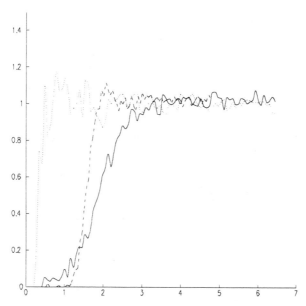

Figure 1. Electron centre-of-mass hard sphere radial distribution function. The dotted line is the hard sphere crystal, with $\rho\sigma^3 = 0.201$. The solid line is for the fluid at the same density, and the dashed line is for the fluid at $\rho\sigma^3 = 0.50$. No electron penetration of the hard spheres is possible. The horizontal axis is in bohrs.

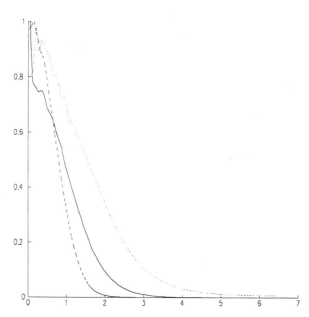

Figure 2. Electron density relative to the electron centre-of-mass. The line notation is as for figure 1.

REFERENCES

Allen, M.P. and Tildesley, D.J., 1987, "Computer Simulation in Liquids", Oxford University Press, Oxford.

Berne, B.J. and Thirumalai, D., 1986, On the simulation of quantum systems: path integral methods, Ann. Rev. Phys. Chem., **37**, 401.

Chandler, D. and Wolynes, P.G., 1981, Exploiting the isomorphism between quantum theory and classical statistical mechanics of polyatomic fluids, J. Chem. Phys., **74**, 4078.

Coker, D.F., Berne, B.J. and Thirumalai, D., 1987, Path integral Monte Carlo studies of the behaviour of excess electrons in simple fluids, J. Chem. Phys., **86**, 5689.

Cruzeiro-Hannson, L., Baum, J.O. and Finney, J.L., A new sampling scheme for path integral calculations, Physica Scripta, submitted.

Feynman, R.P. and Hibbs, A.R., 1965, "Quantum Mechanics and Path Integrals", McGraw-Hill, New York.

Goldstein, H., 1950, "Classical Mechanics", Addison-Wesley, Reading, Mass.

Jordan, H.F. and Fosdick, L.D., 1968, Three-particle effects in the pair distribution function for He^4 gas, Phys. Rev., **171**, 128.

Lévy, P., 1954, "Le mouvement Brownien", Memor. Sci. Math. Fasc., **126**, Gauthier-Villas, Paris.

Metropolis, N., Rosenbluth, A.W., Rosenbluth, M.N., Teller, A.H. and Teller, E., 1953, Equation of state calculations by fast computing machines, J. Chem. Phys., **21**, 1087.

Nicholls, A.L., Chandler, D., Singh,Y. and Richardson, D.M. (1984), Excess electrons in simple fluids. II. Numerical results for the hard sphere solvent, J. Chem. Phys., **81**, 5109.

Pollock, E.L. and Ceperley, D.M., 1984, Simulation of quantum many-body systems by path-integral methods, Phys. Rev. B, **30**, 2555.

Sprik, M., Klein, M.L. and Chandler, D., 1985, Staging: A sampling technique for the Monte Carlo evaluation of path integrals, Phys. Rev. B, **31**, 4234.

COMPUTATIONAL METHODS IN ELECTRONIC STRUCTURE
CALCULATIONS OF COMPLEX SOLIDS

W.M. Temmerman, Z. Szotek, H. Winter[†] and G.Y. Guo,

SERC Daresbury Laboratory, Daresbury, Warrington WA4 4AD, UK

1. INTRODUCTION

In these two lectures I hope to give you a flavour of some of the computational
methods used in electronic structure calculations of complex solids. The methods are concerned with the fully quantum mechanical solution of systems with complicated interactions
which give rise to the structural, chemical, magnetic and superconducting properties of
solids.

A fundamental quantity is the electronic groundstate energy. One imposes a crystal
structure for the ions (bcc, fcc, hcp, etc), or a magnetic structure (ferromagnetic, antiferromagnetic, helical, etc), or a chemical ordering of the different atomic components of
the solid (ordered, disordered, etc) and calculates the electronic total energy. The structure with the lowest total energy is the ground state. To calculate the energy of 10^{23}
electrons moving in these external potentials, one maps the problem into calculating the
energy of one effective electron moving in the external potential and the mean field
created by all the other electrons. This is being determined self-consistently. This gives
rise to the self-consistent field (SCF) methods in solid state physics, whose theoretical
foundation lies in Hartree-Fock (HF) theory or Density Functional Theory (DFT). In
these lectures we will be exclusively concerned with DFT.

The problem of solving an effective one electron Schrödinger equation for a solid, an
infinite periodic array of atoms, is still a formidable task. There are two approaches, one
concerns the expansion of the wavefunction in appropriate basis functions and a varia-

---

[†] Kernforschungszentrum Karlsruhe, INFP, Postfach 3640, D–7500 Karlsruhe, FRG.

Supercomputational Science
Edited by R.G. Evans and S. Wilson
Plenum Press, New York, 1990

287

tional principle determines a set of secular equations. In the other approach the scattering matrix of the solid is calculated and the power of scattering theory is used in the determination of the appropriate physical observables.

Instead of explicitly calculating the total energy of all possible ground states, the possible occurrence of a state with lower symmetry can be investigated through applying an external field and determining whether the system becomes unstable with respect to this perturbation. A linear ansatz is made: linear response theory can be applied. We will be particularly interested in the spin susceptibility which relates to a possible magnetic transition. In the static case a spin density wave, a charge density wave, a concentration wave refer to modulations in the magnetic structure, in the crystal structure, in the chemical structure of the solid. This approach determines the ordering vector (or q vector) of a possible instability, and it is the only way to evaluate the q vector of an incommensurate instability (no periodicity is present).

The outline of these lectures is as follows. The next section deals with performing SCF calculations in a basis set approach, the third section deals with multiple scattering methods and the fourth one with spin susceptibility calculations. These techniques are applied in the fifth section to the study of La_2CuO_4, a parent of the high T_C materials, and to a closely related system La_2NiO_4.

2.   THE LMTO-ASA BAND STRUCTURE METHOD AND CODE

The foundation of DFT are two theorems due to Hohenberg and Kohn (HK) (1964). They can be stated as follows (in atomic units):

$$H = T + U + V$$

$$= \sum_{i=1}^{N} (-\nabla_i^2) + \frac{1}{2} \sum_{i \neq j}^{N} \sum_{j=1}^{N} \frac{2}{r_{ij}} + \sum_{i=1}^{N} v_{ext}(r_i) \tag{2.1}$$

where r_i is a position vector of an electron, $r_{ij} = r_i - r_j$, H is the Hamiltonian of a system of N interacting electrons, T their kinetic energy, U the electron-electron Coulomb repulsion and V some external potential, for example the Coulomb attraction of the nuclei. First HK showed that the external potential is a unique functional of the electron density $\rho(r)$, and hence the properties of the groundstate Φ of an inhomogeneous interacting electron gas are unique functionals of the electron density. Secondly, they showed that $<\Phi|H|\Phi> = E[\rho]$ is a minimum for the true electron density. Kohn and Sham (1965) then showed that this minimization leads to N effective single-particle Schrödinger equations:

$$(-\nabla^2 + V(\underline{r}) - \varepsilon_i)\,\psi_i(\underline{r}) = 0$$

$$\rho(\underline{r}) = \sum_i |\psi_i(\underline{r})|^2\, \theta(\varepsilon_F - \varepsilon_i) \tag{2.2}$$

$$V(\underline{r}) = 2\int d\underline{r}'\, \frac{\rho(\underline{r}')}{|\underline{r}-\underline{r}'|} + \frac{\delta E_{xc}[\rho]}{\delta\rho(\underline{r})} + v_{ext}(\underline{r}) \tag{2.3}$$

$E_{xc}[\rho]$ is the unknown exchange and correlation functional of the charge density. In the local density approximation one writes:

$$E_{xc}[\rho] \approx \int d^3\underline{r}\; \rho(\underline{r})\, \varepsilon_{xc}^{(h)}(\rho(\underline{r})) \tag{2.4}$$

where $\varepsilon_{xc}^{(h)}(x)$ is the contribution of the exchange and correlation to the total energy (per electron) in a homogeneous, but interacting, electron gas of density $\rho(\underline{r})$. This quantity $\varepsilon_{xc}^{(h)}$ (von Barth and Hedin 1972) can be determined to a sufficient accuracy.

It follows then that in solids, Equation (2.2), which is a set of self-consistent equations in the charge density, has to be solved for a periodic arrangement of external potentials. This can be simplified by making use of the lattice periodicity. However, this still leaves us with a formidable numerical problem which we will further simplify by assuming that the potential $V(\underline{r})$ is spherically symmetric within overlapping Wigner-Seitz spheres. This is the so-called atomic sphere approximation or ASA (Andersen 1975, 1984, 1985, Skriver 1984).

If we then choose a linear combination of the solutions φ of the radial Schrödinger equation in the ASA, which are called the muffin-tin orbitals, and their energy derivatives $\dot{\varphi}$ in an expansion of the wavefunction, then application of the variational principle leads to the following generalised eigenvalue problem for the energy eigenvalues $\varepsilon_{\underline{k},n}$ and wavefunctions $\psi_{\underline{k},n}$ where $\underline{k}$ refers to the $\underline{k}$ point in reciprocal space and n to the band index:

$$(H_{LL'}^{\underline{k}} - \varepsilon_{\underline{k},n}\, O_{LL'}^{\underline{k}})\, a_L^{\underline{k},n} = 0$$

and

$$\psi_{\underline{k},n}(\underline{r}) = \sum_{i,L} [\, A_L^{\underline{k},n}(\varepsilon_{\underline{k},n})\, \varphi_{v,L}^i(\underline{r}) + B_L^{\underline{k},n}(\varepsilon_{\underline{k},n})\, \dot{\varphi}_{v,L}^i(\underline{r})\,]\, Y_L(\hat{r})$$

The indices L and L´ are the angular momentum and magnetic quantum numbers ℓ,m. The index i sums over the different atomic spheres which make up the unit cell. The Y's are the spherical harmonics, $\varphi^i_{v,L}$ is the solution of the radial Schrödinger equation in the atomic sphere (AS) i, for the energy ε_v and angular momentum ℓ, $\dot{\varphi}$ is the energy derivative of φ. For the detailed form of the Hamiltonian H, the overlap matrix O and wavefunction coefficients A and B we refer the reader to formulae (5.46), (5.47) and (6.30) of Skriver's book (1984).

The advantage of this particular basis set method is that the matrices are small. Because of the ASA, the matrix elements of H and O are analytical functions of the logarithmic derivatives of a single atomic sphere wavefunction, φ, and the solid state effects enter through the structure constants which depend only on the crystal structure. We note that the basis functions φ and $\dot{\varphi}$ in (2.5) are independent of principal quantum number. In circumstances where one wants to generate the band structure over an energy range which would include bands of different principal quantum number, such as is the case for the calculation of occupied and unoccupied bandstructures, one should include in the basis set the basis functions corresponding to these different principal quantum numbers. The size of the generalised eigenvalue problem then scales according to the number of principal quantum numbers included. In that case one might consider non-linear band structure approach, such as the KKR (see next section) which allows the continuous progression from one principal quantum number to another. In this method the matrix size remains constant, but it has a complicated non-linear energy dependence and the eigenvalues are obtained by finding the zeros of the determinant of the KKR matrix.

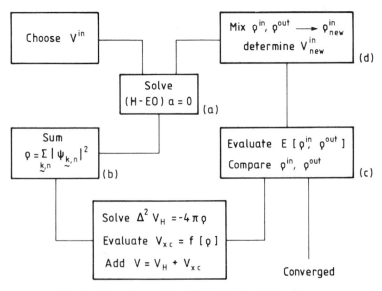

Fig. 1. Flowchart of the SCF-LMTO-ASA program.

Table 1. The analytical expressions for the contributions of a particular tetrahedron, defined by E_1, E_2, E_3, E_4 as energy eigenvalues with the same band index at $\underline{k}$ points 1 2 3 4 which define a tetrahedron, to the density of states and integrated density of states (Temmerman et al 1989).

	Density of states	Integrated density of states $\int_{-\infty}^{E} n(E')dE'$
	$n_1 = \dfrac{3*(E - E_1)^2}{(E_2 - E_1)\,(E_3 - E_1)\,(E_4 - E_1)}\,\theta(E - E_1)$	$I_1 = \dfrac{(E - E_1)^3}{(E_2 - E_1)\,(E_3 - E_1)\,(E_4 - E_1)}\,\theta(E - E_1)$
	$n_2 = \dfrac{3*(E - E_2)^2}{(E_1 - E_2)\,(E_3 - E_2)\,(E_4 - E_2)}\,\theta(E - E_2)$	$I_2 = \dfrac{(E - E_2)^3}{(E_1 - E_2)\,(E_3 - E_2)\,(E_4 - E_2)}\,\theta(E - E_2)$
	$n_3 = \dfrac{3*(E - E_3)^2}{(E_1 - E_3)\,(E_2 - E_3)\,(E_4 - E_3)}\,\theta(E - E_3)$	$I_3 = \dfrac{(E - E_3)^3}{(E_1 - E_3)\,(E_2 - E_3)\,(E_4 - E_3)}\,\theta(E - E_3)$
	$n_4 = \dfrac{3*(E - E_4)^2}{(E_1 - E_4)\,(E_2 - E_4)\,(E_3 - E_4)}\,\theta(E - E_4)$	$I_4 = \dfrac{(E - E_4)^3}{(E_1 - E_4)\,(E_2 - E_4)\,(E_3 - E_4)}\,\theta(E - E_4)$

$E \leq E_1$	0	$E \leq E_1$	0
$E_1 \leq E \leq E_2$	n_1	$E_1 \leq E \leq E_2$	I_1
$E_2 \leq E \leq E_3$	$n_1 + n_2$	$E_2 \leq E \leq E_3$	$I_1 + I_2$
$E_3 \leq E \leq E_4$	$n_1 + n_2 + n_3$	$E_3 \leq E \leq E_4$	$I_1 + I_2 + I_3$
$E_4 \leq E$	$n_1 + n_2 + n_3 + n_4 = 0$	$E_4 \leq E$	$I_1 + I_2 + I_3 + I_4 = 1$

Figure 1 gives a flowchart of the SCF-LMTO-ASA code. We will discuss now the features of the calculation which we found very important in obtaining an accurate and reliable code (Temmerman, Sterne, Guo and Szotek 1989). One starts with an input V^{in}, usually obtained from atomic charge densities which are suitably normalised over the atomic sphere. Given this input potential the generalised eigenvalue problem (a in Fig. 1) is solved via standard numerical techniques (such as Cholesky decomposition) and codes (the EISPACK routines: HTRIDI, IMTQL2 and HTRIBK). This is an adequate procedure for the matrix sizes we are dealing with (of the order of 100). In step b of Fig. 1 we collect all the energy eigenvalues and eigen vectors for a summation over the Brillouin zone

($\underset{\sim}{k}$ sum) and over band indices (n sum) to determine the charge density. To perform the $\underset{\sim}{k}$ sum the irreducible Brillouin zone wedge is divided in tetrahedra. At the vertices of these tetrahedra the energy eigenvalues and eigen vectors are calculated. On the basis of a linear variation of the energy eigenvalues over the tetrahedron (Lehmann and Taut 1972, Jepsen and Andersen 1971, 1984) analytical expressions for the contributions of a particular tetrahedron to the density of states and integrated density of states can be obtained and are given in Table 1. One can derive expressions for the higher energy moments of the density of states: we determined expressions for up to the third moment with the help of the algebraic manipulation package REDUCE. Out of the values I_i^ε from Table 1 we can define weight W, for each point $\underset{\sim}{k}_j$ of the tetrahedral mesh and each band n, as follows:

$$W_{\underset{\sim}{k}_j,n} = \underset{\text{tet}}{\Sigma} \overset{4}{\underset{i=1}{\Sigma}} I_{\underset{\sim}{k}_i,n}^{\varepsilon_f} \delta_{\underset{\sim}{k}_i \underset{\sim}{k}_j}.$$

The first summation is over all the tetrahedra spanning the irreducible wedge of the Brillouin zone and the second summation is over the four vertices of each tetrahedron. The Brillouin zone integrals of the wavefunction coefficient then become the following $\underset{\sim}{k}$ sums:

$$A_L = \underset{n}{\Sigma} \underset{\underset{\sim}{k}_j}{\Sigma} A_L^{\underset{\sim}{k}_j,n} W_{\underset{\sim}{k}_j,n}$$

$$B_L = \underset{n}{\Sigma} \underset{\underset{\sim}{k}_j}{\Sigma} B_L^{\underset{\sim}{k}_j,n} W_{\underset{\sim}{k}_j,n}$$

The charge density for the ith site in the unit cell then becomes:

$$\rho^i(\underset{\sim}{r}) = \underset{L}{\Sigma} [\, |A_L|^2 (\varphi_{v,L}^i(\underset{\sim}{r}))^2 + |B_L|^2$$

$$\times (\dot{\varphi}_{v,L}^i(\underset{\sim}{r}))^2 + (A_L^* B_L + B_L^* A_L)\, \varphi_{v,L}^i(\underset{\sim}{r})\, \dot{\varphi}_{v,L}^i(\underset{\sim}{r})]$$

An alternative method of calculating the charge density via a moment expansion of the density of states (expression (6.41) in Skriver's book (1984) was found to give a substantially slower convergence of at least twice as many SCF cycles. This is because expression (6.41) does not span the Hilbert space defined by φ and $\dot{\varphi}$.

One of the most important ingredients in the rate of convergence is the mixing scheme to obtain from the output charge density ρ^{out} a new input charge density $\rho_{\text{new}}^{\text{in}}$ [step c in Fig. 1]. A vast literature on the subject exists and an excellent review of the various methods is given by Pickett (1989). We found it adequate to implement a generalization of a simple linear mixing due to Anderson (1965). This scheme uses a linear combination of input and output densities of two successive iterations (M-1 and M) to give an optimized input $\bar{\rho}^{in}$ and output $\bar{\rho}^{out}$:

$$\bar{\rho}_M^{in(out)} = \theta_M \, \rho_M^{in(out)} + (1 - \theta_M) \, \rho_{M-1}^{in(out)}$$

and θ_M is determined by minimizing the distance Δ

$$\Delta(\underline{r}) = (\rho^{out}(\underline{r}) - \rho^{in}(\underline{r}))$$

between $\bar{\rho}_M^{out}$ and $\bar{\rho}_M^{in}$ (i.e. convergence is obtained when $\bar{\rho}_M^{out} = \bar{\rho}_M^{in}$) which leads to the following expression for θ_M:

$$\theta_M = \frac{\int d\underline{r} \, [\Delta_{M-1}(\underline{r}) \Delta_{M-1}(\underline{r}) - \Delta_{M-1}(\underline{r}) \Delta_M(\underline{r})]}{\int dr \, [\Delta_M(\underline{r}) - \Delta_{M-1}(\underline{r})]^2}$$

The new input charge density is then obtained from

$$\rho_{M+1}^{in} = \lambda \, \bar{\rho}_M^{out} + (1-\lambda) \, \bar{\rho}_M^{in}$$

where we treat λ like the mixing parameter in the simple linear mixing scheme. More sophisticated mixing methods are available such as Broyden's method (Srivastava 1984).

The quantity which converges first should be the total energy since the functional $E_{total}[\rho]$ is minimized by the true ground state density $\rho(\underline{r})$. However care has to be taken by using a total energy expression which is truly variational. This is especially the case when using a total energy expression which incorporates the one-electron sum which is not a functional of either the input or output density alone (Chelikowsky and Louie 1987, Picket 1989). The LMTO-ASA variational total energy expressions are:

$$E = \int \varepsilon n(\varepsilon)d\varepsilon - \int V_H^{in} \rho^{out} d\underline{r} + \frac{1}{2} \int V_H^{out} \rho^{out} d\underline{r} - \int \mu_{xc}[\rho^{in}] \, \rho^{out} d\underline{r}$$

$$+ \int \varepsilon_{xc}[\rho^{out}] \, \rho^{out} d\underline{r} + \int [\varepsilon_{xc}[\rho^{out}] - \varepsilon_{xc}[\rho_{core}]] \, \rho_{core} \, d\underline{r} + E_{MAD}$$

$$E_{MAD} = \frac{1}{s_{av}} \sum_{ij} [-\frac{1}{2} z_{ion}^i V_{MAD}^{ij} z_{ion}^j + \frac{1}{2} q_{val}^{out,i} V_{MAD}^{ij} q_{val}^{out,j} - q_{val}^{in,j} V_{MAD}^{ij} q_{val}^{out,j}]$$

where Z and q are respectively the charge of the ion core and the electronic charge of the valence electrons. We also made use of an analytical expression for the first moment of the density of states or the one-electron sum.

In summary, we obtain a fast and reliable convergence within the LMTO-ASA scheme by making use of analytical expressions, derived within the linear tetrahedra method, for the Brillouin zone integrals, evaluating the charge density from the wavefunctions, a better than linear mixing scheme, and finally by evaluating the variational expression of the total energy.

3. MULTIPLE SCATTERING THEORY AND KKR

Again we describe the solid as consisting of spherical symmetric potentials situated at each site. However we do not allow these potentials to overlap, they can at most touch each other. In this approximation, the so-called muffin-tin approximation, the potential in the remaining region, the interstitial region, is taken to be a constant. Multiple scattering theory can readily be implemented for this muffin-tin potential, since the incoming wave at any of the spherical symmetric potentials consists of the out-going waves from all the other sites and the out-going wave can be described as a phase shifted spherical wave. A standing wave will describe the allowed solutions. We shall give now a more detailed description (Temmerman and Szotek 1987). Due to the finite range of each muffin-tin potential, we are only interested in "on-energy-shell" scattering describing how an incident wave of a given energy is transformed into a scattered wave with the same energy. The scattering path operator τ^{nm} turns an incident wave at site m into a scattered wave at site n, and which includes the effect of all the scattering in between. Explicitly it reads as:

$$\tau^{nm}_{LL'}(E) = t_{n,L}(E)\, \delta_{nm}\, \delta_{LL'} + \sum_{k \neq n} \sum_{L''} t_{n,L}(E)\, g^{nk}_{LL''}(E)\, \tau^{km}_{L''L'}(E) \qquad (3.1)$$

where the real space structure constants

$$g^{nk}_{LL'}(E) = 4\pi\, \sqrt{E}\, i^{\ell-\ell'+1} \sum_{L''} C^{L''}_{LL'}\, i^{\ell''}\, h^{+}_{\ell''}(\sqrt{E}\,|\underline{R}_n - \underline{R}_k|)\, Y_{L''}(\underline{R}_n - \underline{R}_k) \qquad (3.2)$$

depend only on the spatial arrangement of the scatterers. Here $h^{+}_{\ell''}$ stands for the spherical Hankel function and the Gaunt numbers are defined by:

$$C^{L''}_{LL'} = \int d\Omega\, Y_L(\Omega)\, Y_{L''}(\Omega)\, Y_{L'}(\Omega) \qquad (3.3)$$

where Ω is the solid angle, with Y_L denoting the real spherical harmonics. $t_{n,L}(E)$ are the diagonal "on-energy-shell" matrix elements of the t-matrix, and are related to the scattering phaseshifts $\delta_\ell^n(E)$ through

$$t_{n,L}(E) = -\frac{1}{\sqrt{E}} \sin \delta_\ell^n(E) \exp(i \delta_\ell^n(E)) = t_{n,\ell}(E) \tag{3.4}$$

The phaseshifts are obtained from the requirement that the solutions of the radial Schrödinger equation, regular at the origin ($z_\ell(r,E) \sim r^\ell$ as $r - 0$) join smoothly to

$$z_\ell^n(r,E) = j_\ell(\sqrt{E}\, r)\, t_{n,\ell}(E) - i\, h_\ell^+(\sqrt{E} r) \tag{3.5}$$

at $r = r_{MT}$, the muffin-tin radius. If $\gamma_\ell^n(E) = (\frac{1}{z_\ell^n(r,E)})(\frac{d\, z_\ell^n(r,E)}{dr})$ is the logarithmic

derivative at $r = r_{MT}$ then the phaseshift can be expressed by

$$\cot \delta_\ell^n(E) = \frac{\sqrt{E}\, n_\ell(\sqrt{E}\, r_{MT}) - \gamma_\ell^n(E)\, n_\ell'(\sqrt{E}\, r_{MT})}{\sqrt{E}\, j_\ell(\sqrt{E}\, r_{MT}) - \gamma_\ell^n(E)\, j_\ell'(\sqrt{E}\, r_{MT})} \tag{3.6}$$

Here j_ℓ and n_ℓ are the spherical Bessel and Neumann functions, and j_ℓ' and n_ℓ' are their derivatives. Since the logarithmic derivative can easily be obtained by numerical integration of the radial Schrödinger equation

$$\frac{1}{r}\frac{d^2}{dr^2}[r\, z_\ell^n(r,E)] + [V(r) - E + \frac{\ell(\ell+1)}{r^2}]\, z_\ell^n(r,E) = 0 \tag{3.7}$$

both the phaseshifts and the t-matrix are known. This relatively simple structure of the formalism is due to the muffin-tin nature of the potential.

Equation (3.1) is the fundamental equation of multiple scattering. It is valid for any arrangement of spherical potential wells, even if at each site there is a different potential. The only limitation on its validity is the requirement that the potential wells at different sites may not overlap.

In particular if the sites form a lattice and the lattice sites are occupied by the same potential, then we can lattice Fourier transform Eq.(3.1). Defining

$$\tau_{LL'}(\underline{k},E) = \frac{1}{N} \sum_{n,m} \exp(i\, \underline{k}\, (\underline{R}_n - \underline{R}_m))\, \tau_{LL'}^{nm}(E) \tag{3.8}$$

and

$$g_{LL'}(\underline{k},E) = \frac{1}{N} \sum_{n,m} \exp(i\,\underline{k}\,(\underline{R}_n - \underline{R}_m)) \; g_{LL'}^{nm}(E) \tag{3.9}$$

then we obtain by substituting (3.9) into (3.8) and using Eq.(3.1)

$$\tau_{LL'}(\underline{k},E) = [\, t_L^{-1}(E)\,\delta_{LL'} - g_{LL'}(\underline{k},E)\,]^{-1} \tag{3.10}$$

and substituting (3.10) into (3.8) for the case n = m = 0, we obtain

$$\tau_{LL'}^{00}(E) = \frac{1}{\Omega_{BZ}} \int d\underline{k}\; \tau_{LL'}(\underline{k},E) \tag{3.11}$$

Equations (3.10) and (3.11) are of great physical importance. The poles of $\tau(\underline{k},E)$ determine the energy spectrum in E, $\underline{k}$ space. The denominator of this equation is the matrix of the KKR bandstructure method. Equation (3.11) is a fundamental quantity of the Green function, for $\underline{r}$ and $\underline{r}'$ confined to the same unit cell:

$$G(\underline{r},\underline{r}';\epsilon) = \sum_{LL'} [\, Z_L(\underline{r},E)\,\tau_{LL'}^{00}(E)\,Z_{L'}(\underline{r}',E) - Z_L(\underline{r}_<,E)\,J_L(\underline{r}_>,E)\,\delta_{LL'}\,] \tag{3.12}$$

where r, r' $\leq r_{MT}$. The regular solution of the Schrödinger equation is

$$Z_L(\underline{r},E) = z_\ell(r,E)\,Y_L(\hat{r}) \tag{3.13}$$

and

$$J_L(\underline{r},E) = \tilde{j}_\ell(r,E)\,Y_L(\hat{r}) \tag{3.14}$$

is the solution of the Schrödinger equation irregular at the origin which joins smoothly onto $j_\ell(r,E)Y_L(\hat{r})$ at $r = r_{MT}$. The imaginary part of (3.12) integrated over $\underline{r}$ is the density of states:

$$n(E) = -\frac{1}{\pi}\,\mathrm{Im}\int d\underline{r}\; G(\underline{r},\underline{r},E) \tag{3.15}$$

and the Bloch spectral density defined as

$$A_B(\underline{k},E) = -\frac{1}{\pi}\,\mathrm{Im}\,G_B(\underline{k},\underline{k},E)$$

$$= -\frac{1}{\pi}\,\mathrm{Im}\left\{ \sum_n \exp(i\,\underline{k}\,\underline{R}_n)\,\frac{1}{\Omega}\int d\underline{r}\; G(\underline{r},\underline{r}+\underline{R}_n,E) \right\} \tag{3.16}$$

296

where the r integral runs over the unit cell only. Substituting

$$G(\underline{r},\underline{r}+\underline{R}_n,E) = \sum_{LL'} \left[Z_L(\underline{r},E)\, \tau_{LL'}^{on}(E)\, Z_{L'}(\underline{r}',E) \right.$$

$$\left. - Z_L(\underline{r}_<,E)\, J_L(\underline{r}_>,E)\, \delta_{LL'}\, \delta_{on} \right] \qquad (3.17)$$

into (3.16) we obtain with (3.8)

$$A_B(\underline{k},E) = -\frac{1}{\pi}\, \mathrm{Im} \sum_{LL'} F_{LL'}(E)\, \tau_{L'L}(\underline{k},E) \qquad (3.18)$$

with

$$F_{LL'}(E) = \int d\underline{r}\, Z_L(\underline{r},E)\, Z_{L'}(\underline{r},E) \qquad (3.19)$$

The sigularities of $A_B(\underline{k},E)$ or $\tau(\underline{k},E)$ are the energy eigenvalues of the system.

Inspection of equations (3.15), (3.12) and (3.18) shows that in order to calculate n(E) and $A_B(\underline{k},E)$ we need to evaluate $\tau(k,E)$ and $\tau(E)$. The other quantities depend on the solution of the radial Schrödinger equation for a single muffin-tin sphere which we solved to obtain the phaseshifts. We therefore turn our attention to the evaluation of $g_{LL'}(\underline{k},E)$ in Eq.(3.10) (Stocks, Temmerman and Gyorffy 1979) and to performing the Brillouin zone integral of $\tau(\underline{k},E)$ in Eq.(3.11) (Temmerman and Szotek 1987).

The structure constants of $g(\underline{k},E)$ Eq.(3.9) and (3.2) are slowly converging lattice sums. Application of the Ewald procedure transforms the slowly converging series (3.9) into the sum over two rapidly converging series D^1 and D^2 and a term D^3:

$$g_{LL'}(\underline{k},E) = 4\pi \sum_{L''} C_{LL'}^{L''}\, D_{L''}(\underline{k}\ E) \qquad (3.20)$$

$$D_{L'}(\underline{k},E) = D_{L'}^1(\underline{k},E) + D_{L'}^2(\underline{k},E) + \delta_{L''0}\, D_{00}^3(E) \qquad (3.21)$$

The explicit forms of the three parts are:

$$D_{L'}^1(\underline{k},E) = -\left(\frac{4\pi}{V}\right) e^{E/\eta} \left(\frac{1}{\sqrt{E}}\right)^{\ell''} \sum_n k_n^{\ell''} (k_n^2 - E)^{-1} \exp(-k_n^2/\eta)\, Y_{L'}(\hat{k}_n) \qquad (3.22)$$

$$D^2_{L'}(\underline{k},E) = -(2)^{\ell''+1}\left(\frac{1}{\sqrt{\pi}}\right)\left(\frac{1}{\sqrt{E}}\right)^{\ell''}\sum_s i^{\ell''}\exp(i\underline{k}\cdot\underline{R}_s)\,Y_{L'}(\hat{R}_s)$$

$$\times R_s^{\ell''}\int_{\sqrt{\eta}/2}^{\infty} d\xi\,\xi^{2\ell''}\exp[-\xi^2 R_s^2 + E/4\xi^2] \tag{3.23}$$

$$D^3_{00}(E) = -\sqrt{\eta}\left(\frac{1}{\sqrt{2\pi}}\right)\sum_{j=0}^{\infty}\left(\frac{E}{\eta}\right)^j\left(\frac{1}{j!(2j-1)}\right) \tag{3.24}$$

In Eq.(3.22) V is the unit cell volume, $\underline{k}_n = \underline{K}_n + \underline{k}$, and $k_n = |\underline{k}_n|$, with $\underline{K}_n$ being the reciprocal lattice vectors. The prime on the summation in (3.23) indicates that the term $\underline{R}_s = 0$ is omitted, with $\underline{R}_s$ being the real space lattice vectors. The Ewald constant η will determine how fast (3.22) and (3.23) converge.

These structure constants are independent of the material and dependent only on the crystal structure. Moreover by defining dimensionless units (d.u.) the structure constants can be determined independently of the value of the lattice constant a. The appropriate conversion factors are: Length (d.u.) $=\frac{2\pi}{a}$ length (atomic units), E(d.u.) $=(\frac{a}{2\pi})^2 E(Ry)$. These structure constants are therefore universal enough to investigate if they are amenable to a polynomial fit in $\underline{k}$ and E as a fast way of generating them. Whilst the D^2 and D^3 terms are smoothly varying functions, the D^1 term contains a singularity at $E = (\underline{k}+\underline{K}_n)^2$, and is therefore not immediately amenable to polynomial fitting. However D^1 can be further decomposed over a limited energy range into two terms: one singular D^S and one regular $D^{1,R}$ at $E = (\underline{k}+\underline{k}_n)^2$

$$D^1_{L'}(\underline{k},E) = D^{1,R}_{L'}(\underline{k},E) + D^S_{L'}(\underline{k},E) \tag{3.25}$$

$$D^{1,R}_{L'}(\underline{k},E) = -\left(\frac{4\pi}{V}\right)\left(\frac{1}{\sqrt{E}}\right)^{\ell''} \times \left(\sum_{n\varepsilon A} k_n^{\ell''}(k_n^2 - E)^{-1}\right.$$

$$\left.[\exp(E - k_n^2)/\eta - 1]\,Y_{L'}(\hat{k}_n) + \sum_{n\notin A} k_n^{\ell''}(k_n^2 - E)^{-1}\times\exp(E - k_n^2)/\eta\,Y_{L'}(\hat{k}_n)\right) \tag{3.26}$$

$$D^S_L(\underline{k},E) = -\left(\frac{4\pi}{V}\right)\left(\frac{1}{\sqrt{E}}\right)^{\ell''}\sum_{n\varepsilon A} k_n^{\ell''}(k_n^2 - E)^{-1}Y_{L'}(\hat{k}_n) \tag{3.27}$$

The reciprocal lattice vectors in the set A which are included in the singular term (3.27) are those for which $E - (\underset{\sim}{k}+\underset{\sim}{k}_n)^2 = 0$ or becomes small for any $\underset{\sim}{k}$ in the Brillouin zone and any energy E for which we are going to use the structure constants. The set A contains typically between 10 to 20 vectors. The D can now be written as the sum of a regular and a singular part as

$$D_{L'}(\underset{\sim}{k},E) = D_{L'}^R(\underset{\sim}{k},E) + D_{L'}^S(\underset{\sim}{k},E) \tag{3.28}$$

$$D_{L'}^R(\underset{\sim}{k},E) = D_{L'}^{1;R}(\underset{\sim}{k},E) + D_{L'}^2(\underset{\sim}{k},E) + \delta_{L'0}D_{00}^3(E) \tag{3.29}$$

where D^S is given by (3.27). In Figs.2 and 3 we show D^R as a function of E and $\underset{\sim}{k}$ along an arbitrary direction from the Brillouin zone centre to the Brillouin zone boundary. In Fig.2 no singular term has been subtracted and D^R=D. The structure constant shows a singularity at $E=k_n^2$. In Fig.2. we removed the two reciprocal lattice vectors at (0,0,0) and (-1,-1,-1) from D^R (3.26) and put them in D^S (3.27). We have now obtained a function D^R which is easily fitted, both in E and $\underset{\sim}{k}$, by low degree polynomials. We fitted for each $\underset{\sim}{k}$ direction the D^R in the energy range of -0.2 < E < 1.0 (d.u.) using Chebyshev polynomials of degree five in E and seven in $\underset{\sim}{k}$. To fit polynomials of low degree we also found it useful not only to remove the reciprocal lattice vectors which contribute a singularity in the fit range but also those for which $E-k_{\sim n}^2$ is small. Moreover multiplying each D^R by a factor $(\sqrt{E})^{L''}$ removes the E=0 singularity in (3.26). The singular term

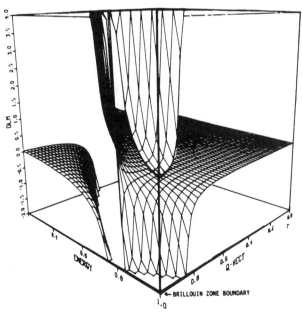

Fig. 2. $D_{00}(\underset{\sim}{k},E)$ plotted as a function of energy and as a function of $\underset{\sim}{k}$ along a line from the Brillouin zone centre to the point (0.482, 0.350, 0.668) on the boundary of an fcc Brillouin zone. No free electron poles have been removed (Stocks et al 1979).

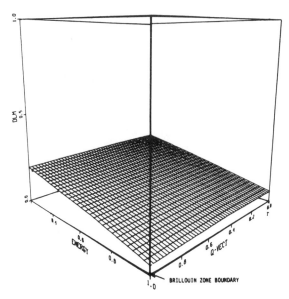

Fig. 3 $D_{0,0}^R(\underline{k},E)$ according to Eq.(3.26) with the set A consisting of the vectors (0,0,0) and (-1,-1,-1) (Stocks et al 1979).

(3.27) can be fitted analytically along a direction in $\underline{k}$ space. We can write the numerator of (3.27) as

$$| \underline{k} + \underline{K}_n |^{\ell} \, Y_L(\widehat{k + \underline{K}_n}) = \sum_{m=0}^{\ell+1} a_m^n k^m \qquad (3.30)$$

where the coefficients a_m^n can be calculated analytically for each direction $\underline{k}$ and reciprocal lattice vector $\underline{K}_n$. Summarizing, there exists a numerical and analytical procedure to fit the structure constants along directions in the Brillouin zone. To fit the D^R in our calculations for Pd we generate a small dataset of about 25000 words: number of directions (21) * number of (ℓ,m) $(\ell_{max}=2)$ (25) * degree of fit in k (8) * degree of fit in E (6). For the singular term we need: number of directions (21)* number of (ℓ,m) (25) * degree of fit in k (5) * number of reciprocal lattice vectors (10) giving an array of about 26000 words.

Up to now we implicitly assumed the energy to be a real quantity, even though the formalism we developed does not depend on that. It turns out that the direct evaluation of (3.11) and (3.10) is greatly helped by adding a small imaginary part of approximately 0.001 d.u. to the energy. Thus the inversion of (3.10) can be accomplished with standard matrix inversion techniques. We found the Gauss-Jordan algorithm very useful to obtain a highly vectorisable code. Consider A: the matrix which needs inverting; B: the unit matrix; C: the inverse of matrix A; N: the dimension of the matrix; TD, AD and BD:

temporary storage arrays of size N each, then our Fortran code is as follows:

```
    DO 1 I=1,N
    DO 2 J=1,N
    TD(J)=A(J,I)/A(I,I)
2 CONTINUE
    TD(I)=(0.0,0.0)
    DO 3 K=1,N
    AD(K)=A(I,K)
    BD(K)=B(I,K)
3 CONTINUE
    DO 4 K=1,N
    DO 5 J=1,N
    A(J,K)=A(J,K)-(TD(J)*AD(K))
    B(J,K)=B(J,K)-(TD(J)*BD(K))
5 CONTINUE
4 CONTINUE
1 CONTINUE
    DO 6 I=1,N
    DO 7 J=1,N
    C(J,I)=B(J,I)/A(J,J)
7 CONTINUE
6 CONTINUE
```

We note that in this code all the do-loops run from 1,N. In the codes based on the Gaussian elimination method for inverting matrices we find nested DO loops of the type

```
    DO 1 I=1,N
    DO 2 J=I,N
```

optimised for scalar computers where we want to reduce the number of arithmetic operations performed. On vector processors we do not want to reset the lower-index I of the inner-loop DO 2 and we want to construct a vector of a fixed length independent of the value of I.

At this stage the evaluation of the integrand of the Brillouin zone integral (3.11) has been optimised by the polynomial fit of the g's and an efficient inversion routine for vector processors. The integral in $\tau_{LL}^{oo}(E)$ (3.11) is a rapidly varying function of $\underset{\sim}{k}$ over the Brillouin zone. Integration techniques which are based on calculating the integral on a fixed $\underset{\sim}{k}$ grid in the Brillouin zone, defining tetrahedra, and then evaluate the contribution of the integrand over this volume-element to the total integral by interpolation are unsuitable. This integrand becomes large at these E and $\underline{k}$ values where the electronic states occur, being small everywhere else and this integrand is therefore not amenable to interpolation.

This Brillouin zone integral will be obtained by writing $\tau^{oo}(E)$ as

$$\tau^{oo}(E) = \frac{1}{\Omega_{BZ}} \int d\,\Omega_{\hat{k}}\,\tau_{\hat{k}}(E) \qquad (3.31)$$

where $\Omega_{\hat{k}}$ is the solid angle and

$$\tau_{\hat{k}} = \int_0^{k_{BZ}} dk\,k^2 \tau(k,E) \qquad (3.32)$$

where τ's are matrices in the angular momentum components, k_{BZ} denotes the Brillouin zone boundary along the direction $\underline{k}$. The integration technique involves the accurate determination of the line integrals (3.32) and finds the set of directions over which we have to sum to obtain the Brillouin zone integral. This approach only makes sense when $\tau_{\hat{k}}(E)$ is a smoothly varying function of the radial direction $\hat{k}$ and we can perform these radial integrals.

For a given direction in the Brillouin zone we ensure the convergence of the one-dimensional integral by concentrating the points at which the integrand is evaluated in those regions where the integrand is large and then we perform the integral analytically using a quadratic interpolation. Depending on the nature of the structure in the integrand, this step will typically require evaluating the integrand at between 100 and 300 points along each direction. A ZOOMIN routine will take the integrand evaluated on a fixed k grid of about 60 points and then generate a denser mesh in those regions where the function is large. It determines this mesh by examining if the differences between the values of the real and the imaginary part of the function at two successive grid points become larger than the fixed quantities CPH and CPH2 respectively and then halves this interval. It keeps halving this interval unless the values of the real and imaginary part of the function between the two successive grid points become smaller than CPH and CPH2 respectively or the interval itself becomes smaller than a fixed quantity APH. Another useful indicator that the integrand will have much structure is that the real part of the integrand will change sign. We will adopt this too as a condition to "zoom in". The choice of the zoomin parameters can vary from APH = 10^{-5}-10^{-6}, CPH=20.0 and CPH2=10.0 where the integrand has very sharp peaks to APH=10^{-3}-10^{-4} with CPH=1.0 and CPH2=0.5 when the integrand is more smeared out. A listing of the FORTRAN code of this subroutine can be found in Temmerman and Szotek (1987). The Brillouin zone integral (3.11) is then evaluated as

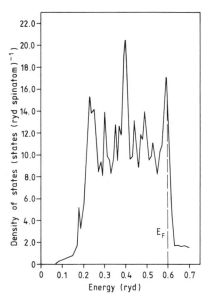

Fig. 4. The density of states of Pd calculated using (3.15) and Im $\varepsilon = 10^{-3}$ Ryd.

$$\tau^{OO}(E) = \sum_{i=1}^{N} w_i \tau_{\hat{k}_i}(E) \qquad (3.33)$$

where i=1... N defines a set of directions and w_i is some weight function. A convenient way is to divide the irreducible wedge of the Brillouin zone in prisms each having its apex at the zone centre and base at the Brillouin zone boundary. The direction along which we perform the one-dimensional integrals are then taken to be the centre of mass lines of the prisms. For the weight function we take the volume of the prisms. Other methods for choosing direction and their weights are discussed in Temmerman and Szotek (1987). In Fig. 4 we show the density of states of Pd evaluated using Eq.(3.15) (Winter, Stenzel, Szotek and Temmerman 1988a). The Brillouin integral was performed using 36 prism directions and on an energy mesh parallel to the real axis with an imaginary part of 10^{-3} ryd. We found that 36 directions were converged since the

Fermi energy ε_F, determined from the integral over this density of states $\int_{\varepsilon_B}^{\varepsilon_F} n(E)dE=N$, where ε_B is the bottom of the band and N the total number of valence electrons, changed by only 2 mRyd in going from 36 to 136 directions.

4.   SUSCEPTIBILITIES

A first principles theory of the spin susceptibility for an extended solid, formulated in terms of local spin density functional approach (LSD) and random phase approximation

(RPA) was described in detail in our previous work (Stenzel and Winter 1985, 1986). Here we give an outline of the formalism in order to get on with a discussion of the numerical evaluation of the formulae (Winter, Stenzel, Szotek and Temmerman 1988, Stenzel, Winter, Szotek and Temmerman 1988). The quantity containing all information, which may most conveniently be calculated, is the lattice Fourier transform, $\chi_q(\rho,\rho',\omega)$, of the dynamical

spin density-spin density correlation function defined by:

$$m(\underline{r};\omega) = \int \chi(\underline{r},\underline{r}';\omega) \, B(\underline{r}';\omega) dr'$$

where $B(\underline{r};\omega)$ is an externally applied magnetic field of frequency ω, $m(\underline{r};\omega)$ describes the magnetization density. For periodic systems

$$\chi_q(\rho,\rho';\omega) = \sum_j e^{i\underline{q}.\underline{R}_j} \chi(\rho,\rho' + \underline{R}_j;\omega) \tag{4.1}$$

where the space coordinates $\underline{r}$ and $\underline{r}'$ are written in the local coordinates ρ,ρ'; with for example $\underline{r}' = \rho' + \underline{R}_j$, where ρ' is measured from the site at $\underline{R}_j$ nearest to $\underline{r}'$.

Within the LSD-RPA approach χ_q is described by the following integral equation

$$\chi_q(\rho,\rho';\omega) = \chi_q^P(\rho,\rho';\omega) + \int d\rho'' \, \chi_q^P(\rho,\rho'';\omega) \, K_{xc}^s(\rho'') \, \chi_q(\rho'',\rho';\omega) \tag{4.2}$$

where ρ,ρ' and ρ'' are the space coordinates in the unit cell, the wave vector q is restricted to the first Brillouin zone. χ_q^P is usually called the non-interacting

susceptibility and can be expressed in terms of the band structure one-particle Green's functions or wavefunctions. It is in particular with the numerical evaluation of χ_q^P that

will be concerned in these lectures. The interaction potentials, K_{xc}^s, are the derivatives of the exchange and correlation potentials with respect to the magnetisation density $\underline{m}$ at $|\underline{m}| = 0$, and may be evaluated using the self-consistent paramagnetic charge densities.

Once χ_q is known, all the relevant quantities may readily be evaluated. Most useful

of them is the diagonal part of the real-space double Fourier transform $\tilde{\chi}(q,q;\omega)$, whose imaginary part goes into the magnetic neutron scattering cross section, and reads:

$$\tilde{\chi}(q,q;\omega) = \int d\rho \int d\rho' \, \chi_q(\rho,\rho';\omega) \, e^{i\underline{q}.(\rho-\rho')} \tag{4.3}$$

The tendency of the system to undergo a magnetic phase transition would be indicated by a large value of $\tilde{\chi}(q,q;0)$ for an appropriate vector q.

The non-interacting static susceptibility χ_q^P can be written in terms of the retarded one-particle Green's function as:

$$\chi_q^P(\varrho,\varrho';0) = \frac{2}{\pi} \, \text{Im} \sum_j \int_{-\infty}^{\varepsilon_F} d\varepsilon \, G(\varrho,\varrho' + \underline{R}_j;\varepsilon) \, G(\varrho' + \underline{R}_j,\varrho;\varepsilon) \, e^{iq.\underline{R}_j} \quad (4.4)$$

The first principles evaluation of this quantity is a formidable task and only recently some progress has been made. The previous section was concerned with the reliable and accurate evaluation of integrals over only one Green's function. In contrast, here we are dealing with the product of two Green's functions which is roughly proportional to the energy derivative of one Green function. Therefore we have to be even more careful in picking up the weight of the integrand, which will vary even more rapidly in energy and - in $\underline{k}$-space. To convince ourselves that we have evaluated (4.4) correctly, we developed two alternative methods to calculate χ_q^P. In the first method we express the Green's function in terms of the multiple scattering quantities $\tau(\underline{k},\varepsilon)$ of section 3, while the second is based on the one-particle energy eigenvalues and the wavefunction coefficients. We shall now discuss both methods, their numerical implementation and application to Pd. The comparison of the results will be the measure of the reliability of the calculational schemes. First,

$$G(\varrho,\varrho' + \underline{R}_j;\varepsilon) = g_s(\varrho,\varrho';\varepsilon)\delta_{oj} + \sum_{LL'} Z_L(\varrho,\varepsilon) \{\tau_{LL'}^{oj}(\varepsilon) - t_L(\varepsilon)\delta_{LL'}\} Z_{L'}(\varrho';\varepsilon) \quad (4.5)$$

where g_s is the single site Green function, Z_L the single scatterer angular momentum eigenstates and $\tau_{LL'}^{oj}$, are the matrix elements of the scattering path operator. Substituting (4.5) into (4.4) χ_q^P can be written as follows:

$$\chi_q^P(\varrho,\varrho';0) = \frac{2}{\pi} \, \text{Im} \int_{-\infty}^{\varepsilon_F} d\varepsilon \, [I_q^{(1)}(\varrho,\varrho';\varepsilon) + I_q^{(2)}(\varrho,\varrho';\varepsilon) + I_q^{(3)}(\varrho,\varrho';\varepsilon)] \quad (4.6)$$

where

$$I_q^{(1)}(\varrho,\varrho';\varepsilon) = g_s(\varrho,\varrho';\varepsilon) \, g_s(\varrho,\varrho';\varepsilon)] \quad (4.7)$$

$$I_q^{(2)}(\varrho,\varrho';\varepsilon) = 2 \sum_{LL'} g_s(\varrho,\varrho';\varepsilon) \, Z_L(\varrho',\varepsilon) \, \tau_{LL'}^{oo}(\varepsilon) \, Z_{L'}(\varrho',\varepsilon) \quad (4.8)$$

$$I_q^{(3)}(\rho,\rho';\varepsilon) = \sum_{LL'L_1L_1'} Z_L(\rho;\varepsilon)Z_{L_1}(\rho;\varepsilon)Z_{L'}(\rho';\varepsilon)Z_{L_1'}(\rho';\varepsilon)S_{LL_1L'L_1'}(q,\varepsilon)$$

and

$$S_{LL_1L'L_1'}(q,\varepsilon) = \int \frac{d\underline{k}}{\Omega_{BZ}} \, \tau_{LL'}(\underline{k},\varepsilon)\,\tau_{L_1L_1'}(\underline{k}+q;\varepsilon) \tag{4.10}$$

With the techniques developed in the previous section $I_q^{(1)}$ and $I_q^{(2)}$ can be evaluated. We turn our attention now to the evaluation of $I_q^{(3)}$ or (4.9). $S_{LL_1L'L_1'}$ contains the product of two τ matrices with different arguments. This integrand exhibits extremely spiky features. Moreover, in general there is no simple relation between the contributions from the individual irreducible wedges of the Brillouin zone, necessitating a $\underline{k}$-integral over the <u>full</u> Brillouin zone. We will use the same integration techniques as in section 3: using discrete directions $\hat{k}_i$ emanating from the Γ point and restricted to a particular irreducible part of the Brillouin zone, named ir_1 in the following, through

$$\tau_{LL'}(O_\alpha \underline{k},\varepsilon) = \sum_{\bar{L}\bar{L}'} D_{L\bar{L}}(O_\alpha^{-1}) \tau_{\bar{L}\bar{L}'}(\underline{k};\varepsilon) D_{\bar{L}'L'}^\alpha(O_\alpha^{-1}) \tag{4.11}$$

Here, O_α is any symmetry operation of the point group of the crystal with D the corresponding rotation matrix in the real spherical harmonics representation. We obtain for S:

$$S_{LL_1L'L_1'}(q,\varepsilon) = \sum_\alpha \sum_{\bar{L},\bar{L}'} \sum_{\bar{L}_1,\bar{L}_1'} D_{L\bar{L}}(O_\alpha^{-1}) D_{\bar{L}'L'}(O_\alpha^{-1}) D_{L_1\bar{L}_1}(O_\alpha^{-1}) D_{\bar{L}_1'L_1'}(O_\alpha^{-1})$$

$$\frac{1}{\Omega_{BZ}} \int_{ir_1} d\underline{k}\, \tau_{\bar{L}\bar{L}'}(\underline{k},\varepsilon)\, \tau_{\bar{L}_1\bar{L}_1'}(\underline{k}+q_\alpha,\varepsilon) \tag{4.12}$$

with $q_\alpha = O_\alpha^{-1} q$ and Ω_{BZ} the volume of the BZ. Whereas the factor consisting of the four rotation matrices does not cause much trouble because it can be applied at the end, the sum over the symmetry operations α necessitates the integration for all different q_α. In the case of O_h symmetry and for q in the (1,0,0) direction this amounts to 6 q_α's.

The $\underline{k}$ regions where $\tau(\underline{k}\hat{k}_i;\varepsilon)$ is large and varies rapidly with $\underline{k}$ do not coincide with with those where this is the case for $\tau(\underline{k}\hat{k}_i + q_\alpha,\varepsilon)$. It is therefore necessary to evaluate $\tau(\underline{k}\hat{k}_i + q_\alpha,\varepsilon)$ independently from $\tau(\underline{k}\hat{k}_i,\varepsilon)$, thus avoiding any interpolation. For this purpose we extended the codes to calculate both the singular and the slowly varying parts of the structure constants for arbitrary finite q_α.

In analogy to the $q_\alpha=0$ case it proved possible to divide this problem into two parts. The first step consists in computing various $\hat{k_i}$- and q_α-dependent quantities only once for a given direction and to use them in a second step for a fast evaluation of τ^{-1} at any desired $\underline{k}$. Relation (4.11) is thereby being employed to obtain τ^{-1} in all the irreducible wedges passed by $k\hat{k_i} + q_\alpha$ as $k\hat{k_i}$ moves from the Γ point to the zone boundary. In addition use of the periodicity of τ^{-1} in reciprocal space has been made.

Moreover, we modified the strategy to determine τ for a sufficient number of adequately distributed $\underline{k}$ points in a given direction as follows: Starting with an equidistant mesh the behaviour of the principal matrix elements of τ^2 serves as the criterion for putting in more points locally. Sign changes of Im τ^2 and Re τ^2 as well as Im τ and Re τ are thereby used as "zoom in" criteria. We perform this step for both $\tau(k\hat{k_i},\epsilon)$ and $\tau(k\hat{k_i}+q_\alpha,\epsilon)$ separately and put the results on a common $|\underline{k}|$ grid to do the radial parts of the Brillouin zone integrals of (4.12).

The angular part of the Brillouin zone integral is performed by multiplying each line integral with the proper weight and summing over directions (see section 3). The final energy integral of $I_q^{(3)}$ would need a mesh of about 3000 non-equidistant energy points

to assure adequate convergence. However the analytic properties of the integrand open up the possibility of deforming the integration path into a contour, C, in the complex plane. Due to its smoother energy dependence in regions sufficiently far away from the real axis the number of energy points can be substantially reduced. Our procedures described above apply to all parts of C down to Im $\epsilon \approx 10^{-3}$ Ryd. Their expenditure diminishes automatically as the structures of the $\underline{k}$ dependent quantities get washed out with increasing distance from the real axis by reducing the amount of zoom in and the number of directions for the evaluation of the Brillouin zone integral.

Applying this to Pd, we use a $\hat{k_i}$ mesh of 36 or 10 space filling prism directions. Three straight pieces, one parallel to the real axis with Im $\epsilon=0.5$ Ryd (marked as piece II) and two parallel to the imaginary axis with Re $\epsilon=0.597$ Ryd (marked as piece I) and Re $\epsilon=0.01$ Ryd (marked as piece III), respectively defined the contour, C. Thirty seven (37) energy points along this contour proved sufficient: 17 along part I, 7 along part II and 13 along part III. At the boundaries of C we approached the real axis to Im $\epsilon=10^{-3}$ Ryd and the procedures turned out to work properly even for these small values.

Figure 5 shows our results for $\chi^P(q,q;0)$, the Fourier transform (4.3) of (4.6). In

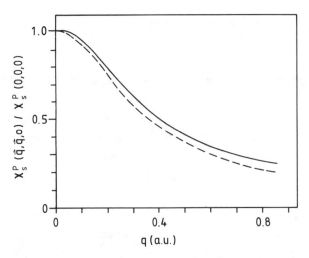

Fig. 5. The comparison of the static wave vector dependent non-interacting susceptibility of Pd for q in (100) direction calculated with the multiple scattering method (full line) and the band structure method (dashed line).

Table 2. Values for the wave vector-dependent static non-interacting susceptibility obtained from the contour integral on (4.6). In columns 3 to 5 the individual contributions defined by (4.7), (4.8) and (4.9) are listed. The value for $\chi^P(0,0;0)$ is 77.5×10^{-6} (EMU mol^{-1})

q (units of $2\pi/a$)	$\chi^P(q,q;0)/\chi^P(0,0;0)$	$\chi^{P(n)}(q,q;0)/\chi^P(0,0;0)$		
		1	2	3
0.0	1.000	-0.006	0.116	0.890
0.1	0.973	-0.006	0.119	0.860
0.2	0.849	-0.006	0.127	0.728
0.3	0.720	-0.005	0.141	0.584
0.4	0.570	-0.005	0.157	0.418
0.5	0.465	-0.005	0.175	0.295
0.6	0.401	-0.005	0.193	0.213
0.7	0.358	-0.004	0.210	0.152
0.8	0.319	-0.004	0.223	0.100
0.9	0.297	-0.003	0.232	0.068
1.0	0.262	-0.003	0.236	0.029

table 2 we list the Fourier transforms of the three individual contributions to $\chi^P(q,q;0)$ coming from $I_q^{(1)}$, $I_q^{(2)}$ and $I_q^{(3)}$ of equation (4.7), (4.8) and (4.9). $\chi^{P(1)}$ should be zero, because g_s is a real quantity on the real energy axis and the corresponding numbers are indeed rather small. The wave-vector dependence of $\chi^{P(2)}$ is weak since it is entirely due to phase factors. The $\chi^{P(3)}$ term dominates and gives rise to the shape of χ^P which peaks at $|q|=0$ and decreases monotonously towards the Brillouin zone boundary giving rise to a smooth and structureless function.

Finaly, the identity $\chi^P(0,0;0) = n(\varepsilon_F)$ is fulfilled to within a 3% accuracy. This discrepancy is mainly due to the fact that while evaluating $\chi^P(0,0;0)$ we have used 36 directions only for nine energies along part I of C and ten directions otherwise, whilst for $n(\varepsilon_F)$ 36 directions were used. In view of the complexity of the computations we consider this to be a reasonable agreement.

Secondly, we use the wavefunctions and energy eigenvalues to write

$$\chi^P(\underline{q},\underline{q};\omega) = \sum_{\lambda\lambda'} \int \frac{d\underline{k}}{\Omega_{BZ}} M_{\lambda\lambda';\underline{k}}(\underline{q}) M^*_{\lambda\lambda';\underline{k}}(\underline{q}) I_{\lambda\lambda';\underline{k}}(\underline{q},\omega) \qquad (4.13)$$

with the summation extending over all transitions from occupied states λ to unoccupied states λ',

$$I_{\lambda\lambda';\underline{k}}(\underline{q},\omega) = \frac{f(\varepsilon_{\underline{k}+\underline{q},\lambda}) - f(\varepsilon_{\underline{k},\lambda'})}{\varepsilon_{\underline{k}+\underline{q},\lambda} - \varepsilon_{\underline{k},\lambda'} - \omega + i\eta} \qquad (4.14)$$

and the site-dependent matrix elements $M_{\lambda\lambda';\underline{k}}$ determined by the Bloch states $\psi_{\underline{k}+\underline{q},\lambda}$ and $\psi_{\underline{k},\lambda'}$ through the relation

$$M_{\lambda\lambda';\underline{k}}(\underline{q}) = \int d\underline{\rho} \, e^{-i\underline{q}\underline{\rho}} \, \psi^*_{\underline{k}+\underline{q},\lambda}(\underline{\rho}) \, \psi_{\underline{k},\lambda'}(\underline{\rho}) \qquad (4.15)$$

The functions $I_{\lambda\lambda',\underline{k}}(\underline{q},\omega)$ vary rapidly over the Brillouin zone and we will now discuss our strategy for evaluating Im $\chi(\underline{q},\underline{q};\omega)$ for a given wave vector $\underline{q}$ and frequency ω.

We need to spot the poles of I in Eq.(4.14) fulfilling the Fermi criterion and we have to consider the rapid variations of their residues. Also the matix elements (4.15) vary significantly and they also have to be determined on a dense $\underline{k}$-mesh. To construct the $\underline{k}$-mesh we divide the irreducible wedge of the Brillouin zone into a space-filling assembly of tetrahedra, whereby the edges of each of them are defined by three rays emanating from the Γ point and cutting at the Brillouin zone boundary. In the case of Pd a total of 136 directions were used, each of them uniformly sub-divided into 100 k-points. In this way we both define the mesh ($M_{\underset{\sim}{k}}$) on which we require the band energies and the state vectors and decompose the tetrahedron entities (T_j) into small prisms (P_j^i). The $\underset{\sim}{k}$-dependent band structure quantities of Eqs.(4.14) and (4.15) were obtained from ab initio calculation, out of which the $\underset{\sim}{k}$+q dependent ones were obtained through linear interpolation. As $\underset{\sim}{k}$+q may fall outside the irreducible Brillouin zone wedge and the whole Brillouin zone zone contributes, we applied symmetry operations on the vectors $\underset{\sim}{k}$+q as well as on the state vector coefficients. We search each individual prism, P_j^i, for contributions to $\text{Im}(\chi_q^P)$. If necessary, a given P_j^i gets further divided into up to 1000 parts in order to adequately trace out the regions providing contributions in cases of a spars occurrence of poles and/or severe restrictions through the Fermi criterion. Due to a linear interpolation of the band energies the partial contributions within P_j^i are evaluated with the help of analytical formulas. For the matrix elements on the other hand it proved sufficient to - use the average over the corners of P_j^i.

We use the results for $\text{Im}\,\chi_q^P$ to evaluate $\text{Re}\,\chi_q^P$ via the Kramers-Kronig relation (Fig. 5). We consider the agreement between the static quantities of the two methods as satisfactory. Their shapes are the same and as a function of q they behave smoothly. For a qualitative comparison we consider the ratio $X^P(q,q;0)/\chi^P(0,0;0)$ and observe that for larger wave vectors the numbers resulting from the bandstructure method are somewhat below those of the multiple scattering method. The inclusion of more conduction bands in the bandstructure method would increase $\text{Im}\,\chi(q,q;\omega)$ in this q range and therefore increase $\chi(q,q;0)$.

Finally, knowing χ_q^P one can solve the integral equation (4.2) for χ_q. How this equation can be converted into a set of matrix equations and then solved by matrix inversion, the reader is referred to Winter, Szotek and Temmerman (1989), and the references therein.

5.   GROUNDSTATE OF La_2CuO_4 AND La_2NiO_4

We demonstrate the applicability of the preceeding sections on a study of the electronic, structural and magnetic properties of La_2CuO_4 and La_2NiO_4. These systems are antiferromagnetic insulators, and La_2CuO_4 becomes a high T_C superconductor upon Sr doping on the La sublattice. The T_C of $La_{1.85}Sr_{0.15}CuO_4$ is approximately 30 K. The study of the electronic properties of $La_{2-x}Sr_xCuO_4$ and a whole family of related systems (the high T_C materials) has been the subject of an unprecedented research effort for the past three years. The bandstructure methods too have been used in the

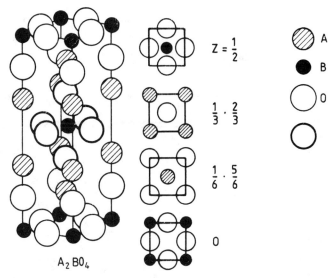

Fig. 6. The atomic arrangements of La_2CuO_4 and La_2NiO_4 in the body centred tetragonal structure.

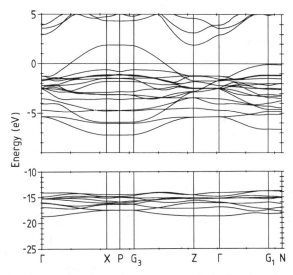

Fig. 7. The LMTO-ASA bandstructure for non-magnetic body centred tetragonal La_2CuO_4 along some symmetry directions; together with the 20 lowest valence bands, the La 5p and the O 2s semi-core states are also plotted.

understanding of the electronic structure of the high T_C materials. In the following I will give a brief sketch of some of our calculations.

In Figure 6 we show the structure of La_2CuO_4 and La_2NiO_4. It forms the body centred tetragonal structure, consisting of CuO_6 octahedra embedded in a La sublattice. These CuO6 octahedra are highly distorted, the ratio CuO_{apex}/CuO_{planar} bondlength is

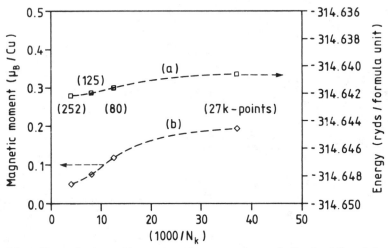

Fig. 8. The self-consistent antiferromagnetic moment on each Cu site (a), and the total energy (b), versus the number of k points inside the irreducible wedge of the Brillouin zone (1/8 of the Brillouin zone) for the body centred orthorombic structure. The lines are merely a guide to the eye.

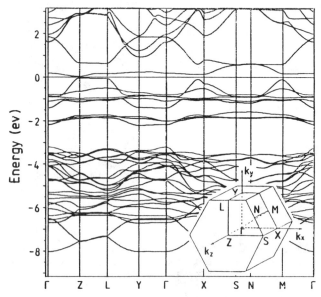

Fig. 9. The band structure of the antiferromagnetic and orthorhombic La_2NiO_4, with the Brillouin zone shown in the inset. Note that k_z and k_x axes are parallel to the NiO_2 planes.

1.28. Moreover these octahedra tilt easily, giving rise to orthorhombic distortions. The energy eigenvalue spectrum (band structure) is shown in Fig.7. We find the Cu d and Op bands highly hybridised and the La d bands essentially unoccupied. The bandstructure accurately describes the bonding properties of La_2CuO_4 such as the p-V curve, Akhtar et al (1988), the structural parameters (Cohen et al 1989), and even the tilting mode (Cohen et al 1989). The Fermi energy cuts a half filled Cu $d_{x^2-y^2}$ - O $p_{x,y}$ anti-bonding band and this half filled band situation is potentially unstable towards a groundstate of lower symmetry. In particular, we allowed the system to be antiferromagnetically ordered and then performed LSD calculations (Guo et al 1988, Temmerman et al 1988) to see if this groundstate is stable or reverts back to the non-magnetic groundstate of Fig.7. In Fig.8 we show the value of the spin magnetic moment of La_2CuO_4, $m=N_\uparrow- N_\downarrow$ where $N_{\uparrow(\downarrow)}$ is the number of spin up (down) electrons. We see that performing more accurate Brillouin zone integrals by decreasing $1000/N_k$ reduces the magnetic moment substantially, whilst keeping total E essentially constant. From these calculations we infer that the band picture predicts incorrectly a non-magnetic ground state, whilst giving an excellent description of the bonding properties. To shed more light on this bandstructure dilema we study La_2NiO_4 which has the same structure as La_2CuO_4. In Fig.9 we show the bandstructure for La_2NiO_4. We note that the Ni bands are well separated from the O bands, with the Ni bands straddling the Fermi energy. This system is stable with respect to an antiferromagnetic groundstate as can be seen from Fig.10. There we plot the magnetic moment with respect to the Ni-O$_{apex}$ to Ni-O$_{planar}$ bondlength ratio R. The experimental value would correspond to R=1.08. We see that on reducing this ratio the system can be driven from a metal to an insulator. Together with this, there is also a

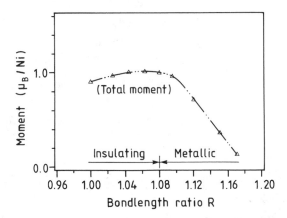

Fig. 10. Total spin moment as a function of the Ni-O$_{apex}$/Ni-O$_{planar}$ bond length ratio in the antiferromagnetic and orthorhombic La_2NiO_4.

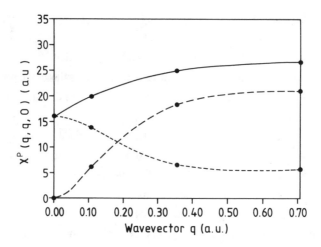

Fig. 11. The static non-interacting spin susceptibility $\chi^P(q,q,0)$ of La_2CuO_4 for q in (110) direction (solid line). Individually drawn are the contributions from the intraband transitions (band 17) ($\cdots\cdots$) and the interband transitions ($-----$).

strong dependence of the magnetic moment on R. The magnetic moment rises sharply to 1 μB in going from metal to insulator and then drops slightly. From this we see that the bandstructure correctly describes the antiferromagnetic insulating groundstate of La_2NiO_4, but not of La_2CuO_4. Therefore we want to investigate how far away we are in La_2CuO_4 from obtaining an antiferromagnetic groundstate. In Fig.11 we show the susceptibility results for La_2CuO_4 in the [110] direction (Winter et al 1989). The q value of (0.5,0.5,0) corresponds to the q vector of the observed antiferromagnetic groundstate. These calculations are based on a generalization of Eq.(4.13) to systems with many atoms per unit cell. In this figure we show the contribution to the susceptibility of the half-filled band which crosses E_f(band 17). We see that this contribution decreases from Γ to the Brillouin zone boundary: therefore we obtain no tendency to antiferromagnetism at all. Including all the other bands changes the shape of the curve: increasing from the Brillouin zone centre to the Brillouin zone boundary. Therefore the antiferromagnetic tendency in La_2CuO_4 comes from all the occupied bands and no single band can be identified as being of greatest importance. Finally the value of the susceptibility at the Brillouin zone boundary is a factor of 3 too small to give rise to an antiferromagnetic instability.

In conclusion, we need to improve our band description of La_2CuO_4 and in particular in our present calculations the Cu d states are too extended. A useful improvement to the LSD, the self interaction correction (SIC) (Jones and Gunnarsson 1989) would correct for this effect and would more localise the Cu d states.

6. CONCLUSIONS

I hope to have given you in these two lectures a flavour of the physical concepts and numerical techniques used in electronic structure calculations with application to the study of La_2CuO_4 and La_2NiO_4. The important concepts were Density Functional Theory out of which followed the foundation of an effective one-electron theory. Then, dividing up the solid in spheres gives rise to powerful techniques to solve the effective one-electron Schrödinger equation for the solid: out of its radial solutions one can construct basis functions (LMTO-ASA) or one applies multiple scattering theory. In the evaluation of the most time consuming bits the codes have been highly vectorised (fitted structure constants or matrix inversion), or the diagonalisation packages (EISPACK) have been made highly efficient by certain computer manufacturers such as FPS and Cray. The codes are highly parallel in character. In order to perform the Brillouin zone integral of the LMTO-ASA method the repeated and independent diagonalisation of Hermitean matrices is needed. Moreover the LMTO-ASA code spends more than 90% of its time doing it. Performing these diagonalisations in parallel on the iPSC/2 hypercube or multitasking on the Cray X-MP/4 leads to substantial time gains. On an empty Cray using 3 tasks we have obtained a speed up in through-put of nearly 3. On the iPSC/2 which allows for 64 nodes the through-puts also scale with the number of processors until a limit is reached where the communications are becoming more expensive than the CPU performed by the processors. With these substantial improvements in through-put we can tackle more complicated systems or improve our approximations. For example, the implementation of SIC which was mentioned at the end of the last section would involve a substantial increase of matrix diagonalisations due to the orbital dependence of the potential.

REFERENCES

Akhtar, M.J., Catlow, C.R.A., Clark, S.M. and Temmerman, W.M., 1988, The pressure dependence of the crystal structure of La_2CuO_4, J. Phys. C: Solid State Phys., 21:L917.

Andersen, O.K., 1975, Linear methods in band theory, Phys. Rev., B12:3060.

Andersen, O.K., 1984, Linear methods in band theory, in: "The Electronic Structure of Complex Systems", P. Phariseau and W.M. Temmerman eds., NATO ASI Series Physics, B113, Plenum Press.

Andersen, O.K., Jepson, O. and Glotzel, D., 1985, Canonical description of the band structure of metals, in: "Highlights of Condensed Matter Theory", F. Bassani, F. Fumi and M.P. Tosi eds., North-Holland.

Anderson, D.G., 1965, Iterative procedures for nonlinear integral equations, J. Assoc. Comput. Mach., 12:547.

Chelikowsky, J.R. and Louie, S.G., 1984, First principles linear combination of atomic orbitals method for the cohesive and structural properties of solids. Application to diamond, Phys. Rev., B29:3470.

Cohen, R.E., Pickett, W.E. and Krakauer, H., 1989, Phys. Rev. Lett., 62:831.

Guo, G.Y., Temmerman, W.M. and Stocks, G.M. 1988, On the metal-semiconductor transition and antiferromagnetism in La_2CuO_4, J. Phys. C: Solid State Phys., 21:L103.

Guo, G.Y. and Temmerman, W.M., 1988, Electronic structure and magnetism in La_2NiO_4, J. Phys. C: Solid State Physics., 21:L803.

Guo, G.Y. and Temmerman, W.M., 1989, Electronic and magnetic properties of La_2NiO_4: the importance of La-O planes, Phys. Rev., B40:285.

Hohenberg, P. and Kohn, W., 1964, Inhomogeneous electron gas, Phys. Rev., 136:B864.

Jepson, O. and Andersen, O.K., 1971, The electronic structure of HCP ytterbium, Solid State Commun., 9:1763.

Jepson, O. and Andersen, O.K., 1984, No error in the tetyrahedron integration scheme, Phys. Rev., B29:5965.

Jones, R.O. and Gunnarsson, 1989, The density functional formalism, its application and prospects, Rev. Mod. Phys., 61:689.

Kohn, W. and Sham, L.J., 1965, Self-consistent equations including exchange and correlation effects, Phys. Rev., 140:A1133.

Lehmann, G. and Taut, M., 1972, On the numerical calculation of the density of states and related properties, Phys. Rev., B54:469.

Pickett, W., 1989, Pseudopotential methods in condensed matter applications, Computer Physics Reports, 9:15

Skriver, H., 1984, "The LMTO Method", Springer-Verlag.

Srivastava, G.P., 1984, Broyden's method for self-consistent field convergence acceleration, J. Phys. A, 17:L317.

Stenzel, E. and Winter, H., 1985, A real-space method for the evaluation of the dynamic spin susceptibility of paramagnetic metals with application to paladium, J. Phys. F: Met. Phys., 15:1571.

Stenzel, E. and Winter,H., 1986, The wave vector dependent dynamic spin susceptibilities of Pd and V and their contributions to the low temperature specific heat, J. Phys. F: Met. Phys., 16:1789.

Stenzel, E., Winter, H., Szotek, Z. and Temmerman, W.M., 1988, On the theory of spin fluctuations in paramagnetic transition metals, Z. Phys. B, 70:173.

Stocks, G.M., Temmerman, W.M. and Gyorffy, B.L., 1979, in: "Electrons in Disordered Metals and at Metallic Surfaces", P. Phariseau, B.L. Gyorffy and L. Scheire eds., NATO ASI Series Physics, B42, Plenum Press.

Temmerman, W.M. and Szotek, Z., 1987, Calculating the electronic structure of random alloys with the KKR-CPA method, Computer Physics Reports, 5:174.

Temmerman, W.M., Szotek, Z. and Guo, G.Y., 1988, A local spin density study of antiferromagnetism in La_2CuO_4 and $YBa_2Cu_3O_6$, J. Phys. C: Solid State Phys., 21:L867.

Temmerman, W.M., Sterne, P.A., Guo, G.Y. and Szotek, Z., 1989, Electronic structure calcualtions of high T_C materials, Molecular Simulation, 4:153.

Winter, H., Stenzel E., Szotek, Z. and Temmerman, W.M., 1988, On the evaluation of spin susceptibilities within multiple scattering theory, J. Phys. F: Met. Phys., 18:485.

Winter, H., Szotek, Z. and Temmerman, W.M., 1989, A study on the dynamical spin susceptibility of paramagnetic La_2CuO_4, submitted to Z. Phys. B,

IMPLEMENTATION OF A NUMERICAL SEA MODEL

ON A CRAY X-MP SERIES COMPUTER

A M Davies

Proudman Oceanographic Laboratory
Bidston Observatory
Birkenhead
Merseyside L43 7RA
United Kingdom

R B Grzonka

Atlas Centre
Rutherford Appleton Laboratory
Chilton
Oxfordshire OX11 0QX
United Kingdom

Present Address

Sowerby Research Centre
British Aerospace PLC
PO Box 5
Filton
Bristol BS12 7QW
United Kingdom

INTRODUCTION

The modelling of three-dimensional sea regions, consists of the solution of a set of partial differential equations, subject to set of initial and boundary conditions, for fields which describe the hydrodynamics and other physical phenomena of interest, as functions of time. Numerical techniques consist of the usual transformations of a continuum description to a discrete description by: finite differences; finite elements; functional expansions; or some combination of these (e.g., Davies (1980)).

The physical space corresponding to a sea is divided into three regions: sea, land and boundary. The fields are defined to be zero for all time on land, leading to some measure of computational redundancy. Therefore, because of the variety of different sea geometries ('many' to 'few' land areas with different spatial distributions), a computationally efficient program would incorporate at least two different data structures.

Supercomputational Science
Edited by R.G. Evans and S. Wilson
Plenum Press, New York, 1990

We have implemented a mixed explicit/implicit forward time integration scheme for an idealised sea to evaluate parallel vector processing on a Cray X-MP series computer. The explicit component corresponds to a finite difference scheme over the horizontal extent of the sea and the implicit to a functional expansion over the vertical extent. This scheme was chosen for it's high level of data independence (relative to completely implicit schemes), allowing us to gain an insight into the computation-communication trade-offs that are inherent in parallel processing. Furthermore, the resulting 'prototype' program is designed to provide the basis for the implementation of other (possibly more data and control dependent) solution schemes with the development of more realistic descriptions of seas in mind.

PROGRAMMING FRAMEWORK

A set of conventions have been used for program control and data scope, that will enable any parallelism to be maintained as much as possible and hopefully increased, whenever the program is modified or extended. This is because, the control and storage dependencies are defined. These conventions are based on the OLYMPUS system (Roberts (1974)).

The conventions, along with a set of field data structures, define our initial programming framework for a global organisation of data via FORTRAN COMMON blocks. Combined with the use of the Cray FORTRAN 'microtasking' facility (Cray 1988) for the parallel execution of independent DO-loop iterations, the above corresponds to the sharing of data between parallel processes or tasks. In Cray terminology, parallel processing is referred to as 'multitasking'. Changes to shared data are only made inside 'critical sections', in which only one Cray X-MP central processing unit (CPU) executes.

Our current multitasking strategy, within the programming framework, is to adhere to the FORTRAN standard, which is allowed by the exclusive use of microtasking. Microtasking is implemented by FORTRAN comment based directives, which indicate sections of the program that have been manually structured and data scoped for parallel execution. The program with the microtasking directives is then processed by a pre-compiler utility before processing by the FORTRAN compiler. This method of implementing parallel processing within standard FORTRAN programs has been recently automated with the introduction of 'autotasking' (Cray (1989)).

The use of microtasking corresponds to a self-scheduling strategy for the tasks (Snelling (1986)). Different iterations of a DO-loop are assigned at execution time to different CPUs. A CPU, when it has completed an iteration, will select the next uncompleted iteration. Therefore, each CPU may process a different number of iterations. For a number of iterations equal to an integer multiple of the number of CPUs, with equal amounts of work, the workload is equally distributed amongst the CPUs and the program is said to be balanced.

We hope that these initial conventions and data structures will eventually evolve to form a set of parallel processing conventions for the development and maintenance of programs capable of effectively exploiting future generations of parallel vector processors. We are motivated by the successful exploitation of such computers in meteorological modelling (Dent (1986)).

DATA STRUCTURES

A data structure is defined to be an organisation of data elements determined both by their relationships and access functions. The concept of a data structure, unifies the computation and communication (transfer of data between the CPU, memory and disc) aspects of program design. FORTRAN data structures, for general scientific applications, which do not require access to all the resources of a computer (e.g., the problem being solved is small, so that the storage of the results of intermediate computations in disc files is unnecessary), tend to be relatively simple.

The basic data organisation in our program is, of course, the array, for the storage of discrete field values. For arrays which store field values over the entire finite difference grid, we refer to a finite difference grid (FDG) data organisation, which is appropriate for a sea region where the amount of sea relative to land is large. For arrays which only store field values participating in the computation of field finite differences, we refer to a packed participative point (PPP) data organisation, which is appropriate for a sea region where the amount of land relative to sea is large. The arrays are two-dimensional, for both FDG and PPP data organisations and are indexed by horizontal domain FDG and PPP indices, respectively in the first dimension. In the second dimension, indexing is by vertical domain functional expansion indices. This indexing is chosen for vector processing over the horizontal domain and parallel processing over the vertical domain.

The different access functions (e.g. sequential indexing with a mask, strip-mining and indirect addressing via index lists) that can be devised then define a set of data structures. The nature of the access function, in terms of it's access patterns to the Cray X-MP's memory, determines the computational efficiency of a particular algorithm and data structure, for a fixed data organisation. Note that, an algorithm with it's data dependencies can almost completely determine the data structure and the definition of computational efficiency can be extended to include the economies or charges of computation, communication and storage on a particular computer. That is, a program may be portable, but it's carefully designed computational efficiency may not be, because of differences in computer architectures and charging algorithms.

COMPUTER BENCHMARK

We consider the wind induced flow in a closed rectangular basin, of dimensions 400 km in the x-direction, 800 km in the y-direction and a depth of 65 m, with a suddenly imposed and maintained horizontal wind stress of -1.5 Pa in the y-direction. The dimensions of the basin approximate the geometry of the North Sea. The finite difference grid has 225 points in the x-direction and 418 points in the y-direction, some of which at the edges of the grid, represent the sea-model boundary. Since the basin is closed, flow field values for points on the sea-model boundary are zero for all time, as are flow field values on points on a closed sea-land boundary. The number of basis functions for the vertical representation of flow is 16. The time differencing is 30 s with 3200 forward time steps from the imposition of the wind stress.

This simple 'North Sea Basin' is used for the development of three-dimensional mathematical and numerical formulations and represents a 'benchmark' for their quality. Sufficient complexity is included in the physical description for an effective benchmarking of the data structures, for a particular algorithm.

Our objectives are to maximise the program's throughput (the reciprocal of the elapsed real time in a batch or dedicated environment) and to minimise the memory requirement. These performance metrics usually determine a large scale project's computer productivity and therefore, influence the scientific productivity. In a batch environment, where the Cray X-MP executes a number of programs in parallel, the availability of Cray X-MP CPUs is determined by the operating's systems scheduling strategy (usually for maximum overall system throughput). For a microtasking program in a batch environment, each CPU may be dedicated to the program for differing amounts of time, in line with this strategy, leading to variations between program executions at different real times. Therefore, our performance metrics are derived from program execution in a dedicated environment, i.e., where only one program executes, to ensure reproducibility. Performance data from a single program execution in a batch environment may be derived from a weighted mean of the metrics for each CPU, where the weights are the CPU times. This weighted mean may also be used for a program in a dedicated environment which is slightly unbalanced.

The throughput of a multitasking program in a dedicated environment can be estimated from Amdahl's Law for the multitasking speed-up over a single task,

$$S = [(1 - s)/n + s + c(n)]^{-1} \ ,$$

where s is the fraction of sequential (scalar and vector) program processing time spent in critical sections, n is the number of CPUs used and $c(n)$ is a cost function ($c(1) = 0$, $c(n) > 0$, $n > 1$), introduced by the use of multitasking. Note that, the cost function does not only depend on n, it also depends on the program's algorithm and the relative speeds of computation and communication on the computer. That is, on a Cray X-MP the cost function includes a measure of the effect of memory access conflicts (when a program is multitasking, there are a number of CPUs competing for access to the shared central banked memory (Oed and Lange (1986))), as well the multitasking overheads of task initiation and synchronisation, for a particular algorithm. The effect of memory access conflicts can usually only be measured, while the multitasking overheads can be both estimated and measured.

For our prototype program, assuming a cost function that is zero for all n, we estimate the maximum masked FDG speed-up to be $S = 3.39$, for $n = 4$ and $s = 0.06$ (from single CPU measurements). For $n = 8$ and 16, with the same fraction of critical section time, we have the maximum speed-ups of 5.63 and 8.42. This indicates that if computers, such as the Cray Y-MP series with eight CPUs, evolve to 64 CPU machines, the development of new numerical formulations, with much smaller critical sections in the corresponding algorithms, will be necessary. We hope to begin this development using the following measurements as a guide.

Measurement of program metrics on the Cray X-MP are by calls to the hardware performance monitor (Cray (1987)). Our measurements are only of the program kernel, which corresponds to 98 to 99% of the program's CPU time. That is, to remove the possibility of perturbation of the metrics, by program compilation, load, initialisation and I/O, we respectively start and stop measurement at the beginning and end of the kernel execution.

Program metrics for execution in a dedicated environment are given in Table 1. Estimates of the cost function, derived from estimates of the critical section times are given in Table 2. The program is well balanced, except for several seconds relative to the real time in a few four CPU cases.

DISCUSSION OF BENCHMARK RESULTS

The masked FDG data structure is a trade-off of unnecessary work being done at a high computational rate (and a low communication overhead because of the sequential addressing of memory banks) against more memory. That is, all field values are stored and computation occurs over land regions, but is always masked to give zero field values. The PPP data structure is a trade-off of only doing necessary work at a lower computational rate (and a high communication overhead because of the 'random' indirect addressing of memory banks) against less memory. That is, only field values which participate in the computation of field finite differences are stored and computation only occurs over sea regions and the sea-land and sea-model boundaries. Unsurprisingly, the metrics for the FDG data structure are independent of a particular distribution of land and sea. The dependence of the metrics for the PPP data structure on the geometry of the sea region demonstrates that the performance of a numerical sea model program is influenced by a choice of data structure.

Our hypothesis for the performance loss for four CPUs, as indicated by the estimates for the multitasking cost function, is that the number of memory banks on the Cray X-MP used (thirty-two) is insufficient to support CPU-memory system communication when highly vectorised tasks are simultaneously executing in four CPUs. This hypothesis is motivated by a 'bandwidth balance' argument. The CPU system to memory system bandwidth is equal to the number of CPU memory ports (sixteen) divided by the machine clock period. The memory system to CPU system bandwidth is equal to the number of banks (thiry-two) divided by the bank access time (four clock periods), neglecting the equal distribution of the banks into four sections to reduce the complexity of the CPU-memory interconnection network. Therefore we have:

(32 words)/(4 clock periods) < (16 words)/(1 clock period) .

For a sixty-four bank Cray X-MP, the bandwidths are balanced. Note that the Cray X-MP is a vector 'pipelined' CPU-memory machine and not just a pipelined CPU machine.

For this program, it is important to note that the main computational 'bottleneck' comes from the critical section time. Nevertheless, multitasking with four CPUs is still worthwhile, particularly if the entire central memory is required, as the program has over three times the throughput in a dedicated environment, relative to a single CPU program.

To test the above hypothesis, Cray Research (UK) Ltd. have kindly offered to benchmark our program on a Cray Y-MP series machine, which has a greater number of memory banks than a Cray X-MP series. A full account of our work (we have considered other data structures and program metrics) and a comparison with a Cray Y-MP will be produced elsewhere.

CONCLUSION

The performance of a program on a computer capable of parallel processing is determined by the fraction of execution time that is spent in sequential processing and the particular data structure that has been chosen to manage the storage and accessing of data within the memory system. Our program's sequential execution times of between 6 and 10% are much too high; we clearly have only begun to develop truly parallel numerical sea models.

There are a number of motivations for developing large scale programs which can exploit parallel processing. Two are 'financial' and 'scientific'. The financial motivation corresponds to the desire to utilise scare and expensive resources effectively. The scientific motivation corresponds to the desire to maximise the quality and the quantity of science that can be produced within the usual knowledge, resource and time constraints. These two motivations sometimes can be in conflict.

Another motivation which can be said to combine the other two motivations is 'competition'. A research group who has invested in program development, all other things being equal, may enjoy a considerable advantage over a competing group who has not.

ACKNOWLEDGEMENT

The program development and benchmarking were carried out on the Joint Research Council's Cray X-MP series computer, located at the Atlas Centre, Rutherford Appleton Laboratory. The authors would like to thank the Atlas Centre for the provision of facilities and the scheduling of dedicated computer time.

TABLES

Table 1. Program Performance Metrics

The characteristics of the input data sets can be summarised by:

Sea 1. #land/boundary points = 1286   #grid points = 94050
Sea 2. #land/boundary points = 43944 #grid points = 94050

Sea 1 has no land distribution. The land distribution for Sea 2 is a central 'diamond' shaped island with two smaller rectangular islands centred between the sea-model boundary and the central island on a basin diagonal. This peculiar sea is used to give varying distributions of vector lengths to simulate CPU-memory workloads of real seas. The benchmark used the Cray FORTRAN CFT77 3.0 compiler and the Cray operating system COS 1.17.

Table 1(a) Data Structure 1

Data Organisation: FDG Access: Sequential Indexing/Mask

	n	CPU time/s	Real time/s	MFLOPS	Speed-up
Sea 1	1	1001	1001	176	1.00
	2	1066	533	331	1.87
	4	1268	318	555	3.15
Sea 2	1	1001	1001	176	1.00
	2	1066	533	331	1.87
	4	1263	326	558	3.07

Table 1(b) Data Structure 2

Data Organisation: PPP Access: Indirect Addressing

	n	CPU time/s	Real time/s	MFLOPS	Speed-up
Sea 1	1	1494	1494	98	1.00
	2	1664	832	176	1.80
	4	2105	524	278	2.83
Sea 2	1	807	807	98	1.00
	2	904	452	175	1.79
	4	1147	288	277	2.82

Table 2. Multitasking Overheads

The percentage multitasking cost function is estimated from Amdahl's law, using the data in Table 1 and a measurement of the percentage critical section time.

		Data Structure	
		1	2
		$s = 6\%$	$s = 10\%$
n	2	0.2%	0.6%
	4	2.3%	2.8%

REFERENCES

Cray, 1989, Cray Channels, Spring 1989, 2-3.

Cray, 1988, Multitasking Programmer's Reference Manual, SN-0222.

Cray, 1987, Programmer's Library Reference Manual, SR-0113.

Davies A M, 1980, Computer Methods in Applied Mechanics and Engineering 22, 187-211.

Dent D, 1986, in Hoffman G R and Snelling D F, 1988, Editors, Multiprocessing in Meteorological Models, 369-381, Springer-Verlag, Berlin.

Oed W and Lange O, 1986, Parallel Computing 3, 343-358.

Roberts K V, 1974, Computer Physics Communications 7, 237-243.

Snelling D F, 1986, in Hoffman G R and Snelling D F, 1988, Editors, Multiprocessing in Meteorological Models, 237-253, Springer-Verlag, Berlin.

FLOOD PREDICTION : A STUDY IN FORTRAN OPTIMISATION AND CONNECTIVITY

B. J. Ralston and F. Thomas

IBM UK Ltd., 378 Chiswick High Road, London W4 4AD

H. K. F. Yeung

Rutherford Appleton Laboratory, Chilton, Oxfordshire OX11 0QX

INTRODUCTION

The application of some simple techniques has allowed a FORTRAN program for river simulation to run about twenty times faster. Since some of these techniques may be useful in other programs, the main steps taken are outlined below.

The application needs a lot of CPU time and its progress usefully monitored graphically. This led to an exercise in connecting a supercomputer (an IBM 3090 Vector Facility) to a Unix workstation (an IBM 6150). This is also described.

RIVER SIMULATION

River simulations predict the behaviour of river networks under various flow conditions. The total river system may contain junctions, weirs, sluice–gates and reservoirs with water running in steady or unsteady state, confined or spilling out of the system. The results of the simulation may be used in the design of drainage, irrigation or flood alleviation schemes as well as water resource planning studies and catchment development planning.

The flow of water in an open channel in comparison to other fluid flow simulations is sometimes seen as a trivial problem. When considering the effect on the environment of a badly designed flood protection system or the wastage in a costly river diversion or draining system involving several million pounds then doing a good simulation justifies itself. River simulations are carried out widely in the UK by the National River Authority.

A large river system can involve thousands of nodes and take several hours to run on a mainframe computer. It is a recent example of the application of vector processing to another new area.

Supercomputational Science
Edited by R.G. Evans and S. Wilson
Plenum Press, New York, 1990

From the users point of view, displaying the changes of the key variables (water level, velocity, water flow) at a dedicated workstation as the simulation proceeds timestep by timestep on the batch mainframe improves both the user's productivity and his understanding of the river system.

THE ONDA PACKAGE

Onda is a modern river simulation Fortran program used by several UK National River Authority regions. It is written and supported by the water division of the engineering consultancy, Sir William Halcrow and Partners, Swindon.

The open channel system consists of units delineated by nodes. The program reads characteristic data for every unit as well as the initial conditions for every node. The program then operates in a time–stepping mode during the computational phase. Its steering systems route the computation through a set of subroutines appropriate to the physical units given in the data set. Each subroutine produces linearised equations describing the behaviour of a particular unit and the resultant set of equations is solved by a sparse matrix routine. Iteration is used to deal with non–linearities (about 6 iterations per timestep). The units currently available are as follows:

a) river reach

b) junction (3 to 10 way)

c) reservoir

d) weir

e) sluice

f) localised hydraulic loss

g) lateral in– and out–flow

h) flow–stage control unit

i) stage–flow, stage–time, flow–time and tidal boundary conditions

j) over bank spills.

OPTIMISATION PROJECT RESULTS

Onda and a medium–sized test case of 256 nodes was supplied for investigation into its potential for vectorisation. Work was carried out on the IBM 3090 at the Rutherford Atlas Centre. Within one man–month the program was shown to be vectorisable. It was first necessary, however, to perform considerable scalar optimisation. The program now performs around 19 times faster than in its original form on an IBM 3090.

The timings achieved for this test case are currently.

	CPU time	Ratio
IBM 3090–180E (original)	25 mins	1
IBM 3090–180E (best scalar)	150 secs	10
IBM 3090–180E (best vector)	80 secs	19

For comparison, the program took 42 minutes on a Hitech–10 Whitechapel workstation, 87 minutes on an IBM 6150 Model 125 and over 600 minutes on a Sun 3/60 workstation.

OPTIMISATION CARRIED OUT

The changes made to achieve these times are listed below.

i)   Increase the level of automatic optimisation of the VS Fortran compiler from 0 to 3.

This was trivial to implement but can have dramatic effects for sites (unlike Rutherford) that do not use OPT(2) or (3) as default.
(Gain 950 seconds)

ii)   Replace nested IF tests by a table look–up.

A hotspot analysis revealed that a large part of the CPU time was spent in a set of nested do loops involving complicated IF–THEN–ELSE constructs. These could readily be replaced with a table–look up algorithm.
(Gain 195 seconds)

iii)   Remove time–independent calculations from timestep loop.

To save space, several variables which were dependent only upon the geometry of the network were recalculated at every timestep. Many applications written in the days of small memory systems can be adapted to use more memory in order to improve execution speed.
(Gain 150 seconds)

iv)   Improve algorithm, remove function call overhead.

A function was called with eight arguments to return a logical true value if two lines crossed. This was replaced by a simpler, in–line test on whether two differences had the same sign.
(Gain 32 seconds)

v)   Replace divides by multiplies and avoid calls to generalised exponentiation.

Divides are usually slower than multiply (perhaps by an order of magnitude) and $X^{**}1.5$ was found much slower than $X^*SQRT(X)$. At the same time some results, slow to calculate, were saved for later re–use and a call to a specialised exponentiation routine was replaced by inline code.
(Gain 21 seconds)

vi)   Re–use previous interpolation results.

Linear interpolation was performed for several functions over the same x range. By saving the x interpolation results, rescanning of the x range was avoided.
(Gain 14 seconds)

vii)　　　Replace solver by vectorised version.

The program uses the Harwell Library routine MA28. A vectorised version, MA48, is being developed by Ian Duff of Harwell which takes advantage of matrix factorisation to reduce the calculation to several calls to the ESSL dense matrix solver routines.
(Gain 40 seconds)

viii)　　　Restructure the code for vectorisation.

This involved reorganising the way nodes were referenced internally so that all units of a particular type were stored together. Node types occurring frequently were then processed together within one DO loop instead of one node per subroutine call.
(Gain 21 seconds)

CONNECTIVITY

The IBM 6150 Unix workstation was already connected over the site Ethernet onto the IBM 3090 via the mainframe's 8232 adaptor. This was the way the workstation shared resources with the IBM 3090. By taking advantage of the TCP/IP software running under VM/XA on the mainframe, communication with the IBM 6150 was set up. Direct access to the mainframe could also be achieved using the 3278 emulation utility on the workstation.

Using NFS (Network File System) working under TCP/IP, a CMS minidisk was MOUNTed as an auxiliary device to the IBM 6150. The graphics program running on the IBM 6150 could then pick up and display data as it was being produced on the IBM 3090. It should also be possible to use X–Windows to run a graphics program on the IBM 3090 displaying data on the IBM 6150. Programs running on the two machines could also communicate with each other using the Remote Procedure Calls (RPC) facility.

The connectivity study was carried out by one of the authors, (HKFY). Because the program can also be parallelised, he is investigating adapting the program to run on a Transputer network connected to an IBM 6150.

CONCLUSIONS

Some general points can be drawn.

i)　　　Need for hotspot analysis.

Program optimisation cannot be achieved effectively without doing detailed execution time analysis. The VS Fortran Version 2 Interactive Debug provides detailed program timings.

ii)　　　Vectorisation can only be effective on efficient scalar code.

The vectorisable content of this program was initially 7% and appeared inappropriate for running on a vector processor. After optimising the scalar component, the vector component became 70%. This is worth the effort of vectorising.

iii)   Mainframes are good for program development.

One outcome of this project was a more efficient simulator for the workstation. Each test compile and run of the program on the workstation takes about 50 times longer than on the mainframe. The mainframe program development tools are very helpful.

iv)   Workstations and mainframes work well together.

Using the number–crunching advantages of the mainframe in co–operation with the interactive capabilities of the Unix workstation introduces some very useful possibilities.

SUPERCOMPUTING –

A FORWARD LOOK

B.W. Davies

Rutherford Appleton Laboratory
Chilton, OX11 0QX, U.K

INTRODUCTION

In this talk I will take the term "supercomputing" to cover high–performance numerically–intensive computing used mainly for scientific/engineering applications. Also, I will take it to include the use of computers which can enable an individual in the course of one day to perform about as much computation as he could by accessing a shared state–of–the–art supercomputer.

The second of the above comments might seem somewhat imprecise since what a user gets from a shared supercomputer depends among other things on how many people are sharing it. But the general point is that some users might be able to do as much useful work per day on an advanced workstation dedicated to one user as on a minisupercomputer of ten times the power shared between ten users or on a supercomputer of one hundred times the power shared by a hundred users. So we should look at all these options in our review.

USING TODAY'S SUPERCOMPUTERS

Let us begin by looking at what actually happens on large supercomputers as currently used by the academic community in the UK. Specifically, at the Atlas Centre we have two powerful machines, a Cray X–MP/48 and an IBM 3090–600E/6VF. The peak performance of the Cray is quoted as 940 MFLOPS and the IBM as 696 MFLOPS. The Cray has four processors and the IBM six. It is interesting to compare the peak performance figures with what users actually achieve.

The first observation is that users tend not to embark on multiprocessing unless they can see clear benefits in doing so. This is a reasonable attitude; multiprocessor use requires the users to do work on their codes and the cost of this work and the likely machine–dependence of the resulting code have to be offset against the perceived benefits which may be marginal or even negative for jobs which are well within the supercomputer's capabilities. The benefits start to accrue when real–time considerations come into play or when dealing with large–memory jobs which on the Cray could result in a single user blocking all four processors while using only one. These factors are now coming into play and some of the Cray users are achieving excellent performance (>500MFLOPS) by harnessing all four processors.

Supercomputational Science
Edited by R.G. Evans and S. Wilson
Plenum Press, New York, 1990

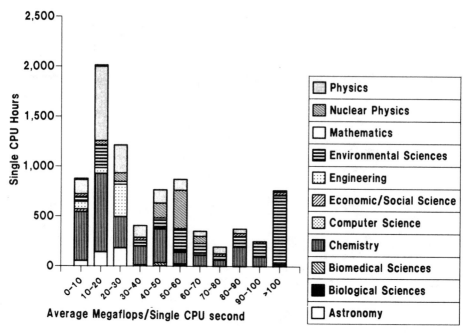

Fig.1. Performance actually achieved on a single processor of the Atlas Centre Cray X–MP/48 in different areas of computational science.

The second observation is that real sustained performance is well below the peak figures quoted by the suppliers. This is entirely to be expected since peak performance can be attained only in highly artificial circumstances in which all the relevant functional units are operating simultaneously flat out. Real problems seldom provide such circumstances.

Fig 1. shows the MFLOP performance actually achieved on a single processor of the Atlas Centre Cray X–MP/48. The range extends beyond the 100 MFLOPS level but the average is around 50 MFLOPS against a peak of 235 MFLOPS. Incidentally these figures are good by world standards; 50 MFlops corresponds to about 70% of the executed code being vectorised and 100 MFLOPS to about 90% vectorised. It is relevant to note that the groups getting 100 MFLOPS have put a lot of effort into optimising their software. Moving nearer the peak 235 MFLOPS would require ever increasing work on optimisation and there is bound to be some limit beyond which further vectorisation is impossible.

We can conclude from these observations that today's supercomputers can indeed deliver high performance (vector and parallel) on real codes, but that in general the user has to do a significant amount of work to attain it because of the complexity of the supercomputer hardware. We are some considerable way from the desirable state of having transparent access to the underlying high performance potential of these machines. If supercomputers have to become more complex in future to provide ever increasing power then it may become ever more difficult to extract their potential performance unless there are major improvements to the software aids available to the user.

It may be useful at this point to examine in a little more detail the two main techniques by which modern supercomputers attain their high peak performance.

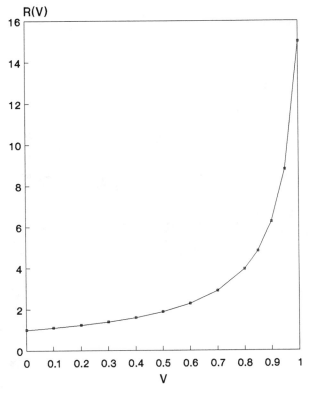

Fig. 2. Plot of the function R(V) for r=15.

VECTORISATION AND PARALLELISM

The MFLOP ratings obtained at the Atlas Centre are an illustration of Gene Amdahl's well known "law" that determines the speed up that is attainable for work of a given vector content. If V is the fraction of code amenable to vector processing and the vector unit is r times faster than the scalar unit then the overall speed up R(V) is

$$R(V) = 1/((1-V) + V/r).$$

It is instructive to plot this equation for a variety of parameters. Fig 2 shows a particular example for r=15, a plausible starting point for the designer of a vector processing machine. It shows that one has to have code of which more than about 80% is vectorisable before one sees substantial improvement over the basic scalar performance of the machine.

Surveys of "real workloads" by computer suppliers and others show that a lot of work falls in the 30–60% vectorisable band. This leads most supercomputer suppliers to conclude that although it is important to strive for the highest possible vector performance, it is at least as important to ensure that the scalar performance is also as high as possible, otherwise their products will be attractive only to that group of customers whose workloads consistently run with very high vector content.

The exploitation of parallelism follows the same algebraic law as vectorisation. If P is the fraction of a workload that is amenable to parallel processing and there are N processors available for use then the speed–up ratio R(P) is

$$R(P) = 1/((1-P) + P/N).$$

Again the conclusion is that a computing workload with high degree of parallelism is needed before substantial gains over serial processing are obtained.

An interesting consequence for designers of general purpose supercomputers is illustrated in Fig. 3. This shows a comparison of performance across the parallelism spectrum for two types of design; one in which there are 16 processors each of 1 unit of power and the other in which there are 4 processors each of 4 units of power. In each case the maximum performance is 16 units, attainable with a workload that is 100% parallel. For any workload with less than 100% parallel content the performance is greater with a small number of powerful processors than with a larger

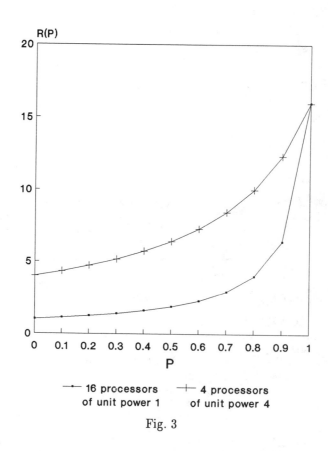

Fig. 3

number of less powerful ones. Note that this conclusion does not take into account the relative costs of the two types of design; it is possible that a large number of less powerful machines will be cheaper, and we will return to this when we consider massively parallel machines later.

From the above we conclude that if the objective is to build a powerful general purpose supercomputer one should aim to provide the power through the smallest possible number of processors and to ensure that the scalar performance of each processor is as high as possible. Vector performance should also be as high as possible but it may not generally be cost effective to aim for extreme vector performance at the expense of scalar performance.

NEXT GENERATION SUPERCOMPUTERS

The established contenders in the supercomputer market at present are Cray (which recently split into two companies), Hitachi, Fujitsu and NEC. IBM is fast re—establishing itself in the high performance marketplace and has sold a large number of its vector facility add—ons to 3090 mainframes. There is also a relatively new company, SSI, started by former Cray designer Steve Chen, which receives IBM funding. A substantial and influential supercomputer company, ETA, pulled out of the business in mid—1989.

All these suppliers, except ETA, have well advanced plans for future products. The general aim is to move into the tens of GFlops peak performance area in the early 1990s. Most are taking further gradual steps into multiprocessing architectures though it is noticeable that the Japanese suppliers in particular are also placing a lot of emphasis on raising substantially the performance level of individual processors.

Available memory sizes are likely to move through hundreds of Mwords to around a Gword by about 1993. In order to feed such powerful engines it is clear that substantial advances in peripheral devices will be needed, in particular for faster I/O bandwidth. While it is likely that the other obvious need, higher storage capacity, might be met via 'routine' advances in storage media within the data processing industry at large, the development of the very high speed peripheral facilities may to some extent be a supercomputer—specific activity.

A significant trend is the expressed intention of all suppliers to adopt the Unix[1] operating system either as their only offering for supercomputing or as a major option.

Table 1 is a convenient summary, taken from the July 15, 1989 issue of Datamation, of the likely offerings of the supercomputer suppliers in the next two or three years.

[This table is reproduce with the permission of Datamation © Reed Publishing, USA, 1989]

Table 1

	Cray Y-MP	Cray C-90	Cray Cray-3	SS1 SS-1	NEC SX-X	IBM 3090/600S VF	Hitachi 5-820/80	Fujitsu VP-2600/20
Base Technology	Silicon	Silicon	Gallium Arsenide?	Gallium Arsenide?	Silicon	Silicon	Silicon	Silicon
Clock Cycle	6 nsec	4 nsec?	2 nsec?	1 nsec?	2.9 nsec	8 nsec	4 nsec	4 nsec
Memory Capacity	128 megawords	256 MW?	1,024 MW?	2,048 MW?	256 MW	32 MW	64 MW	256 MW
Architecture	Vector	Vector	Vector	Vector	Pipeline	Vector	Vector	Vector
Processors	1-8	?-16	?-16	16-64	1-4	1-6	1	1
Peak Performance	2.7 GFLOPS	16 GFLOPS?	16 GFLOPS?	?	22 GFLOPS?	8 GFLOPS	3 GFLOPS	4 GFLOPS
Operating System	UNICOS, COS, CTSS	UNICOS, COS, CTSS	UNICOS, COS	UNIX	UNIX	MVS, AIX, VM/CMS	Proprietary OS, HIUX	Proprietary OS, UTS/M
Number of Applications	750	750	500	?	50	1,250	?	?
Availability	1988	1990	1990-1991	1991-1992?	1990	1988	1988	1990-1991
Price	$5-25 million	$5-30 million?	$25 million?	$30-75 million?	$4-25 million	$2-20 million	?	?

Source: Datamation 15 July 1989
Dataquest Superperformance Computing Service, Argonne National Laboratory

MASSIVELY PARALLEL MACHINES

The attraction of massively parallel architecture computers is the ability to exploit the rapid advances in chip technology which enable one to put together large ensembles (hundreds or thousands) of interconnected processors, each with local memory. The nominal aggregate power and memory can exceed that of the most powerful supercomputers; in a sense they are unlimited since one can always add further processors into the ensemble. The basic hardware price of such ensembles can be considerably less that that of conventional supercomputers of the same nominal power.

That being the case, the obvious question is why such machines have not put conventional supercomputers out of business. The answer, at least so far, is that while the advances of hardware technology make it easy to develop and implement new computer architectures, the advances in software that are needed to enable the average user to exploit such architectures are proceeding much more slowly. A new hardware generation might occur every year or two; new software generations occur more nearly every decade or two.

In other words many of the issues confronting the users of conventional supercomputers in adapting to multiprocessing appear writ large with massively parallel machines. Around the world a lot of skilled effort is being applied to the task of making massively parallel machines easy to use and to hide the intricacies of the hardware from the sort of scientist who wants to use the machine as a tool without having to get involved in computer science. Progress is being made in this direction and there are also some spectacular measurements of performance beginning to emerge for work in several scientific disciplines.

Much of the current debate about parallel architectures is about whether they can cover the needs of general purpose numerically intensive computing workloads or whether their role will be mainly confined to specific niches of the marketplace in which their architecture matches particular types of problem. On the one hand one can argue that since most scientific phenomena are intrinsically parallel (eg the advance of a wavefront) then parallel computers ought to be widely applicable. The counter argument is that although this is true in general there are often dependencies between different spatial or temporal domains of real parallel problems with the consequence that the processors assigned to different aspects of the problem need to intercommunicate and transfer data from one to another. This can generate overheads, depending on the design of the machine, and the argument is about the extent to which these overheads can be minimised.

The case that overheads can dominate the overall performance has been set out recently by Amdahl (1988). He considers a hypercube architecture in which every processor runs until it finishes its currently assigned task, at which point it switches to a new task for which code and data may have to be transferred across communication lines.

For a machine with N processors, and for a particular optimistic assumption about the distribution of code and data (see the definition of p below), he derives the speed up R(N) over the performance on a single processor to be:

$$R(N) = N/(1 + cpN \; lnN/w(1+p)ln2)$$

where

$c =$ task switch and interlock time across one edge of the hypercube

$p =$ probability that the next task is on a neighbouring node, p^2 two nodes away, p^3 three nodes away...

$N =$ number of processors over which the workload is distributed

$w =$ the workload computation time

This expression has a maximum at

$$N_{max} = w(1+p) \; ln2/cp,$$

at N_{max} the speed up is

$$R_{max} = N_{max}/(1+lnN_{max}),$$

and in general

$$R(N) = N/(1+(N/N_{max}) \; lnN).$$

The quantity N_{max} is characteristic of the machine architecture and of the workload. It represents the maximum granularity into which it is worthwhile splitting the workload; it is a measure of the "problem size".

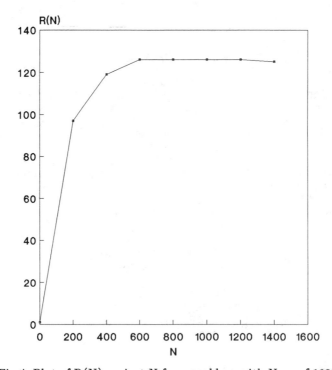

Fig 4. Plot of $R(N)$ against N for a problem with N_{max} of 1000.

In the expression for R(N) the term $(N/N_{max})lnN$ is a measure of the communication overhead and it is possible for this to exceed the original workload which is represented by 1.

Fig 4 shows a plot of R(N) against N for a problem with N_{max} of 1000. It can be seen that the maximum predicted performance is only about 125 times that of a single processor. Also, the shape of the curve is such that although the peak performance occurs with 1000 processors there is little practical benefit in running with more than about 250 processors.

From the expression for R(N), it is clear that the only way to make R(N) approach the ideal N is to make c tend to zero (ie aim for zero task switching time) or to make p tend to zero (when code and data required for the next task is always in a processor's local memory). The contention of the supporters of this argument is that these conditions cannot generally be met.

These arguments put forward a pessimistic future for the widespread use of massively parallel machines outside special niches. More optimistic notes are struck by performance measurements at the Sandia Laboratories last year in which a 1000 fold speed up was reported for certain jobs running on a 1024 processor machine. Furthermore, returning to the discussion in the second section, as some problems scale upwards in size the serial content becomes a smaller fraction of the total and so the option to use parallel architectures looks increasingly attractive.

I believe it will be some years before these the outcome of these arguments is clear. during that time the suppliers of conventional machines will gradually increase their numbers of processors and there may be a convergence of ideas and techniques around a few hundred processors.

MINISUPERCOMPUTERS

Minisupercomputers typically offer a tenth of the power of a supercomputer for about the price of a minicomputer, and often incorporate vector and multiprocessor architectures similar to those of supercomputers. Because they are not aiming at the extreme performance of supercomputers the designers of minisupercomputers can exploit technology which is less costly and less demanding in terms of the support environment. For example, the Convex C–1 used 8000 gate per chip technology by which the processor and 128 Mwords of memory could be packaged into a single 19 inch rack and the total power dissipation was a few kilowatts. By contrast the Cray X–MP machines use 16 gate–per–chip technology and the power dissipation is over 100 kilowatts, requiring complex and expensive cooling plant.

Minisupercomputers are very effective machines for groups of scientists within a department or a laboratory; as well as providing computing power they provide it under local control, the machines can be relatively easily connected to high speed local area networks and to graphics facilities.

From the technical viewpoint there is no reason why minisupercomputer vendors should not continue to exploit the advances in technology to develop more powerful and more cost effective machines. The difficulties they face are much more concerned with sustaining a clearly defined marketplace into which to sell. The minisupercomputer performance level is being squeezed from above and below. From above the supercomputer suppliers are realising that there could be a market for slower and cheaper entry–level versions of their existing machines, while from below the suppliers of advanced workstations are pushing up towards the performance offered by minisupercomputers. In the past few months a number of minisupercomputer suppliers have gone out of business or have otherwise gone in for radical restructuring, and it is not clear that the shake–out is yet complete. It may be that the likely outcome will be a small number of companies with firm financial backing.

SUPERCOMPUTING WORKSTATIONS

Extremely powerful graphics workstations started to appear on the market in 1988, the major impact being made by two companies Ardent and Stellar which have recently announced that they will merge with one another. Their products combined very high performance graphics with the computational power of a minisupercomputer. The list price was over $100K and they were single user machines (one screen and one keyboard). While it was not clear how big the market would be for single user machines at that price level, the undoubted attractiveness of the facilities that were on offer and the expected improvement in price/performance have opened up a new market into which some of the more established graphics and workstation suppliers are beginning to move.

Table 2 shows the main characteristics of four systems available in mid 1989. No doubt there will be rapid developments in this area.

Table 2

	Apollo 1000VS	Ardent Titan	Silicon Graphics Power Server	Stellar GS1000
Number of Processors	Up to 4	Up to 4	Up to 4	1(4 str.)
Main memory (MB)	8-128	8-128	8-128	16-128
Cache memory (instr/data-KB)	128/64	16/16	64/64	1 MB
Internal bus (MB-sec/width)	150/64	256/64	64/32	380/N.A.
Operating System	Aegis	-	IRIX	Stellix
MIPS	15-30	10-35	10-20	14-25
Dhrystones	31,000	19,000	43,000	n/a
Linpack 100x100DP (Single Proc)	5.8	6.0	3.0	7.0

[Reproduced, with permission, from the Spang Robinson Report, March 1989; © J. Wiley, New York, 1989]

A somewhat related development is opened up by the availability of very powerful processor chips which can be added to inexpensive personal computers. Examples are the latest Intel chip or the recently announced next generation transputer both of which can offer tens of MFLOPS peak performance. The very attractive prices of such devices will drive forward the investigation of new ways of harnessing their potential. In some ways a PC with tens of MFLOPS may be seem a highly desirable facility. On the other hand the I/O capabilities of the typical PC may be in a different league and so the production of balanced configurations capable of sustaining the processor performance may not be easy to attain.

THE SUPERCOMPUTING ENVIRONMENT

In the context of this discussion supercomputing is a means to an end, the end being productive science. Supercomputers, or any other high performance computing engines used for simulation and modelling in science, can produce vast quantities of output, the essence of which is often pictorial rather than numerical. So the availability of high quality facilities for visualisation is becoming a critical factor in the exploitation of these machines. Furthermore pictorial information usually has a high data content and therefore the means of shipping large quantities of data from the compute engine to the visualisation device is vital.

The graphics workstation takes these problems in—board; such a device is designed with graphics and fast internal data transfer in mind. But a graphics workstation has only a limited amount of power and cannot be expected to cope with problems greater than a certain size. A major challenge is how we can provide something approaching this level of graphics and data transmission when one is working with a departmental minisupercomputer through a local area network or, even more challenging, with a national supercomputer across a long distance network.

As we noted earlier most supercomputer suppliers are adopting Unix as their mainstream operating system. Also Unix is the operating system predominantly used on advanced workstations and on many minisupercomputers. High speed Unix to Unix communication across local and national networks is therefore emerging as a key requirement. The technical means of providing this is fairly clear. The challenge is to the funding bodies to be able to respond with the funding and other necessary pre—requisites that can turn the ideas into reality in the near future.

[1] Unix *is a registered trademark of AT&T*

REFERENCE

Amdahl, G.M., 1988, The International Journal of Supercomputer Applications, Vol. 2, No. 1, pp 88–97.

Contributors

D.J. Baker, Rutherford Appleton Laboratory, Chilton, Oxfordshire OX11 0QX.

J.O. Baum, Rutherford Appleton Laboratory, Chilton, Oxfordshire OX11 0QX.

A.R. Bell, Plasma Physics Group, Imperial College of Science, Technology and Medicine, London SW7 2BZ.

K. Berrington, Department of Applied Mathematics and Theoretical Physics, The Queen's University of Belfast, Belfast BT7 1NN.

L. Cruzeiro–Hansson, Birkbeck College, Malet Street, London WC1E 7HX.

A.M. Davies, Proudman Oceanographic Laboratory, Bidston Obervatory, Birkenhead, Merseyside L43 7RA

B.W. Davies, Rutherford Appleton Laboratory, Chilton, Oxfordshire OX11 0QX.

J.J. Du Croz, The Numerical Algorithms Group Ltd., Wilkinson House, Jordan Hill Road, Oxford OX2 8DR.

R.G. Evans, Rutherford Appleton Laboratory, Chilton, Oxfordshire OX11 0QX.

T.P. Flores, Laboratory of Molecular Biology, Department of Crystallography, Birkbeck College, Malet Street, London WC1E 7HX.

R.B. Grzonka, Rutherford Appleton Laboratory, Chilton, Oxfordshire OX11 0QX.

G.Y. Guo, Daresbury Laboratory, Warrington WA4 4AD.

I. Haneef, The Astbury Department of Biophysics, The University of Leeds, Leeds LS2 9JT.

L. Heck, Physics Department, The University, Durham DH1 3LE

P.J. Knowles, School of Molecular Science, University of Sussex, Falmer, Sussex

P.J.D. Mayes, The Numerical Algorithms Group Ltd., Wilkinson House, Jordan Hill Road, Oxford OX2 8DR.

D.S. Moss, Laboratory of Molecular Biology, Department of Crystallography, Birkbeck College, Malet Street, London WC1E 7HX.

D. Moncrieff, ANU Supercomputer Facility, Australian National University, GPO Box 4, Canberra ACT 2601, Australia.

H.M. Quiney, Department of Theoretical Chemistry, University of Oxford, 5 South Parks Road, Oxford,

B. Ralston, IBM UK Ltd., 378 Chiswick High Road, London W4 4AD.

W.G. Richards, Physical Chemistry Laboratory, University of Oxford, South Parks Road, Oxford

V.R. Saunders, Daresbury Laboratory, Warrington WA4 4AD.

J.B. Slater, Bath University Computing Service, University of Bath, Claverton Down, Bath, Avon BA2 7AY.

Z. Szotek, Daresbury Laboratory, Warrington WA4 4AD.

W.M. Temmerman, Daresbury Laboratory, Warrington WA4 4AD.

F. Thomas, IBM UK Ltd., 378 Chiswick High Road, London W4 4AD.

S. Wilson, Rutherford Appleton Laboratory, Chilton, Oxfordshire OX11 0QX.

H. Winter, Daresbury Laboratory, Warrington WA4 4AD.

H.K.F. Yeung, Rutherford Appleton Laboratory, Chilton, Oxfordshire OX11 0QX.

INDEX

ADA, 27
Alliant FX series, 109
Amdahl/Fujitsu/Siemens VP series, 109, 338
Amdahl's Law, 8, 14, 15, 322, 335ff
Array processors, 17
Atlas Centre, 333, 334
Atomic collision processes, 147ff
Atomic structure calculations, 159ff, 185ff

Basic Linear Algebra Subroutines, 23, 110ff
Beeman method, 247–248
Binary tree topology, 71
Black box testing, 37–38
BLAS, 23, 110ff
Bond angles, in the definition of potential energy functions for molecular dynamics simulations, 254
Bond potential, 254
Boundaries, treatment of, in molecular dynamics simulations, 258

C, 27, 69
Cause effect graphing, 38
CDC Cyber 205, 109
CDC Cyber 990, 109
CDC STAR–100, 5
CDC 6600, 4,5
CDC 7600, 4,5
CMOS, 9
COBOL, 27, 49
Collision processes in atoms and molecules, 147ff
Comparison errors, 51
Complex solids, 287ff
Computation errors, 50
Computation partitioning, 83ff
Condensed matter, excess electrons in, 275ff
Configuration interaction method, 211ff
Constant temperature and pressure, in molecular dynamics simulations, 261, 262

Constrained dynamics, in molecular dynamics simulations, 260, 261
Continued fractions, 190
Control flow graphs, 82ff
Control–flow errors, 51, 52
Conventional architectures, 3ff
CONVEX C–1, 109
CONVEX C–2, 55, 109
Counting/Queuing semaphores, 61, 62
CPC, 69
Cray C–90, 338
Cray X–MP, 10, 55, 68, 87, 109, 155, 183, 319, 323, 324, 333, 334
Cray Y–MP, 55, 109, 324, 338
Cray–1, 5, 16, 109
Cray–2, 8, 109
Cray–3, 9, 338
Cross terms, in the definition of potential energy functions for molecular dynamics simulations, 255, 256
Cube architecture, 18

Daisy chain topology, 71
DAP, 17
DAP Fortran, 23
Data driven parallelism, 21
Data declaration errors, 50
Data farming, 70
Data partitioning, 86
Data reference errors, 50
Data structures, 58, 59, 321
Debugging, 41–43
Desk checking, 48
Development cycle of software product, 30–33, 45–47
Dirac–Hartree–Fock equations, 164ff, 185ff
Dispersion terms, in the definition of potential energy functions for molecular dynamics simulations, 256–257
Distributed Array Processor (DAP), 17
Distributed Memory Architecture, 19, 20
Documentation, 33, 43–44
Drug design, 269ff

Duplication, 48

ECL, 9
Electron correlation
  in atoms and molecules, 201*ff*
  in small molecules, 211*ff*
Electrostatic terms, in the definition of
    potential energy functions for
    molecular dynamics simulations,
    258
ENCORE systems, 55
Energy minimisation, 235*ff*
Equivalence partitioning, 38
Error function, 89–97
Error guessing, 39
ETA–10, 9

Fast Fourier Transforms, 122–127
Ferranti ATLAS1, 4
Flood prediction, 327*ff*
Fluid codes, for plasma simulations,
    138*ff*
Fokker–Planck simulations of plasmas,
    143*ff*
FORTNET Harness, 72*ff*
FORTRAN, 27, 49, 65, 69, 82, 87, 320
FORTRAN 8X, 23
FPS M64 series, 109
Free energyies of perturbation, 265,
    266
Fujitsu VP series, 8, 10
Full configuration interaction, 219–222
Full configuration space, 214–217

GaAs, 9, 11
Gallium Arsenide, 9, 11
Gear method, 248
Gene sequences, 273
Gould NP1, 109
Grid topology, 71

Harvard architecture, 3, 4
Hierarchical architecture, 19
Hitachi S–820/80, 338
Householder diagonalization, 155*ff*
Hydrogen bonds, in the definition of
    potential energy functions for
    molecular dynamics simulations,
    258
Hypercube, 18, 71

IBM FORTRAN, 50
IBM 3090, 55, 109, 333*ff*
IBM 360/195, 4, 5
ICL DAP 510, 17
IMSL, 23
Incomplete beta function, 188*ff*
Inmos T800, 67, 68
Input/output errors, 53
Inspections, 48–49
Interface errors, 52,53

Languages for parallel programming,
    23
Linear algebra, 110*ff*
LMTO–ASA Band structure method,
    288*ff*
Local data structures, 58

Many–body perturbation theory,
    179–182, 201*ff*
Massively parallel machines, 339–349
Matrix multiplication, 98–105
MBPT, 185*ff*
Meiko systems, 69*ff*, 152
Memory management, 105–107
Memory speed limitation, 4, 5
Mesh architecture, 18
MIMD, 16, 17
Minisupercomputers, 341–342
MISD, 16
Models of parallelism, 70
Molecular dynamics methods, 243*ff*
Molecular ynamics of protein
    molecules,251*ff*
Monte Carlo testing, 39
Multiconfiguration self–consistent field
    method, 222–227
Multiple images, example of the use of,
    62–63
Multiple scattering theory, 294*ff*

NAG, 23, 69, 109*ff*
NAS 9160, 109
NEC SX series, 109, 338
NMR structures, solution of, 262–264
Non bonded interactions, 256
    calculation of, 259–260
Non–computer based testing, 45*ff*
Novel architectures, 13*ff*
Numerical Sea Model, 319*ff*

OCCAM, 23, 65*ff*
Opacity Project, 153–154
Ordering/Queuing semaphore, 63

Parallel computing, 13*ff*, 82*ff*
Parallelism, models of, 70*ff*
Parallel processing, 55f, 201*ff*
Parallel processors, 17
Parity Non–Conservation (PNC), 159
Particle code for simulating plasmas,
    132*ff*
Pascal, 69
Path integral simulation,275*ff*
Peer review, 48
Plasmas, computer simulation of, 131*ff*
PL/I, 49Pragmatic testing, 40–41
Potential energy function, 253–258
Process parallelism, 21*ff*
Programming models for parallel
    computing, 21*ff*
Programming techniques, 25*ff*

Program testing, 28*ff*

Quadrature, 119–122
Quantum Electro–Dynamics (QED), 159

Random Number Generators, 118–119
Relativistic atomic structure calculations, 159*ff*, 185*ff*
Relativistic quantum mechanics, 160*ff*
Repulsive terms, in the definition of potential energy functions for molecular dynamics simulations, 257
Ring topology, 71
R–matrix method, 147*ff*
River simulation, 327*ff*

SCHEDULE tool, 82
Semaphores, 60–63
SEQUENT systems, 55
Serial computer, 16
Shared data structures, 58
Shared locked data structures, 58
Shared memory architecture, 19, 20, 56*ff*
Shared memory, Multi–user systems, 55*ff*
Silicon Complementary Metal Oxide Semiconductor, 9
Silicon Emitter Coupled Logic, 9
SIMD, 16
Simulated annealing, 240–241
Simulation of plasmas, 131*ff*
SISD, 16
SSI SS–1 system, 338
Stellar GS1000, 109
Strategy for testing, 39–40
Structure factor refinement, 235*ff*
Supercomputational science, 2
Supercomputing workstation, 342–343
Susceptibilities, 303*ff*

Task farming, 71*ff*
Test case design methodologies, 35*ff*
Thermodynamic perturbation method, 249–250
Thinking testing, 43
Torsions, proper, in the definition of potential energy functions for molecular dynamics simulations, 254, 255
Transputer, 67*ff*, 152

Unisys ISP, 109
UNIX, 11, 337

Vector processing, 5–11, 16, 201*ff*
Vector processing computer, 16
Verlet method, 246–247
Very Long Instruction Word, 10
VLIW, 10
von–Neumann architecture, 3, 4

Walkthroughs, 47–48
White box testing, 36–37
Workstations, 11, 13, 342

X–ray crystallographic data, refinement of, 264–265
X–windows, 11